Queer Dance

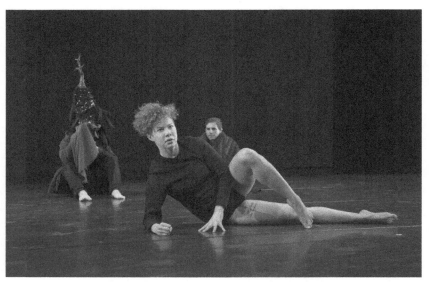

From left to right: Anna Martine Whitehead with Efren Cortez Cruz and Anthony Alterio in Whitehead's "Memory Loser." Photo by Sarah Nesbitt.

Queer Dance

Meanings and Makings

Edited by

CLARE CROFT

OXFORD
UNIVERSITY PRESS

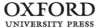

Oxford University Press is a department of the University of Oxford. It furthers
the University's objective of excellence in research, scholarship, and education
by publishing worldwide. Oxford is a registered trade mark of Oxford University
Press in the UK and certain other countries.

Published in the United States of America by Oxford University Press
198 Madison Avenue, New York, NY 10016, United States of America.

CIP data is on file at the Library of Congress
ISBN 978–0–19–937733–6 (pbk)
ISBN 978–0–19–937732–9 (hbk)

9 8 7 6 5 4 3 2

Paperback printed by Webcom Inc., Canada
Hardback printed by Bridgeport National Bindery, Inc., United States of America

Contents

PART II: *Dancing toward a Queer Sociality*

PART III: *Intimacy*

Acknowledgments

Queer Dance: Meanings and Makings has been generously supported by a number of entities. The Congress on Research in Dance, which supported the initial 2012 conference as a special topics conference, was a tremendous force in moving this conversation forward. The University of Michigan, with its commitment to feminist and queer studies, has been the ideal incubator for *Queer Dance*. In particular at Michigan, the School of Music, Theatre, and Dance (SMTD); the Department of Dance; the Institute for Research on Women and Gender (IRWG); and the University of Michigan Office of Research (UMOR) have supported the project many times over—through all of the residencies required for the live performance series, as well as the collection of the performance documentation and the interviews with artists. A host of other Michigan departments, programs, and initiatives have supported *Queer Dance*: the ADVANCE Program; Arts at Michigan; the Center for Southeast Asian Studies; the Center for World Performance Studies; the Confucius Institute; the Departments of Afroamerican and African Studies, English, Musicology, Theatre and Drama, and Women's Studies; the King-Chavez-Parks Visiting Professor Program; the Institute for the Humanities, the International Institute; LGQRI; Latina/o Studies Program; the Lieberthal-Rogel Center for Chinese Studies; Rackham Graduate School; the Stamps School of Art and Design; the Sally Fleming Master Class Series; the Spectrum Center; University Musical Society (UMS) Community Engagement; and the University Research Opportunity Program (UROP).

This book also required tremendous administrative help. Carla Mickler-Konz and Megan McClure provided superb guidance and troubleshooting—all with good humor. I will never write a book without the expert skills of Tara Sheena in all things archival and photographic. The Website would have been only a dream without the work of the entire crew of the Duderstadt Video Studio and Sharad Patel's patient editing.

This is also a project that has been tremendously challenged and shaped by the presence of a great number of students—in the classroom, in performances, and sitting with me in audiences. First and foremost, I thank all the students at the University of Michigan who have worked together to make my Dancing Women/Dancing Queer courses an incredible ground for feminist and queer artmaking and scholarship. Our conversations affected so much of how I conceptualized this work. I also want to thank the team of students who helped create *we* [still] *queer here 4.5*. A special thank you to Anthony Alterio for his work as my research assistant on *Queer Dance*.

Thank you to thomas defrantz, Judith Hamera, and Ramon Rivera-Servera for serving as an internal review board; your comments were invaluable in moving the essays to deeper places. For their *many* conversations and readings and re-readings of the Introduction, I am grateful to Jessica Del Vecchio, Kareem Khubchandani, S.E. Kile, Petra Kuppers, Sara McClelland, Patrick McKelvey, Jennifer Monson, and Emily Wilcox. Thank you, too, to Oxford's anonymous reviewers for seeing the themes emerging across the project. Norm Hirschy deserves a huge "thank you." He told me this book needed to exist before I knew it did. May all editors be as supportive of queer work as you have been.

There is no support that will ever come close to what Sara McClelland offers every day. Thank you for teaching me what it means to ask real questions. (Please find the boat.)

Finally, my most boundless gratitude goes to the people who have written and performed *Queer Dance* into existence. This is truly a co-authored project. I don't have words for how honored I have been to witness your performances, read your drafts, talk with you, think with you, and dream with you. We have done too much work to think of this project as a beginning. I hope—in fact, I am sure—that we are in the middle of something, and I hope it spreads in directions we can't yet imagine.

List of Contributors

Angela K. Ahlgren is Assistant Professor in the Department of Theatre and Film at Bowling Green State University. Her writing has been published in *Contemporary Directions in Asian American Dance* (University of Wisconsin Press, 2016), *Women & Music: A Journal of Gender and Culture*, and the *Journal of Dramatic Theory and Criticism*, and she is at work on a monograph, *Drumming Asian America: Taiko, Performance, and Cultural Politics.*

Jennifer L. Campbell specializes in twentieth-century American music, focusing on composers Aaron Copland, Virgil Thomson, and Paul Bowles. She frequently undertakes interdisciplinary projects, exploring connections between music, dance, art, politics, and cultural identity and has published on such topics in the journal *Diplomatic History* (2012) and in the volume *Paul Bowles—The New Generation Do You Bowles?* (2014).

Peter Carpenter (MFA, PhD) is Associate Professor of Dance at Columbia College Chicago where he teaches courses in choreography and dance studies. His choreography focuses on developing the political potential of the concert dance event.

Julian B. Carter is Associate Professor of Critical Studies at the California College of the Arts. He is a critical historian and performance theorist whose work focuses on normativity, embodiment, and the collective construction and maintenance of identity systems. He is the author of *The Heart of Whiteness: Normal Sexuality and Race in America, 1890–1940* (Duke University Press, 2007) and sits on the editorial board of the *Trans Studies Quarterly.*

Sandra Chatterjee (PhD, UCLA) works at the intersection of theory and artistic practice with a focus on queer, postcolonial, and migration studies. A choreographer and researcher, she has worked as a postdoctoral researcher on two projects at the Department of Music and Dance Studies, University of

Salzburg (*Traversing the Contemporary (pl.)*, Austrian Science Fund (FWF) P 24190-G15, and *Dance and Migration*, Austrian Science Fund (FWF) WPK 32) and is a co-founder of the Post *Natyam* Collective. http://www.sandrachatterjee.net.

Clare Croft is a dance historian, theorist, dramaturg, and curator. She is the author of *Dancers as Diplomats: American Choreography in Cultural Exchange* (Oxford, 2015), and the editor and curator of *Queer Dance: Meanings and Makings*. Croft is Assistant Professor at the University of Michigan.

thomas f. defrantz is Professor and Chair of African and African American Studies at Duke University, and director of SLIPPAGE: Performance, Culture, Technology, a research group that explores emerging technology in live performance applications. Books: *Dancing Many Drums: Excavations in African American Dance* (University of Wisconsin Press, 2002), *Dancing Revelations Alvin Ailey's Embodiment of African American Culture* (Oxford University Press, 2004), *Black Performance Theory*, co-edited with Anita Gonzalez (Duke University Press, 2014), *Choreography and Corporeality: Relay in Motion*, co-edited with Philipa Rothfield (Palgrave, 2016). Creative: *Queer Theory! An Academic Travesty* commissioned by the Theater Offensive of Boston and the Flynn Center for the Arts, and *Monk's Mood: A Performance Meditation on the Life and Music of Thelonious Monk*, performed in Botswana, France, South Africa, and New York City. He convenes the Black Performance Theory working group. In 2013, working with Takiyah Nur Amin, he founded the Collegium for African Diaspora Dance.

Nicholas Gareiss is a dancer and dance researcher creating work at the intersection of percussive dance, traditional music, and queer ethnography. He has concertized for over fifteen years with many of the luminaries of traditional Irish music and dance and continues to perform and teach internationally.

Doran George has a PhD tracing the historical development of Somatic training in contemporary dance. A funded artist, they research accessibility in dance to disabled people, and deconstruct identity in bodily performance. Doran is also published in journals and anthologies, produces symposia and conferences, and teaches in universities, art colleges, and in professional dance.

Lou Henry Hoover is a choreographer and performer that utilizes drag, dance, theater, and spectacle to make work that is celebrated internationally for being both comedic and heartfelt. Lou is best known for collaborative work as duo Kitten N' Lou.

Kareem Khubchandani is the Mellon Assistant Professor in the Department of Drama and Dance at Tufts University teaching at the intersections of queer studies and performance studies. He received his PhD in performance studies from Northwestern University and is working on a book project titled *Ishtyle: Labor, Intimacy, and Dance in Gay South Asian Nightlife.*

Hannah Kosstrin, PhD, is a dance historian who researches Jewishness and gender in modern and contemporary dance. At the Ohio State University, she is Assistant Professor in the Department of Dance and affiliated faculty with the Melton Center for Jewish Studies.

Cynthia Ling Lee (MFA, UCLA) creates interdisciplinary choreography and scholarship that instigate postcolonial, queer, and feminist-of-color interventions in the field of experimental South Asian performance. Cynthia is a member of the Post *Natyam* Collective and Assistant Professor of theatre arts at the University of California at Santa Cruz. http://www.cynthialinglee.com

Anna Martine Whitehead is a movement artist and writer interrogating the poetics of space, time, and loss at the limits of performance. They write about black performance in the contemporary art world and have contributed chapters to several texts on queer dance, performance, and social practice.

Patrick McKelvey is Visiting Assistant Professor of theatre studies at Florida State University. His current book project is *Crip Enterprise: Disability Goes to Work in U.S. Performance.*

Raquel L. Monroe (PhD, UCLA) is Associate Professor in Dance at Columbia College Chicago.

Jennifer Monson is a choreographer and performer. She is the artistic director and founder of iLAND –interdisciplinary Laboratory for Art Nature and Dance and Professor of dance at the University of Illinois Urbana Champaign.

Justin Torres is the author of the bestselling novel *We the Animals*, and his honors include a Stegner Fellowship, a Radcliffe Institute Fellowship, and a Cullman Center Fellowship. Named one of the National Book Foundation's 2012 "5 under 35," he is Assistant Professor of English at UCLA.

Emily E. Wilcox is Assistant Professor of modern Chinese studies in the Department of Asian Languages and Cultures at the University of Michigan. Her research focuses on dance and cultural history in Asia, with a focus on the People's Republic of China.

How to Use the *Queer Dance: Meanings and Makings* Website

The *Queer Dance: Meanings and Makings* website (www.oup.com/us/queer-dance, username: Music3, password: Book3234) is an integral part of engaging with the this project. On the website, you will find two sets of videos.

The first set of videos focus on performance itself, and include ten videos: five short works, one music video, and three evening-length works. The shorter works feature the work of Lou Henry Hoover, the Post *Natyam* Collective, Nicholas Gareiss and Cleek Schrey, Peter Carpenter, and Anna Martine Whitehead. The music video, "Sari," is the work of LaWhore Vagistan and collaborator Auntie Kool Jams, with direction by Kareem Khubchandani. One of the evening-length works, Jennifer Monson and DD Dorvillier's piece, *RMW(a) & RMW*, appears twice, so viewers can see how the improvisational structure shifted over two performances, filmed two nights in a row. The other evening-length works feature the collaborative ensemble SLIPPAGE with direction by thomas f. defrantz in *theory-ography 4.5: we* [still] *queer here* and *Right & Left*, choreographed by Gu Jiani.

The second set of videos focus on interviews with the artists who created and, in some cases, performed in the works documented. The conversations, conducted by *Queer Dance* editor and curator Clare Croft, track a wide range of topics, including the creation and the performance of the works, the works' invitations to audiences to imagine queer dance, and the artists' larger investments in dance as a political practice and a way to wrestle with identities. All of the interviews are segmented into chapters, arranged by topic, to make them easier to move through and to use in the classroom.

Video Material Table of Contents

Video material available online at
Web address: www.oup.com/us/queerdance
Username: Music3
Password: Book3234

Introduction

Clare Croft

Dancer Cynthia Ling Lee of Post *Natyam* Collective struggles into a pair of butch jeans; her *dupatta*, the scarf usually worn while dancing kathak, flips about her neck, underscoring the physical frustration of her labor. In one sock and one cowboy boot, Peter Carpenter limps with a sense of defiance, his off-kilter swagger slowly becoming a gay man's weapon against Ronald Reagan's voice, the primary sound in his solo's sonic accompaniment. Anna Martine Whitehead's legs churn with fury and strength, as the velvety deer head she wears—part mask, part fantastic accessory—bears down on two boys who yell, "Have you seen her?" Partial visibility becomes a tool of Black queer power; even as she wears a puppet, she is the puppeteer. Nicholas Gareiss cuts his eyes right, coyly challenging fiddler Cleek Schrey with his feet and his gaze. Together Gareiss and Schrey shape an avant-garde Irish score: lilts and squeaks, scrapes and knowing grins. Drag king Lou Henry Hoover falls and drops a plastic baby, then falls and drops it again. The precisely choreographed, repeated failure seems to eventually give birth to a central prop in the work: a mug that says, "#1 Dad."

This collage of images bears some of the sensibilities of something we might call "queer dance." The pleasures *and* difficulties of moving between multiple, layered identities. Frustration and diminishment physically reframed as strength. Images that do not immediately make sense, but that somehow gather force. A slyness, a sexiness, or a joke arriving fast, sideways, and deep all at once. No single entity marks something as queer dance, but rather it is how these textures press on the world and against one another that opens the possibility for dance to be queer.

All these choreographic moments appeared in *Confetti Sunrise*, an evening of dance I curated in Ann Arbor, Michigan in 2015. The range of work and the emergence of a layered sense of politics make *Confetti Sunrise* an ideal entrée into *Queer Dance: Meanings and Makings*—this anthology, the performances and interviews documented on the *Queer Dance* website, and the ongoing performance series. In *Queer Dance*, "queer" emerges from specific contexts. It is not a label to be categorically applied or agreed upon, but rather it is a force of disruption that simultaneously draws on historical genealogies of queer and freshly imagines "queer" in the contemporary moment. In its insistence that queer *does* (rather than *is*), *Queer Dance* recognizes the links between dance and legacies of queer activism: the work activists did in the eighties and nineties to recuperate "queer" from a heckle of hate into a proclamation of power and the work queer activists are doing in the twenty-first century within, for instance, the United States's Black Lives Matter movement and movements for trans rights. In all these arenas, "queer" signals a coalitional sensibility—one that brings LGBTQ identities into provisional, strategic unity. As a coalitional force, queer activism demands visibility and respect for a range of people and communities *and* demands that receiving respect should not be predicated on behaving in a certain way, a "normal" way. "Queer" in *Queer Dance* then, in addition to focusing on LGBTQ identity and community, also draws on a more expansive notion of "queer," a broader challenge to social norms. In this project, LGBTQ life and queer politics are not separate.[1] Through making dance, watching dance, and studying dance, *Queer Dance* examines the performance of a wide range of genders and sexualities (onstage and off) as a challenge to social norms.

Dance has potential to have a particular power within queer work because dance emphasizes how public, physical action can be a force of social change.[2] Dance, as it is taken up by artists, teachers, administrators, and scholars, produces a field for discussing and imagining how bodies in motion offer alternative meanings and ways of being. Some dance makers, audiences, and thinkers have long embraced queer possibilities of coalition, anti-normative critique, and social disruption. In other realms, more could be done to imagine how queer dance might productively challenge conservative arenas. *Queer Dance: Meanings and Makings* considers both terrains: what has been done and what needs to be done. How have people forged representations, institutions, and practices that press us into more open, creative possibilities in dance? What obstacles prevent queer work in artmaking, in scholarship, in teaching, and in institution building?

Queer Dance, in its many meanings and makings, emerges in encounters across difference, in spaces of heterogeneity. *Queer Dance* refuses monolithic signification and instead forges a politics from the productive frictions among identities (gender and sexuality, yes, but also race and ability, nationality and diaspora). Representing this range of ways of being and knowing requires that *Queer Dance* comes in multiple formats: written, filmed, and performed. *Queer Dance* is this book: a collection of writing in the form of scholarly articles, artist manifestos, and personal essays. *Queer Dance* is the website: a collection of nine films of performance (including the works from *Confetti Sunrise*) and interviews with the artists who created each work.[3] And *Queer Dance* is an ongoing live performance series. Just as the works performed in *Confetti Sunrise* produced multiple definitions of queer as they comingled, so, too, do all the formats, all the pieces of *Queer Dance: Meanings and Makings*. No one thing is *the* thing. The thing, the "queer," is what emerges among, across, and between.

Queer Dance: Driving Forces

While many conversations and, I hope, debates will arise from readers' and viewers' engagement with *Queer Dance*, I curated and edited this project to demand that queer dance, as it is made manifest, must be broadly inclusive of the LGBTQ community, specifically in terms of identity and geography; and to note how queer dance, at its best, is in conversation with and often in productive overlap with feminist, anti-racist, and anti-colonial artmaking, activism, and scholarship. These broader goals take shape in the project as five specific stances on what queer dance might be: (1) that women and feminism are central to any queer project; (2) that social dance and concert dance hold equal import; (3) that, through anti-racist and anti-colonial labor, queerness must always work to challenge white privilege; (4) that queerness has to challenge the entrenchment of the gender binary; and (5) that queer dance happens across an expansive map, both global and regional.

My insistence that *Queer Dance* demonstrate why and how queer dance must be deeply tied to feminism is where this project began. The people who introduced me to the existence of something called "queer performance" were women—all feminists, mostly lesbians—in Texas. In the classrooms and theaters these women led, I first aligned myself with queer politics, both in terms of my emerging lesbian identity and my desire to imagine multiple ways of being in public.[4] In the arts, this is a relatively familiar story: artistic and intellectual arenas offer many a first glimpse of ways of being other than the dominant modes of being straight, being a man, being white, and so on. And, too, the arts often offer a relatively safe space—stage even—to try on new identities and other modes of relating. What was not necessarily typical about my passage into LGBTQ politics and community was the degree to which my local world was women-centered. This means, for me, women have always been central to queer community, and, too, these female forces shielded me from the frequent misogyny of queer spaces. Given this lesbo-centered entrée into queer life, I was surprised to find the subhead, "Where are the women?" in the foundational dance studies text connecting dance and sexuality, Jane Desmond's essential edited collection *Dancing Desires* (2001).[5] I thought, "Wasn't everyone interested in queerness because of all the women? Their sexiness? Their feminism?" From this slightly naïve, but earnest mix of desire and politics emerged my commitment to make any queer dance space I shaped one where people who identified as women were many and in leadership.

There is a tension in my autobiographical anecdote between what is imagined, hoped, and desired for queer dance (in this case, a centrality of feminism and women) and what queer dance might be in practice (sometimes misogynist). This entanglement of imagination and practice is key to all of *Queer Dance*. Sites of social dance have been vital for queer dance (and scholarship about queer dance) because the social dance floor is very much a place for a simultaneous imagining, rehearsal, and performance of queerness—a space where there is a moment-to-moment navigation of desire and physical enactment borne out across a group. As dance studies scholars Ramón Rivera-Servera, David Román, and Fiona Buckland have described,[6] this overlay of dreaming and doing allows bodies to come together into many configurations of coalition and collectivity. This unsettles the primacy of the heterosexual male/female couple (and the nuclear family we imagine it "naturally" creates) as society's foundation.[7] While the dance floor is not immune to heteronormativity,[8] its enactment of other ways to relate, valuing temporary attachments and meaningful relationships that extend beyond couples, opens possibilities for imagining how people can and do connect.

It is worth noting that not all queer dance floors exist in the darkness of a club. Other social dance spaces offer queer possibility, too. For instance, as thomas defrantz describes, the intergenerational dance floors of Black family gatherings, with a supporting circle of cousins, grandchildren, uncles, and mothers clapping along and people taking turns in a circle's center, invite a more expansive sense of movement that does not always pose biological family connections as at odds with queer possibility.[9] The boundaries of private and public, protagonist and antagonist, constantly shift, making physical an insistence on instability and fluidity.

Queer dance floors sometimes offer relief from the pains of living in a sexist, racist, heteronormative world, but those respites are usually temporary. Comfort and pleasure, as important as both are to queer politics, cannot be the only drivers of any coalitional movement, as Black feminists have long described.[10] Dance floors are not utopias. What was once a lesbian space is no longer when the straight men start coming to the bar, watching the women as though they are there for the men's entertainment. Queer dance clubs remain, in many cities, racially segregated, often populated predominantly by white people. Where white people feel emboldened, queer people of color might not even feel welcome. The 2016 shooting at a Latin Night at Pulse nightclub in Orlando, Florida, brought the role of race in queer nightlife into national attention in the United States. Forty-nine people were killed and fifty-three injured; most were Latinx, many Puerto Rican. The event reverberated through Black and Brown queer communities, worsening as press coverage of the event often called it terrorism, rather than naming its homophobic, xenophobic, and racist dimensions.[11]

Queer Dance keeps race central; there are no parts of this project that are "about race." Here queer is always about race. *Queer Dance* works to avoid the common situation theorists E. Patrick Johnson and Mae Henderson have critiqued: that "queer" has too often become a moniker for whiteness, disaggregating LGBTQ subjectivity from race.[12] The artists and writers in this anthology and represented throughout the performance series and its documentation bring the voices and dancing of a range of identities—Black, Latinx, and those of the Asian diaspora—to the forefront of imagining queerness.

The predominance of whiteness in queer performance is often implicitly tied with an imagination of queer as of "the West." So many narratives of sexual identity posit the United States or the "West" as centers of liberation. *Queer Dance* unsettles this. Writing and performances throughout the volume move in the vein postcolonial theorists Gayatri Gopinath and Jasbir Puar, among others, have charted. They highlight gaps in queer studies where scholars have failed to examine the experience of those moving in diasporas of all kinds, and in performances beyond the "West."[13] This has particular relevance for imagining queer dance because the pairing of white privilege and Euro-American centrism limits the range of dance forms categorized as queer, focusing on ballet and modern dance as though those are the only norms to queer. As Alyson Campbell and Stephen Farrier note in their reflection on queer performance dramaturgies, "[T]hat which is radically queer in one context can be less so in another."[14] *Queer Dance* examines dance broadly, including Irish step dance, kathak, Bollywood performance, and contemporary dance from Beijing, tracing queer in its global, intersectional circulation. In this expansion, artistic and written contributions to *Queer Dance* explore questions of race, the postcolonial, and gender as informing one another, especially as they move into performance and pedagogical strategies, transferring ideas body-to-body. Emphasizing physical transmission in global circulation seems especially exciting in terms of what Campbell and Ferrier call the "translocal," the ways that global economies shape local practices and vice versa. All this said, however, most of the scholars and artists in *Queer Dance* are US-based, even if their gaze or life history extends outward. Much more work needs to be done to examine queer dance within global migration and translation. *Queer Dance* begins this work, looking beyond the US-centered dance world and dance practices, including those practices and sites already mentioned, as well as looking at dance in the United Kingdom, France, and Bangalore by way of Ghana.

Another narrative *Queer Dance* resists is one of the gender binary, the notion that "men" and "women" are opposites and are the only categories available for thinking about gender. Focusing on the performances documented on the website, it quickly becomes obvious just how ludicrous a supposition it is that "male" or "female," "masculine" or "feminine" would be sufficient for discussing the wide range of gender presentations in dance. Trans studies has increasingly shed light on these binaries' limitations, and the central tenets of that field bear great weight here. *Queer Dance* is deeply invested in the questions of identitarian and community formations that helped form both queer studies and transgender studies, yet, too, both fields have broader implications. Trans studies has particularly worked to undermine the power of the gender binary as institutional force and linguistic limitation. This project draws on a post-1990s understanding of the term "transgender," what trans studies theorists Susan Stryker and Paisley Currah describe as "a broad class of phenomena related to historical shifts in how sex, sexuality, gender, identity, and embodiment are thought to be conjoined and how—and to what ends—they may be reconfigured."[15]

Dancing queerly challenges dance communities of all kinds to overcome unimaginative categorizations that conceptualize gender difference as an essentialized, physical difference. To take full advantage of queer possibility, these assumptions—often unspoken or implied—which shape and limit our work as artists and scholars, dancers and teachers, must be confronted. The stories told through dance—narrative and otherwise—are enacted everyday by groups of people coming together to dance in classes, in rehearsals, and on dance floors. As a practice, dance highlights assumptions about the relationship between one's body and one's gender expressions.When people assume, for instance, that men lift and women are lifted, they forget it is training, not genitalia, that creates physiques in all their strengths and weaknesses. Too, these superficial ideas limit the relationships imagined, the choreographies made, and how classrooms can be inhabited.[16] For instance, if we stop forcing gay men to perform a caricature of heterosexual masculinity, they could contribute to imagining broad, varied physical forms of masculinity slipping among a range of sexualities.[17] If femininity is conceptualized as something other than an ideal no one can inhabit or a sign of weakness, it could be more readily available as a platform for power.[18]

The ways power moves and takes hold in dancing can only be understood by attending to the vantage point from which one considers joining the dancing. What makes some feel comfortable jumping into the mix leads others to opt out. A map of queer dance has to consider Arizona and Alabama as potentially hosting as much queer dance as New York or San Francisco are assumed to do. This geographical range presses back on what Jack Halberstam has called the queer narrative of metronormativity: the idea that queer people constantly move away from more rural settings to urban centers and, specifically, some particular urban centers.[19] Artists in this project hail from cities across the United States: Chicago; Greensboro, North Carolina; New Orleans; Roanoke, Virginia; Boston; Seattle; and Long Beach, and, of course, New York and San Francisco. The pragmatics of fundraising mean, of the artists on the website, only Gu Jiani and Kareem Khubchandani live or were born outside the US. But still, *Queer Dance* broadens the map of identities, of genders, of dance forms, and of geographies.

Productive Frictions/Promiscuous Engagements

I hope people feel productively disturbed by their encounters with the capacious archive that is *Queer Dance: Meanings and Makings*. I also hope viewers and readers will not just gravitate to the artists, forms, or scholars they already know, but will instead read and watch promiscuously, opening themselves to new possibilities, pleasures, and curiosities. The various platforms—those live audiences have experienced and will experience in the future, as well as the videos on the *Queer Dance* website and the essays in this book—work together in productive friction. No one thing is the central object here; it is how the elements rub, collide, and comingle that constitutes queer dance.

If all you do is read the essays in this book, you will have missed several opportunities. The written, the spoken, and the danced all intermingle here, sometimes destabilizing one another, and never settling into a comfortable hierarchy. This project takes seriously feminist calls to imagine many ways of knowing, putting the voices of artists and audiences side-by-side. Throughout this book, you will find links to the *Queer Dance* website, which features eight filmed dance performances, as well as interviews I conducted with the artists who created and performed in each of the works. The dance works do not illustrate the points of the writers. Neither the essays nor the interviews explain the dance works. All three of these formats—the interview, the text, and the performed—are potential entry points, and exist alongside one another, offering audiences multiple ways to come into queer association, queer theory, and, especially, queer dancing. Over half of this book is written by makers, those who either make art with explicitly queer artistic intentions or who relish their work living explicitly in a queer frame. Makers do not, however, hold complete purchase on cultural objects' meanings, as the writing of the many historians, ethnographers, and critics within *Queer Dance* attests. Audiences bring their own desires to this work, queering even the most mainstream, canonical performances.[20]

I have been the most privileged audience of this material—disturbed and inspired by all that has been written and performed as I got to watch each work grow and change. It is, however, the collage that makes *Queer Dance*. All the work presented could absolutely stand on its own, but it is all the better for the mixing. The way these pieces come together (and the queer pleasure of their unorthodox pairings) is really this project's work. *Queer Dance* is, in essence, a vision for seeing, reading, and dancing queerly—without privileging any of these modes over another.

The introductory thoughts in the remainder of this essay suggest some paths through this project—both this book and *Queer Dance* in total. First I discuss the project's extension of key trajectories in defining and redefining queer. The next section extends what I have discussed in these opening thoughts, beginning with *Queer Dance*'s central tenets, and then issuing broader challenges to dance and queer studies. In these two sections, the portions focused on definitions and on challenges, I ground my thinking in performance analysis, discussing works that moved me during the years I developed *Queer Dance*. These performance analyses, of US American choreographer Kyle Abraham's *Live! The Realest MC* (2011) and Filipino choreographer Eisa Jocson's *Macho Dancer* (2013), offer examples of making queer meaning from performance, as I hope many will do with the online performance documentation and with performances beyond those featured in *Queer Dance*. In the final portion of the Introduction, I provide an overview of the volume's elements, this book and the performance and conversational material available online, offering possible paths toward promiscuous engagements.

Queer Dance: Named, Felt, Recognized

Queer Dance builds upon three key concepts within the now three-plus decades of the recuperation of "queer": queer activism and queer studies as invested in the body, queer as a critique of normativity, and queer as an embrace of heterogeneity. I first explain why these concepts animate *Queer Dance*, and then

I discuss how dance extends those lines of thinking. I do the latter through a close analysis of Kyle Abraham's *Live! The Realest MC*, a work that defines queerness by playing with the edges of visibility and legibility.

"Queer," as it moves in this project, is a term borne of physical, collective action. Activists recuperated "queer" in the 1990s through moving with their bodies and shouting with their voices, as a group, in public. As a physical action, activism shifted what a word meant and who had the power to define the word. Language is not just a descriptor of the physical; the physical produces and changes linguistic meaning.[21]

In *Queer Dance* "queer" arises from a critical entanglement of gender and sexuality within a larger call for resisting normativity.[22] "Queer" functions as an umbrella term for LGBTQ people and recognizes non-normativity more broadly. All the essays and performances in this volume stage queer by way of engaging with challenges to normative understandings and presentations of sexuality and gender. This is not, however, merely a reorganization of gender and sexuality categories. These reorientations of gender and sexuality are a path toward imagining expansive social possibilities, moving toward horizons of queer potential and revolution.[23] *Queer Dance* focuses on what queer does, rather than imagining queer as having an essential referent or marker within an individual or a relationship. That said, for many their manifestation of gender and sexual identity is a crucial mode for staging queer critique.[24] To lay claim to "queer" as one's identity, as many do in the twenty-first century, often denotes a non-normative gender or sexual identity and that one is not invested in more mainstream LGBT policies. This is an example of how a label can take on a queerly performative function, undoing even what we think a label does.

Queer Dance's "queer" insists on heterogeneity. In the years since 1995, when David Halperin first formulated his now iconic linking of "queer" to an expansive rejection of normativity, what was once an openness that invited heterogeneity in 2016 too often feels like a false veil barely concealing a monolithic core. One now encounters "queer" within more assimilationist agendas, for instance, the US activism around allowing gay people to marry or join the military. And, too, queer, as discussed earlier, often connotes only gay, white, largely affluent men. Claiming queer's non-normative possibilities requires different work in the twenty-first century, as it has moved into more general circulation. It means fighting harder to relish multiple perspectives from outside mainstream institutions and agendas. "Queer" in *Queer Dance* wants what Eve Kosofsky Sedgwick imagined queer could be, a space that does not just allow, but values, even encourages, practices in which "meanings and institutions can be at loose ends with each other."[25]

Queer is a wide-ranging set of notions and practices that collide: a state of conflicting, generative modes of existence. Dance, with its poetic porosity and generative failure to convey direct meaning, engages productively and provocatively with queer's slippery, shapeshifting sensibility. Bodies never do one thing or mean one thing. By embracing a messy, heterogeneous, even possibly contradictory queer, dance forges community, not in spite of, but through and with challenges and contradictions.[26] With no apologies to Lady Gaga, one is not born queer. Instead, to borrow again from Sedgwick, one chooses queer as a commitment to "political adventures" that refuse easy categorization.[27]

How does dance manifest a theory of queerness? Many dance scholars, including Valerie Briginshaw, Fiona Buckland, thomas defrantz, Jane Desmond, Petra Kuppers, Marta Savigliano, and Ramón Rivera-Servera,[28] have worked to answer this question. I want to approach it, as several of these scholars have done, through close analysis of dance, moving into my own poetic, messy engagement with moving bodies to challenge and focus perceptions of queerness. Close attention to the details of performance drives my analysis. I examine choreography; elements of the mise en scène: lights, costume, set; and the historical and cultural contexts in which work was made and in which it is performed.

While watching Kyle Abraham's *Live! The Realest MC* in New York at The Kitchen in its 2011 premiere, I had one of my most visceral experiences of dance as a way to imagine queerness.[29] I saw the work amidst a moment of rampant US media coverage of LGBTQ suicides, specifically Rutgers student Tyler Clementi's suicide, a reaction to relentless homophobic bullying by a classmate. In this context, *Live!* landed hard, and made a powerful statement of Black, queer power. Dancing with smoothness and intensity, Abraham and the dancers of his company, Kyle Abraham/Abraham.In.Motion (A.I.M.), lead the audience toward an experience of queer as simultaneously concealed and fabulously revealed. In the work, Abraham asks the cast to explore—by way of the Pinocchio story, hip-hop lessons, and virtuosic dancing—what it means to be a "real boy." Throughout the evening-length piece, there is a paradoxical sense of legibility, even clarity, though that clarity is always fleeting, bouncing among and between shifting elements.

The juxtaposition of and friction between the multiple elements of any performance—dancing, costuming, sets, sound, and so on—makes performance ideal for embodying the contradictions and disruptions that produce queer possibility. The stage set for *Live!* is relatively bare, making the dancers' costumes, mostly riffs on Adidas track suits—an iconic emblem of hip-hop— a crucial element of the visual landscape. Light also plays a central role in the work, often serving as illumination, sometimes as container in which private, difficult experiences manifest. Sequins that appear throughout the work often connect the tracksuits and the lights. The sequins function as an almost obvious symbol of gay subculture, but they also do queer work as, edging the dancers' bodies, they refract the light.

Of the whole evening, *Live!*'s last image struck me most. It centers a body simultaneously visible but also beautifully beyond my visual or kinesthetic grasp: a paradox crucially made possible through Abraham's performance of Blackness and queerness. *Live!* ends with Abraham alone onstage.[30] He is the figure with whom the audience has journeyed through the piece, the one onstage the most and the one most central, although he often cedes the stage to his mix of male and female dancers and to a series of videos ranging from humorous to poignant. As the piece comes to its end, however, these other elements vanish. Abraham dances alone center stage wearing a black tracksuit; a lone microphone stands downstage in a pool of light. Abraham finishes his final solo with his signature blend of hip-hop and contemporary dance vocabulary at once hard and full of edges, but also smooth, like jazz oozing out of a radio. As his full-bodied motion subsides, he slowly turns away from the audience, unzips his jacket, and with a markedly masculine strut walks to the microphone. But once he arrives—in the light, at the microphone—he does not speak words as we might expect (he spoke last time he came here), but instead he turns his back to us. He lets the jacket go and reveals a bank of starry gold sequins that fall across a billowing black shirt beneath. The wall of sequins seems almost to jump up to the light, leaping to be reflected as the sequins begin to slowly move. Abraham has begun to slide his shoulder blades up and down. The light, now set into motion courtesy of his sequined body, invites a sensuous kinesthetic absorption that speaks volumes even as the microphone's presence underscores the absence of sound. Here is "queer" in dancing terms: at once legible, but also refusing exact referent, at once overwhelming and unmarked. Abraham's body will not speak into the microphone, but will speak otherwise with light, motion, and a gentle fabulosity. Queer chose its spotlight moment, and I saw it in its utterly bare, sexy physicality.

Earlier, in *Live!*'s opening solo, the sequins create a shimmering pool of light around Abraham that allows him to try out new physical possibilities, a new identity—a reference to Pinocchio but also a moment I read as a queer becoming.[31] Testing the new identity has to precede coming out. The next time dancers appear in sequins the costuming seems to be a marker of gay male attraction, offering the performers' desire as a central path into the work. The moment is brief—the two men wearing sequins among a non-sequined crowd do not touch or even see one another. But before the lights fade on the section, we know they are a couple, or at least those "in the know" will suspect their sequins, flashing in the light, suggest a pleasurable outsider-ness. Visibility is not necessarily sought widely, but rather from those who know the code, who know what sequins falling luxuriously across a man's body might mean. A partial audience is enough.

Abraham's third and penultimate sequined appearance is the most difficult to watch because of its display of violence, but, even more important, its display of violence as having emotional, psychical, and physical impact. His sequins here frame a dance of absent presence and the potential pain of visibility. In this solo, the other time in the piece Abraham uses the microphone featured in the work's final moment, he does speak words. He quickly vacillates between a deep, hypermasculine voice, asking iconic emcee phrases like "How ya'll feeling?" and a pained, high-pitched young man's voice, telling his mother of homophobic abuse, repeating, shakily, "They held me down." Abraham's quick shifts merge the two distinct timbres, thus merging the possibilities and hardships of gay, Black, male life. This shifting has physical effect. He shakes. His hands tremble. He works to hail an audience that won't hear him—or at least won't hear the whole story.

The gripping, terrifying monologue ends. Abraham steps to the border of the pool of light. Suddenly we see his sequins. They edge the black tracksuit,

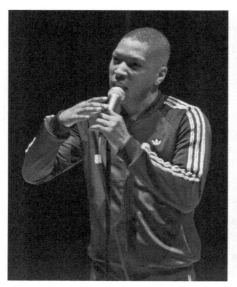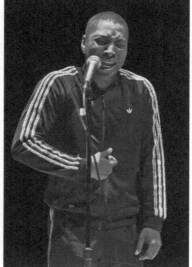

FIGURES I.I AND I.2 Kyle Abraham of Abraham.In.Motion in *Live! The Realest MC*. Photo by Steven Schreiber.

tracing the outside of his arms and legs with a faint glow. Now barely in the light, his body recedes, almost disappears. Only the sequined outline is visible. At once this is a chalk outline at a crime scene and a queer angel—perhaps drawn from the opening solo's swarming stars of protection and queer becoming. He is not visible, and he is shockingly visible to those who want to see. A queer presence and absence at once: beautiful and sad. Importantly, this is not the kind of aestheticized death of an "Other" we see so often in performance—the Ophelia, the woman only truly seen in her beautiful death. Instead, this is a body still dancing, its queerness making it visible despite (or perhaps because of) the lights' limits.

In the sliding of Abraham's shoulders and the glittering of the sequins in the work's final image, all these moments—of opening, of desiring, and of surviving—coexist. The queer layers come together, but resist a single narrative. Queer as it is danced here is a process, a series of actions; a desiring at the edge of visibility; and a feedback loop of violence and survival. Queer holds space for multiple meanings, clashing and unstable, always in motion, much like a dance.

What Does Queer Dance Challenge Us Toward?

To ask "what is queer dance?" is to create a proliferation of potential disturbances that ripple beyond this project. I turn here to these ripples, noting the ways this project seeks to challenge dance and queer studies. In queer studies, these challenges include displacing the primacy of text and acknowledging queer's predecessors in queer activism, the civil rights movement, and feminism. In the dance world, artists and scholars, teachers and students need to expand the language and opportunities for discussing gender and sexuality. Thinking across these two worlds, I finally turn, through an analysis of Eisa Jocson's *Macho Dancer*, to queer dance's broadest avenue for affecting publics: its disorientation and reorientation of audiences.

Queer dance challenges a narrative that overly celebrates written text. The year 1990, when Judith Butler, David Halperin, and Eve Kosofsky Sedgwick all published now iconic queer scholarship, is frequently marked as the watershed moment in queer theory.[32] Queer dance argues, instead, that queerness emerged in action, in protests, and on stages (as well as in writing), demanding a physical history that provocatively moves theorizations of self and sexuality, nation and assimilation alongside written histories and theorizations of queer moments. It is not that scholarly voices are not important. They are, and I hope this volume joins the now robust body of writing about queerness. There are great stakes in proclaiming one's queerness in writing and spoken language—these labels and categorizations have power within and beyond one's community. But there is also great power in claiming queerness in the press of bodies touching or in the exceeding of the body best measured in sweat and exhaustion. The slide of a hand across a hipbone might be just as much an act of coming out as an announcement offered in words. How does queerness exist in the realm of affect and touch, and what then might we find out about queerness through these pleasurable and complex bodily ways of knowing?

Queer dance challenges us to document the role of these physical actions in our pasts, recognizing what people have been able to do with their bodies. Queer dance's investment in bodies as sites to imagine, practice, cultivate, and enact social change is not just an aspiration. It is a documented outcome of our queer dancing pasts. We need only to recall the notable events within activist history—the high-kicking at Stonewall, the gender bending of Weimar cabaret, the fire-eating of the Lesbian Avengers, and the fierce parading in the streets of Ugandan LGBT activists—to know this. These events and more help us know that queer activists have successfully used their bodies to remind dominant cultures of the necessity of recognizing and supporting difference. As dance theorist Susan Foster notes, when ACT UP members piled themselves into tangled masses, die-ins, during protests in the late 1980s and early 1990s to demand the US government address the AIDS epidemic, those human piles did more than insist upon visibility for queer life and death. The activists' physical proximity—bodies closely touching, piled atop one another—kept the police from arresting individual protesters.[33] This was a choreography at once visible and impenetrable to the state. The police could not avoid the very real spectacle of bodies, the living channeling the dead, nor could they separate the group into easy-to-control individuals.

Looking to the past, too, forces us to remember that queer is not —in the 1990s nor now—a new political stance, but is instead intertwined with feminism, particularly Black feminism, as well as anti-racism, disability rights, and postcolonial work.[34] Queer developed from critical political antecedents and must be in conversation with them to remain responsive to the great breadth of dance-making and scholarship today. Within a US context, it is important to note that the physicality of queer protest is learned from—or at least related to—the strategies of the civil rights movement and radical feminism, movements where activists of color and women used their bodies to make radical calls for change in hostile environments.[35] Too, we need to think much more about the debt queer theory owes Black feminist theory and artmaking with their continued investments in multiple ways of knowing and the power and importance of lived experience. Hortense Spillers should be invoked in our teaching and scholarship just as often as Judith Butler; Pearl Primus and Katherine Dunham should be mentioned as often as Merce Cunningham.[36] The celebration of self-described queer voices cannot be a project that erases equally political, disruptive voices, and we have to be especially vigilant for when celebration of queerness is really a white erasure of Black and Brown people and communities.

While dance draws on these powerful legacies of knowing the body makes meaning and change, we still need more languages in dance—physical, written, and spoken—to discuss gender and sexuality in our dancing. Too often we talk of the body as an instrument or machine, disregarding the myriad ways bodies produce and respond to pleasure, desire, and normalizing forces. Treating bodies like instruments rather than social forces forecloses queer possibility, which is often intertwined with the unspoken and the felt. Not speaking about sexuality in robust ways allows homophobia to thrive in our dance institutions and representations. Treating queerness and homosexuality as only existing in the nonverbal realm marginalizes both.

It is key, too, to address sexism and homophobia together. So often homophobia arises from misogyny—a disgust with femininity no matter the body performing it. Femininity in dance is often seen as either an idealized category to which most can only aspire or a sign of weakness. Unless we conceive of femininity as aligned with strength and understand it as a broad, open category, rather than simply as a nymph that dreams of being carried around, our queer dance project will always be stymied in dance.

We need more language for and astute critique of sexuality and gender in dance because we have to hold tight to what drew many, especially so many LGBTQ-identified people, to dance in the first place: the pleasurable strangeness than can proliferate because of dance's often marginal status. This is crucial as some forms of LGBT life gain tolerance in mainstream society.[37] For instance, as artist/scholar Nicholas Gareiss discusses in his essay, traditional Irish dance and music have long held themselves up as bastions of Irish heteronormativity, with gay life largely acknowledged only in that powerful homosexual tool: gossip. Gareiss finished writing his essay in this volume as homosexuality moved into the Irish mainstream. Literally, on the day he wrote the last draft of his essay, Irish citizens voted to make gay marriage legal in Ireland. What it means to be gay thus changed in Ireland, and that will inevitably affect Irish traditional music and dance. It has already affected how one might receive "Lafferty's" (2015), Gareiss's duet with fiddler Cleek Schrey that appears on the *Queer Dance* website. Gareiss and Schrey created "Lafferty's" from the palette of sounds teachers told them were not to be included in Irish traditional dance and music—the squeaks and groans deemed too strange, assaultive to the ear. Gay marriage may bring gains for Irish LGBTQ citizens, and it will do its own queer work of unsettling the enshrinement of home and family in the Irish constitution.[38] But "Lafferty's" might now be seen as a living, sounding queer archive, relishing a strangeness that movements for marriage often mark as something of the past, a long-ago margin no longer needed. Through dancing though, queerness persists.

When we complicate our celebration of legislative gains by confessing to the appeal and possibilities of the margins, we move into the heart of contemporary queer questioning. This double bind is a key point for the field of dance in perhaps one of our most conservative mainstream social institutions: the academy. As dance gains respect as an academic field, we must keep feeding the radical critiques of academic life that dance can make. In the United States, dance studies arose as a field deeply enmeshed in feminism and Black dance studies, which helped it emerge as an area with different methodologies than more text-based humanities, and as a place where scholars and artists might work together. We must continue to infuse dance studies, particularly dance history, with queer sensibilities and to keep the feminist, anti-racist lenses already incorporated in the best of dance scholarship.

In dance studies, queer theory can help us further value the physical, the sexy, the erotic, and the political. Queer dance studies here might join radical feminism and contemporary Black studies to render a subject's worth as an artist or historical figure based on their challenges to the status quo. We could judge artists for their commentary on the erotic, the sexy, rather than judging their respectability or canonical contributions. For instance, we could consider African American scholar/choreographer/dancer Katherine Dunham part of a queer dance history, since she circulated African diasporic dance across US concert stages without refusing erotic possibility and gender radicalism. We could consider the choice to be a sensual, even sexy, Black woman on the concert dance stage as a queer act—an act that asks us to attend to the strictures in which we move and to claim public space for sexuality using the body.

The final large challenge of dancing queerly is its potential to teach us new ways of looking, to help us see beyond the ruts in which we ride. In performance, desires can be remixed and reconfigured, as audiences of all kinds open themselves to experiencing other ways of being.[39] In their writing about queer solo performance, Holly Hughes and David Román offer, as one function of queer performance, the ability to show audiences new ways of looking, sensing, and thinking. Queer performance can thwart an audience's assumptions about bodies, desire, and sex; and walk—or, in its more provocative moments, perhaps seduce or shove—an audience toward sensing differently.[40] In this way, queer performance becomes a kind of pedagogy, teaching someone what it might look like or feel like to refuse norms, particularly those related to gender and sexuality. Queer performance might be a way to promote a gay agenda! Come to our show: feel all the desires you thought you couldn't or shouldn't. How would you move in the world with that taste in your mouth?

Of the many dance works I have seen while shaping *Queer Dance*, no work better taught me the pedagogical power of dance to help me see gender anew than Filipino choreographer/dancer Eisa Jocson's stunning solo, *Macho Dancer* (2013). In the evening-length work, Jocson toys with her audience's gaze, leading us toward multiple ways to see her body and perceive her gender.

When I saw Jocson perform at the TBA festival in Portland, Oregon, in September 2014, her performance already felt slightly queer before she took the stage. I knew Jocson had worked for months with male Filipino macho dancers, who dance the form in clubs, to learn the vocabulary and to build a body that accentuated masculinity in shape and posture. Jocson's *Macho Dancer* cites the already queer gazes macho dancing invites in the Philippines. The form, a mix of snaking hip movements and, sometimes, enactments of bawdy sexual gestures, was once performed largely for gay male audiences. More recently, however, as a result of changing economics in a neoliberal Philippines, clubs opened to both gay male and straight female audiences, drawing both groups together in one club on the same night.[41] This shift means the dancers from whom Jocson learned the trade perform for two audiences, creating a slippage between what might constitute a homoerotic gaze and a heterosexual gaze. This, then, is an excellent example of queer dancing, since it is a dance not invested in or relying on one element to signal an alternative identity. Instead, it is a performance in which multiple alternatives to colonial, patriarchal, heterosexual dance unfold alongside one another.

With the help of macho dancers, Jocson created a body in the gym and in the rehearsal studio that she could use to lead audiences to see codes of masculinity while also seeing physical markers and postures often coded as feminine. For instance, her broad shoulders, built in the gym, pop in performance. In *Macho Dancer*, as she broadens her armpits and flexes her widened neck muscles, her shoulders are more central than her breasts, even when she is shirtless.[42] This is not just a queer performance strategy of a solo female dancer, but a performance that becomes queer through its comingling of sometimes vividly clashing possibilities. Jocson amplifies this queer assemblage, crafting a masculinity with her cisgendered female body through a performance of nonchalant aggression, undoing and repackaging key signifiers of masculinity. She chews gum slowly; strikes her cowboy boots at an

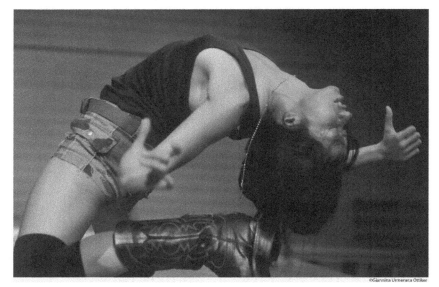

FIGURE 1.3 Eisa Jocson in *Macho Dancer*. Photo by Giannani Ottiker.

off-center, loud angle; and stands with her legs apart so her feet are spread in masculine strength rather than her legs spreading in feminine vulnerability.

The layers of mimicry, persona, and audience engagement/enticement throughout the work are complex. Jocson assumes markers of both hetero- and homo-masculinity that are already complicated within macho dancing. Especially in moments when she stares down the audience with a simulta- neously seductive and uninterested gaze, she confronts the audience into an erotic relationship with her. She creates a strong female persona and a fantasy of male masculinity that simultaneously interrupts a misogynist gaze, invites erotic female gazes, and opens the possibility of a gay male gaze in her echo- ing of the scene in which macho dancing usually unfolds.

As Jocson builds this heightened masculinity for her audience, she does not just denaturalize masculinity for them. *Macho Dancer* is not a drag king performance, but it does do some of the work Halberstam has argued that drag kings do: showing the labor and choices that form masculinity, and thus interrupting masculinity's place as "natural," the gender performance by which other gender performances are measured.[43] Jocson denaturalizes masculinity and points the audience toward her play with a simultaneous per- formance of femininity and masculinity, refusing to allow the audience to easily categorize a body into a gender by foregrounding the erotic. And thus an audience—even a contemporary dance audience that might not come for a queer experience (unlike Filipino macho dance audiences)—is ushered into a moment of public gender-scrambling.

More Than a Book

Just like the word "queer," dance is many things in this volume. The artists who populate this project make solos and group dances, improvisational work and work pre-planned to its last detail. They range widely in their artistic backgrounds; their chosen genres span from taiko drumming to drag kings and queens, solo dance modernism to Irish step dancing. There is not one way of dancing or making dance or studying dance with special access to queer critique—although I hope this project leads to much debate about what conditions of dancing, dance-making, or dance spectatorship invite queer critique.

If you move across and among the essays, the performances, and the interviews, there are many possibilities for queer meaning-making. Watch Gareiss and Schrey's "Lafferty's" and Post *Natyam*'s *rapture/rupture* (2013), the former a traditional Irish dance and music work and the latter a contemporary kathak dance work. Both comment on and resist mainstream modes of training in their respective dance forms—as elaborated upon in the essays written by each of the artists. Or consider different relationships among excess, queerness, and race by watching Lou Henry Hoover's *There Once was a Man* (2014), a drag/burlesque piece that critiques masculinity and whiteness through camp, and reading novelist Justin Torres's meditation on the pleasure of Latin Night at the queer club, a work written in the immediate aftermath of the 2016 Orlando shootings. Or pick up Hannah Kosstrin's queer reading of American modern dancer Anna Sokolow's *Rooms* (1954) after watching Peter Carpenter's performance of "Last Cowboy Standing" (2006); both contributions take up queer solitude as a form of protest. Or watch my interview with improviser and choreographer Anna Martine Whitehead in which we discuss Blackness, queerness, and improvisational practice, and then watch Whitehead's intimate solo/trio, "Memory Loser" (2015) and the gregarious, yet melancholic, *theory-ography 4.5: we* [still] *queer here* (2013), from the SLIPPAGE ensemble. There are so many possible groupings of interviews, performance, and writing in *Queer Dance*. So many. Find yours. There are no wrong ones.

Most of the work in this project, as well as the artists and scholars who produced it, do not fit cleanly—nor do they desire to fit cleanly—into categories presupposed by methods drawn from other academic areas—history or ethnography, for instance. Nor do many of these people fit only into categories of writer or artist. Scholars of queer dance defy traditional disciplinary and methodological divides, refusing divisions among history, ethnography, and theory—camps that have always been underpinned by assumptions about gender, sexuality, and race that should be made visible and reimagined. Too, the writing by artists is one of the strongest aspects of this book, and it is key to note that much of that writing is creative and wide-ranging, not just the kind of instrumental writing, for grants and so on, that has become the primary mode emphasized in teaching writing in arts-oriented programs. Queer approaches to dance scholarship and artmaking make more visible the structures (and limits) imposed on artists and scholars.

While "queer" may seek to defy category, inevitably categorization offers a way to begin. Both the book and the material online appear in suggested groupings. This anthology is organized into three areas: the stage (generally the concert stage), the social (the club, the street, etc.), and the intimate (the solo, the duet, sex). The website is organized in terms of forms of embodied conversation: one set, the eight filmed performances, focuses explicitly on danced interventions in notions of queerness, whereas the other set focuses on spoken conversation and is constituted by interviews I conducted with those performing in each of the documented works.

Queer Text

The book portion of *Queer Dance* begins with essays that define queer dance by unsettling it, exploring and disrupting notions too often central to queer studies and queer performance: white masculinity and Euro-American dance. The book's first part, "Queering the Stage," opens with drag king Lou Henry Hoover's visual and written meditation on the notion of artifice, a long-recognized characteristic of drag queen performance. Hoover flips this association, borrowing from the tricks of artifice long used by queens to create a dance spectacle that blends femininity and masculinity, drag queening and kinging, as well as burlesque. In the next essay, members of Post *Natyam* Collective, a transnational network of performers working with dance of the South Asian diaspora, discuss the process of making *rapture/rupture*, a combination of kathak movement vocabulary, Indian poetic forms, and striking costume changes, the pairing of the traditional *dupatta* with decidedly butch jeans. Choreographer/performer Cynthia Ling Lee and dramaturg Sandra Chatterjee write about the multiple versions of "queer" Post *Natyam* manipulates and reimagines as they moved through their performance research. They first tangled with excess, inspired by San Francisco-based Joe Goode's solo *29 Effeminate Gestures* (1987), but then moved toward thinking about queerness as "not enough" or lack, a formulation that helped them understand queerness at the nexus of South Asian identity, femininity, and diaspora.

In the volume's third essay, Emily Wilcox continues Post *Natyam*'s critique of Western sensibilities, writing about Beijing-based choreographer Gu Jiani's duet *Right & Left* (2014). Wilcox places the female-female duet within the history of women's roles in Chinese contemporary dance, arguing that Gu's choreography challenges heteronormativity's limitations on female performers. The final essay in this opening reassessment of queerness in dance comes from Doran George, who focuses on dances from the 1990s and early 2000s by American choreographers Neil Greenberg, John Jasperse, and Jennifer Monson. George argues that these choreographers, when framed by lenses developed from trans studies, feminist theory, and phenomenology, produce the possibility of what George terms "the hysterical spectator," a figure that moves across multiple gender identities and affinities.

The second half of "Queering the Stage" reimagines dance studies, particularly dance history, from a queer perspective. In an essay about the desires that might drive a queer look at history, Julian Carter traces the motion of the swan across European twentieth-century ballet, following her across time. This engages in what Carter calls "chasing feathers," an approach to dance that sees gender—like dance—as paradoxically ephemeral and lasting, formal and desirous. Jennifer Campbell continues in the realm of ballet, offering a queer reading of early American ballet, including Ballet Caravan's *Filling Station* (1938) and *Time Table* (1941). She argues that queer dance requires an interdisciplinary approach to dance studies. Only by examining the contributions of costume, music, and choreography together (rather than singling out one element) can queer subtext surface. Finally, Hannah Kosstrin concludes Part I with her analysis of Sokolow's *Rooms*. She explores the work in its moment of creation, the period in American history often known as the Lavender Scare when the US government targeted homosexuals under the guise of fighting Communism. In Kosstrin's analysis, *Rooms* becomes a work not generally about urban isolation but one borne of the specific melancholia produced by Cold War homophobia. As Kosstrin floods the piece with one history of its moment of creation, she offers one way to unlock what dance theorist Susan Foster has called modern dance's closet.[44]

In the book's second part, "Dancing toward Queer Sociality," artists and dance researchers examine social spaces that shift normative notions of gender, sexuality, and race. These essays attend to dance as it unsettles notions of relationships between center and margin, practice and product. Part II begins with thomas defrantz's meditation on what a queer ontology imagined from a dancing perspective might be. defrantz writes about working with his collaborators, SLIPPAGE, to create performance that holds queer-ness and Blackness together. He does this as a project that forestalls more utopic notions of worldmaking in favor of material viewings and renderings of bodies in their present moment—recognizing violence alongside possi-bility. defrantz's essay is followed by Torres's celebration of Latin Night at the queer club, an essay originally published in *The Washington Post* days after the massacre at Pulse. Torres lushly demonstrates what it means to resist memo-rialization in favor of celebrating queer life in all its incongruences.[45]

In the next two essays, Nicholas Gareiss and Kareem Khubchandani ex-plore dance forms not often marked as queer—for the former, traditional Irish music and dance, and for the latter, family gatherings in the Indian diaspora. Gareiss thinks across his experiences performing Irish traditional music and dance, examining some artists and audiences' insistence on there being no queer presence or people in the form as proof that queerness exists. Khubchandani takes an autoethnographic eye to his performance as a Bollywood drag performer. Thinking about his work as an Indian-born British citizen living and performing in the United States and India, Khubchandani argues that even as queer does not have a single definition as an identity—an origin one can point to as the root or cause of one's queerness—that does not discount the power, even necessity, of telling queer origin stories.

The last two essays in this part explore queer dance in relationship to activism. Artist/scholar Peter Carpenter discusses his dance-making as he makes work about AIDS and gay masculinity based on his ethnographic work in Los Angeles's gay country-and-western scene. Choreographer/per-former Jennifer Monson concludes Part II by remembering her work as an activist and artist in the early 1990s as the affective and physical landscape from which her choreographic practices have grown. She focuses on her co-creation with longtime collaborator DD Dorvillier, *RMW(a) & RMW* (1993/2004). In a poetic meditation on queer action and objects, Monson discusses the queer transmission between Dorvillier and herself, between artist and au-dience, and between artistry and activism, all of which makes possible a queer becoming of erotics and desire.

In the anthology's final part, "Intimacy," the essays continue themes de-veloped elsewhere, but turn to the personal—to love, to sex, and to friendship. Part III begins from a theater's backstage, as Angela Ahlgren recalls her work as a stage manager, which launched her relationship with the Asian American drumming form of taiko. Her dance as taiko drummer crosses between racial identities, backstage and onstage, and eventually romantic and artistic rela-tionships. Next Raquel Monroe focuses on the spoken word performance of the Punany Poets, Black lesbian activists in Oakland, California, who turned to the stage to offer alternative notions of gender as a way to combat the devastating effects of AIDS in Black hip-hop communities. In her essay, Monroe writes about intimate relationships between masculine and feminine figures that cross a range of stereotypes, shifting larger discourses about intimacy, safety, risk, and gender within Black respectability politics. Patrick McKelvey also challenges notions of risk in his essay, "Choreographing the Chronic," looking at conceptions of bodies and chronic disease in the bugchasing community of gay men, men who actively seek to transform their HIV sero-status to positive. He studies these discursive tropes through the representation of bugchasing in cultural objects, specifically choreographer Octavio Campos's *The Bugchasers* (2007). The anthology ends with a poetic manifesto by artist Anna Martine Whitehead, which reminds us of the challenges and power of physical action as queer: falling as a metaphor and a physical practice that helps recognize and value queer, Black, trans survival.

Emphasizing Performance

The visual portion of *Queer Dance*, the website that houses the performance documentation and filmed interviews, expands the archive of queer dance. All the artists featured on the website appear in the print anthology in some way. Some works preceded this project in their creation, for instance, DD Dorvillier and Jennifer Monson's *RMW(a) & RMW*, a work the two women initially made in 1993 and extended in 2004. This work has been central to my imagination of this entire project. *RMW(a) & RMW* foregrounds relationships between women, whose touching and moving together is, in contemporary dance, stubbornly not read as queer and often marginalized in queer dance spaces. Monson and Dorvillier play with and luxuriate in multiple avenues of desire and the erotic—at once strange and estranging, as well as hot and sexy. Too, the work's first iteration premiered in 1993, a reminder that queer art and queer scholarship have long developed alongside one another.

The second evening-length work featured on the website is a new creation imagined specifically for this project (albeit with some pre-existing elements): *theory-ography 4.5: we* [still] *queer here*, a collective imagining of dance as queer theorizing. thomas defrantz and his collaborative ensemble, SLIPPAGE, including Gina Kohler, Kevin Guy, and James Morrow (with me as dramaturg), descended on Ann Arbor, Michigan in 2013 to create the improvisational work, part of a longer series of dance research projects SLIPPAGE has undertaken to explore the relationship between contemporary theory and performance. This piece, which also featured University of Michigan students, began by engaging José Muñoz's *Cruising Utopia* (2009), asking what it means to create queer now, and how that might always be a project of and for a queer future.

The remaining works featured on the website are small, intimate works—solos, duets, and trios. In many ways, this is a reflection of some of the persistent logistics and thematics of queer performance. For reasons having to do with a lack of resources, queer performance has often tended toward solo work. The solo has become iconic of queer work, too, as Hughes and Román have noted, because queer performance often cuts close to the personal, refusing to rely on critical distance to secure its artistic credibility.[46] The people performing lay bare their actual lives. When I began this project, I wanted dance to be part of the conversation around queer solo performance, which tends toward text-driven work or the "body art" genre of performance art. What might it mean to think of solo dance work—long a hallmark of feminist interventions in dance—as having queer politics?

As I solicited solo works from artists, I got phone calls I now think of under the rubric: "let me tell you about the people in my solo." I began to wonder about the solo as a concept, as much as it is a description of a number of bodies onstage. Queer solo work is often an explicit conversation about self and other, where the queer body is always dancing with its own abjection, making public its multiple, even conflicting desires. This multivocality is an identifying marker of queer solo dances: making one's queer self visible becomes a necessarily social act that sometimes results in other performers on stage. The solo/not solos that constitute much of *Queer Dance*'s performance archive are queer acts because the queer soloist makes these other presences manifest: queer bodies are not relegated to the periphery in stories told about them; they tell their stories.[47] Too, the insistence of these artists that their solos required other performers highlights queer artists as often intensely invested in art making as an act for one's community and as a gesture toward building community. To be queer is perhaps always to be looking for partners and allies, making space with others in a world that would ask you to be alone and quiet.

There is only one actual solo among the queer solos: Peter Carpenter's "Last Cowboy Standing." The solo is an excerpt from Carpenter's evening-length piece *My Fellow Americans* (2009), a work developed (as Carpenter discusses in his essay in this anthology) from his research about AIDS, Ronald Reagan, and country-western gay bars. Both Carpenter and Post *Natyam* Ensemble's *rapture/rupture* explicitly engage with text in their performances: Carpenter with archived speeches given by Reagan and Post *Natyam* with poetry spoken onstage by director Shyamala Moorty as Cynthia

Ling Lee, who wrote the poetry, dances. The effect in the latter "solo" is one of doubling, a sense that Moorty and Lee might together be meditating on the same question. They seem to ask, "How are femininity and queerness in South Asian dance always in conversation with lack?" Both Post *Natyam*'s work and Lou Henry Hoover's drag king/burlesque/modern dance performance work, *There Once Was a Man* (an excerpt from an evening-length work), subvert gender binaries that frame women as lacking, a disruption that unsettles a common LGBTQ trope of identifying only men with fantastic camp sensibilities of excess. Hoover's surprisingly sparse spectacle triangulates Hoover's masculine persona, also named Lou Henry Hoover, with the Texas-sized femininity of Hoover's real-life wife and burlesque partner Kitten LaRue and the world's buffest cockroach and Hoover doppelganger/ nemesis, a role danced by trans performer Elby Brosch. Drag continues to be reimagined in the music video "Sari" (2016), featuring Bollywood drag artist LaWhore Vagistan (Kareem Khubchandani) and Auntie Kool Jams. Vagistan draws on longer traditions of drag queens as sassy, biting figures, as she remixes Bollywood and drag queen excess in a parody of pop star Justin Bieber's "Sorry" (2015).

The final documented performances return to the duet form, and might be profitably placed alongside Monson and Dorvillier's *RMW(a) & RMW* as dances of desire but also as dances of self and other. Beijing-based dancer and choreographer Gu Jiani performs her *Right and Left* with dancer Li Nan, a study in slight differences between two women—a slightly different haircut or a slight difference in movement— that push similar appearances and unison looks toward homoerotic desire. In "Lafferty's," dancer Nicholas Gareiss and musician Cleek Schrey bend queer performance toward an intervention in nation through a flirtatious play with the relationship between the Irish dancer and musician, Irish arts and the state. Scrapes, squeaks, and long-held gazes make legible the subtexts of a supposedly heteronormative, nationalist form. The question of visibility is most intensely taken on by Anna Martine Whitehead, who performs much of the solo/not solo, "Memory Loser," underneath a large blanket and deer head as two other performers shout, "Can you see her?"—a question Whitehead compels them to yell as they listen to instructions through headphones during the performance. The aerobic work, danced to yelling and Michael Jackson, tests the boundaries of seeing and being seen, looking for the queer edges that thwart easy ideas of visibility as they relate to race, gender, and sexuality.

All of the choreographers speak at length online about their works, often joined by their collaborators. Like the duets, these interviews are their own set of performances: of desire, collaboration, and discussion. Too, they serve as a reminder that, while dance is often described as nonverbal, it is deeply embedded in the conversations we have in studios, in theaters, and in a myriad of spaces beyond the concert stage or dance floor.

Onward!

Dancing queerly is a challenge. Dancing—when we are doing it and when we are watching it—can challenge us to put our bodies into motion together and to imagine other ways to live in and move through this world. Too often, we are told there is only one (correct) way to live. But dancing is a concrete, physical path through which we experience different ways of touching, loving, seeing, and being together. As we explore the world and our bodies' potential through dancing, we can bump against and refuse the limitations embedded in the spaces in which we learn to move. We can't always overturn these limitations—at least not immediately: social norms are deeply sedimented—but we can indict norms as arbitrary and punitive. We can trust what dancing itself teaches: that we can and do imagine other possibilities through fleshy, politically charged contact, and that cultivating the capacity to imagine otherwise is at the heart of any queer project.

Dancing queerly is never done alone; there's always someone else in my solo. We have to remember that our daily claims to live otherwise are group choreographies of differing focus: sometimes composed against a norm and sometimes forged shoulder-to-shoulder. When we engage in dance as a daily practice and when we build institutions, as teachers, mentors, and administrators, we invite some physical connections and not others, value some ways of moving over others. Audiences also bring queer desires to their spectatorship as they look back on now canonical work, when they imagine queer possibilities even within the most mainstream work, or when they share desirous pleasure with performers as they watch in spaces of all kinds. Queerness travels on the waves of our desires and actions, constantly composed and recomposed by artists and audiences together as a way to make specific, located challenges to constrictive and limited notions of power.

Queer dance could be the wildest, sexiest, most ferocious desiring of the imagination made flesh. When queer desires and action manifest in dance, we are, first and foremost, challenged to remember and recognize people's bodies doing work. Dancing queerly, when we respect it as a politics that always (at least partially) eludes clear definition, challenges us to think of queer as social action consciously entangled with fantasy, desire, and physical practice. As we dance, dreaming and doing are not separate.

Notes

1. This volume moves in the predominant mode of queer studies, which refuses a notion that queerness has any specific referent, a conception Jack Halberstam, José Muñoz, and David Eng have described as a "subjectless critique" that "disallows any positing of a proper subject of or object for the field by insisting that queer has no fixed political reference." Halberstam, Muñoz, and Eng define this subjectless critique in opposition to what they see as gay and lesbian studies "positivist" stance toward certain kinds of people and lives being at the center of the mode of study, theorization, and historical analysis. This volume questions the degree to which this shift from a supposedly positivist stance toward the subjectless critique might have moved queer studies into what I term a "body-less critique," in as much as the refusal to identify queer with any particular group or individual then—perhaps inadvertently—leads to bodies being only metaphors, never actual, concrete material substances that can make meaning and make change, see David L. Eng with Judith Halberstam and José Esteban Muñoz, "Introduction: What's Queer about Queer Studies Now?" *Social Text* 23, no. 3–4 (2005): 1–16.

2. The emphasis on different kinds of physical embodiments, done in public, as social force is key to dance studies but is also a central force of Lauren Berlant and Michael Warner's now iconic essay (and a major first inspiration for this collection) "Sex in Public," *Critical Inquiry* 24, no. 2 (1998): 547–66.

3. The necessity of incorporating artists, as both performers and writers, into this project builds upon a legacy in dance of artists being some of the first to chart the experience of LGBT life in dance. For exemplary autobiographical writing in this vein, see Bill T. Jones and Peggy Roggenbuck Gillespie, *Last Night on Earth* (New York: Pantheon Books, 1995); and Elizabeth Streb, *How to Become an Extreme Action Hero* (New York: Feminist Press, 2010).

4. For one of the most important early essays about centering women, particularly lesbians, in queer dance, see Ann Cvetkovich, "White Boots and Combat Boots: My Life as a Lesbian Go-Go Dancer," in *Dancing Desires: Sexualities On and Off the Stage* (Madison: University of Wisconsin, 2001): 315-348.

5. "Introduction," in *Dancing Desires: Sexualities On and Off the Stage* (Madison: University of Wisconsin, 2001): 3-34. For more important early work on feminist and queer sensibility in dance, see Ann Cooper Albright, *The Body and Identity in Contemporary Dance* (Middletown, CT: Wesleyan University Press, 1997).

6. For more on the radical possibilities of the club dance floor, as well as the normative strictures that remain in those spaces, see Fiona Buckland, *Impossible Dance: Club Culture and Queer World-Making* (Middletown, CT: Wesleyan University, 2002); David Román, "Theatre Journal: Dance Liberation," *Theatre Journal* 55, no. 3 (2003): 377–94; and Ramón Rivera-Servera, *Performing Queer Latinidad: Dance, Sexuality, Politics* (Ann Arbor: University of Michigan Press, 2013).

7. Michael Warner, "Introduction," in *Fear of a Queer Planet: Queer Politics and Social Theory* (Minneapolis: University of Minnesota Press, 1993), xxii–xxiii.

8. For discussions of heteronormativity in dance clubs, see Cindy Garcia, "'Don't leave me, Celia!': Salsera Homosociality and Pan-Latina Corporealities," *Women & Performance: A Journal of Feminist Theory* 18, no. 3 (2008): 199–213; and Ramón Rivera-Servera, "Choreographies of Resistance: Latina/o Queer Dance and the Utopian Performative," *Modern Drama* 47, no. 2 (2004): 269–89.

9. thomas f. defrantz, "Foreword: Black Bodies Dancing Black Culture—Black Atlantic Transformations," in *EmBODYing Liberation: The Black Body in American Dance*, ed. Dorothea Fischer-Hornung and Alison D. Goeller (Hamburg: Lit, 2001), 11–16.

10. For more on the necessity of discomfort in coalitional politics and the roots of such coalitional work in feminism and Black feminism, see Bernice Johnson Reagon, "Coalition Politics: Turning the Century," in *Home Girls: A Black Feminist Anthology*, 2d ed., ed. Barbara Smith (Camden, NJ: Rutgers University Press, 2000), 343–56.

11. In the immediate wake of the Orlando shootings, several Latinx queer dance and performance scholars spoke with the press about the ways in which the reporting about the shooting extended these racist, homophobic, and xenophobic strands by overlooking questions of identity and also offered alternate perspectives on the shooting that foregrounded the lives of Latinx people. For works that exemplify this scholarly activism as its best, see Spencer Kornhaber, "The Singular Experience of the Queer Latin Nightclub: An Interview with Ramón Rivera-Servera," *The Atlantic*, June 17, 2016, http://www.theatlantic.com/entertainment/archive/2016/06/orlando-shooting-pulse-latin-queer-gay-nightclub-ramon-rivera-servera-intrerview/487442/; and Juana Maria Rodriguez, "Voices: LGBT Clubs Let Us Embrace Queer Latinidad; Let's Affirm This," NBC News. June 16, 2016, http://www.nbcnews.com/storyline/orlando-nightclub-massacre/voices-lgbt-clubs-let-us-embrace-queer-latinidad-let-s-n593191.

12. Mae Henderson and E. Patrick Johnson, "Introduction," in *Black Queer Studies: A Critical Anthology* (Durham, NC: Duke University Press, 2005): 21-51.

13. Gayatri Gopinath, *Impossible Desires: Queer Diasporas and South Asian Public Cultures* (Durham, NC: Duke University Press, 2005); Jasbir Puar, *Terrorist Assemblages: Homonationalism in Queer Times* (Durham, NC: Duke University Press, 2007).

14. Alyson Campbell and Stephen Farrier, "Introduction," in *Queer Dramaturgies: International Perspective on Where Performance Leads Queer* (London: Palgrave McMillan, 2015), 8.

15. "Introduction," *TSQ: Transgender Studies Quarterly* 1, nos. 1–2 (2014): 1–18.

16. Many scholars discuss how the gender binary pervades dance training across multiple dance pedagogical settings, especially as it confuses gender expression and the body, see Judith Hamera's discussion of how gender is embedded into

American ballet studios, in which she notes that "boys" are asked to spend their time differently than "girls," in *Dancing Communities: Performance, Difference, and Connection in the Global City* (New York: Palgrave 2007), 60–76; and Kareem Khubchandani on the gender norms of male and female entrées into different Indian dance practices, especially as certain "moves" are taught to boys and certain ones to girls within Indian dance teams, in "Lessons in Drag: An Interview with LaWhore Vagistan," *Theatre Topics* 25, no. 3 (2015): 287. For more on the challenges disability studies and disabled dancers make to Euro-American approaches to contemporary dance pedagogy, as well as how those challenges are always bound to questions of gender, see Lliane Loots, "'You don't look like a dancer!': Gender and Disability Politics in the Arena of Dance as Performance and as a Tool for Learning in South Africa," *Agenda* 29, no. 2 (2015): 122–32.

17. For more about the codes through which homophobia is transmitted in American dance training, see Doug Ri1sner, "Rehearsing Heterosexuality: 'Unspoken' Truths in Dance Education," *Dance Research Journal* 34, no. 2 (2002): 63–78.

18. For more on the detrimental modes of femininity entrenched in dance, see Clare Croft, "Feminist Dance Criticism and Ballet," *Dance Chronicle* 37, no. 2 (2014): 195–217.

19. Judith Halberstam, *In a Queer Time and Place: Transgender Bodies, Subcultural Lives* (New York: New York University Press, 2005), 36. For more recent discussions of queer and American regionalism explicitly as an alternative narrative to metronormativity, see Martin F. Manalansan IV, Chantal Nadeau, Richard T. Rodriguez, and Siobhan B. Sommerville, "Queering the Middle: Race, Region, and a Queer Midwest," *GLQ: A Journal of Lesbian and Gay Studies* 20, nos. 1–2 (2014): 1–12. For writing about queer life in rural spaces, see Scott Herring, *Another Country: Queer Anti-Urbanism* (New York: New York University Press, 2010).

20. Alexander Doty's now iconic proposal of the possibility of a broad move into queerness from the position of audience member/viewer—that "'queerness' [is] a mass culture reception practice that is shared by all sorts of people in varying degrees of consistency and intensity"—remains a touchstone for this volume, see *Makings Things Perfectly Queer: Interpreting Mass Culture* (Minneapolis, MN: University of Minnesota Press, 1993).

21. While many performance theorists have since written about the performativity of language, I remain indebted to Judith Butler's analysis of the relationship between speech and physical action in *Speech Acts: A Politics of the Performative* (New York: Routledge, 1997).

22. For one of the most careful outlines of "queer" across multiple time periods and competing developments, see "Queer," Siobhan Sommerville, *Keywords for American Studies*, ed. Bruce Burgett and Glenn Hendler (New York: NYU Press, 2007), 182–90. For further outlines of queer's etymologic and historical development, see Annamarie Jagose, *Queer Theory: An Introduction* (New York: NYU

Press, 1997). For discussion of queer studies' emergence from gay and lesbian studies, see "Introduction," in *The Lesbian and Gay Studies Reader*, ed. Henry Abelove, Michele Aina Barale, and David Halperin (New York: Routledge, 1993): xv–xiii.

23. As I discuss the notion of queer horizon, I am invoking Josè Muñoz's notion of queerness as "squinting at the horizon," see *Cruising Utopia: The Then and There of Queer Futurity* (New York: NYU Press, 2009), 22, 117.

24. As David Halperin writes: "Queer is by definition *whatever* is at odds with the normal, the legitimate, the dominant. *There is nothing in particular to which it necessarily refers.* It is an identity without an essence . . . demarcate[ing] not a positivity but a position *vis-à-vis* the normative . . . [describing] a horizon of possibility whose precise extent and heterogeneous scope cannot in principle be delimited in advance," *Saint = Foucault: Towards a Gay Hagiography* (New York: Oxford University Press, 1995), 62.

25. Sedgwick articulates the reasons we need queer's insistence on heterogeneity as she explains why Christmas in the United States can be so awful, noting that Christmas is a time when too many narratives align as public and private; church, family, and state all rally around one message, thus shutting down imagination and possibility, particularly if one lives in opposition to Christianity, capitalism, and/or heteronormativity. It's worth quoting Sedgwick at length. She writes:

> 'Queer' can refer to . . . the open mesh of possibilities, gaps, overlaps, dissonances and resonances, lapses and excesses of meaning when the constituent elements of anyone's gender, of anyone's sexuality aren't made (or *can't* be made) to signify monolithically. The experimental linguistic, epistemological, representational, political adventures attaching to the very many of us who may at times be moved to describe ourselves as (among many other possibilities) pushy femmes, radical faeries, fantasists, drags, clones, leatherfolk, ladies in tuxedoes, feminist women or feminist men, masturbators, bulldaggers, divas, Snap! Queens, butch bottoms, storytellers, transsexuals, aunties, wannabes, lesbian-identified men or lesbians who sleep with men, or . . . people able to relish, learn from, or identify with such.

Sedgwick's description usefully describes or invites an image of queer performance space as she begins by thinking about multiple ways meanings collide— lapse and excess work together, for instance—and, too, her list of those who might populate queer space is one marked somewhat by identity, but primarily by practice, "Queer and Now," in *The Routledge Queer Studies Reader*, ed. Donald E. Hall and Annamarie Jagose with Andrea Bebell and Susan Potter (New York: Routledge, 2013), 7.

26. For more on the challenge to the notion of anti-normativity as falsely treating norms as monolithic and stable, see Robyn Weigman and Elizabeth Wilson, "Queer Theory without Antinormativity," *Differences* 26, no. 1 (2016): 1–25.

27. Sedgwick, "Queer and Now," 7.

28. These texts are where much of this project began, see Buckland, *Impossible Desires*; Desmond, *Dancing Desires*; Rivera-Servera, *Performing*; Valerie Briginshaw, *Dance, Space and Subjectivity* (New York: Palgrave, 2001); thomas f. defrantz, "Blacking Queer Dance," *Dance Research Journal* 34, no. 2 (2002): 102–5; Petra Kuppers, "Vanishing in Your Face: Embodiment and Representation in Lesbian Dance Performance," *Journal of Lesbian Studies* 2, no. 2–3 (1998): 47–63; Marta Savigliano, "Notes on Tango (as) Queer (Commodity)," *Anthropological Notebooks* 16, no. 3 (2010): 135–43.

29. I am grateful to playwright Tina Satter for talking with me about her play, *Ancient Lives* (2015), and her approach to making queer performance. Satter is the one who first talked to me about simultaneous concealment and revelation as central to queerness.

30. All performance descriptions are composites drawn from seeing the work live when it appeared at The Kitchen in New York City in its December 2011 premiere and also from a video of those performances provided by Abraham. in.motion. Many thanks to Hillary Kooistra for making access to the latter possible.

31. For more on "becoming" as a key idea in queer performativity, see Judith Butler, *Gender Trouble: Feminism and the Subversion of Identity*, 10th anniversary edition (New York: Routledge, 1999), 33.

32. The year 1990 saw the publication of three now iconic volumes in queer studies: Judith Butler's *Gender Trouble*, David Halperin's *One Hundred Years of Homosexuality*, and Eve Sedgwick's *The Epistemology of the Closet*. While this volume draws intensely on much of the work in these books, it resists a narrative of these books as the watershed moment in queer theory and, instead, seeks to craft a notion of queer history as moving from the streets and artmaking into the academy and also notes how many artists today are studying queer theory as one part of their artmaking practices. See also Judith Butler, *Gender Trouble: Feminism and the Subversion of Identity* (New York: Routledge, 1990); David Halperin, *One Hundred Years of Homosexuality and Other Essays on Greek Love* (New York: Routledge, 1990); and Eve Kosofsky Sedgwick, *Epistemology of the Closet* (Berkeley: University of California Press, 1990).

33. Susan Foster, "Choreographies of Protest," *Theatre Journal* 55, no. 3 (2003): 404.

34. For more on feminist and anti-racist theoretical and historical contributions to queer studies, see Mae Henderson and E. Patrick Johnson, "Introduction," in *Black Queer Studies: A Critical Anthology* (Durham, NC: Duke University Press, 2005), 21–51; and Heather Love, "Introduction," *GLQ* 17, no. 1 (2011): 1–14.

35. Foster, "Choreographies," 2–4; Rebekah Kowal, "Staging the Greensboro Sit-Ins," *TDR* 48, no. 4 (2004): 135–54.

36. For an overview of the theory of intersectionality as it has moved within and from Black feminist and critical race theory, as well as a discussion of what

it offers and sometimes limits in coalitional organizing, see Jennifer C. Nash, "Re-thinking Intersectionality," *Feminist Review* 89 (2008): 1–15; too, it is useful to mark that much of the concept of gender performativity that ignited what is now known as queer theory—the disjuncture among one's body, how one moves in the world, and how one is described in language as a force of social norms—is elaborated in Black feminist theorist Hortense Spillers iconic essay, "Mama's Baby, Papa's Maybe," which precedes Judith Butler's more often cited (and, of course, important) work in the late 1980s and early 1990s. For more, see "Mama's Baby, Papa's Maybe: An American Grammar Book," *Diacritics* 17, no. 2 (1987): 64–81.

37. For more on this historical shift in "tolerance" for the LGBT community and its negative implications for LGBTQ equality, see Suzanna Danuta Walters, *The Tolerance Trap: How God, Genes, and Good Intentions are Sabotaging Gay Equality* (New York: NYU, 2014).

38. For more on queer performance and queer performativity in Ireland, particularly following the decriminalization of homosexuality in 1993, see Fintan Walsh, "Flaming Archives," *Queer Notions: New Plays and Performances from Ireland* (Cork: Cork University Press, 2010).

39. Jill Dolan discusses feminist performance, especially solo performance, as it invites audiences to consider others' perspectives by way of experiencing that perspective as an audience member watching a performer speaking from a background other than one's own, which, in Dolan's words, can be an experience of "finding our feet in one another's shoes," see *Utopia in Performance: Finding Hope at the Theater* (Ann Arbor: University of Michigan Press, 2005), 63–88. As queer dance moves such notions into more explicit embodied sensibilities though, I also consider Susan Foster's charge to be suspicious of empathetic projects as they threaten, sometimes, to eradicate the unique specificities of underrepresented speakers in favor of making space for the experience of audiences from dominant backgrounds, see *Choreographing Empathy: Kinesthesia in Performance* (New York: Routledge, 2010), 11.

40. Holly Hughes and David Román, *O Solo Homo: The New Queer Performance* (New York: Grove Press, 1998), 5.

41. For more on Jocson's work and touring, see her website, https://eisajocson. wordpress.com/. For more on macho dancing within a Filipino context and a queer context, see Rolando B. Tolentino, "Macho Dancing, the Feminization of Labor, and Neoliberalism in the Philippines," *The Drama Review (TDR)* 53, no. 2 (2009): 77–89.

42. All movement descriptions in this writing are drawn from my attendance at two performances of *Macho Dancer* in Portland, Oregon, in September 2014 as part of the Portland Institute of Contemporary Art's TBA Festival, where I was in residence as a guest scholar. The descriptions are also supported by viewing

documentation, shared with me by Jocson, of a 2013 performance at the contemporary dance festival Impulstanz in Vienna, Austria.

43. Judith Halberstam, *Female Masculinity* (Durham, NC: Duke University Press, 1988), 234.

44. Susan Leigh Foster, "Closets Full of Dances," *Dancing Desires: Sexualities On and Off the Stage* (Madison: University of Wisconsin, 2001): 147–207.

45. I borrow the term "memorialization" from Jack Halberstam, who argues for being suspicious of memorialization as the key work queer art can do and resisting the ways in which memorialization cleans up "disorderly histories," see *The Queer Art of Failure* (Durham, NC: Duke University Press, 2011), 15.

46. Hughes and Román, *O Solo Homo*, 6–8.

47. David Gere, *How to Make Dances in an Epidemic: Tracking Choreography in the Age of AIDS* (Madison: University of Wisconsin Press, 2004), 12.

PART I

Queering the Stage

1

To be a Showboy

Lou Henry Hoover

▶ "There Once Was a Man"
▶ in conversation with Lou Henry Hoover, Kitten LaRue, and Elby Brosch

I make performances about me.

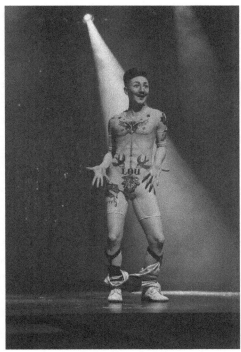

FIGURE I.I Lou Henry Hoover. Photo by Tuula Ylikorpi.

Sometimes that looks like a slow motion walk down the street wearing a white leotard with the word "queer" printed across it. Sometimes that looks like eleven drag and dance artists in summer camp uniforms singing Tiffany's version of "I Think We're Alone Now" around a campfire. Or two vogueing clowns. Or a merman trapped in a net. Or a woman eating potato chips.

I make performance about how I am mostly like you and also a little bit unlike you. I am continually invigorated by my repeated discovery that the moments and emotions that feel most personal in life are also the most universal—most every human has a coming of age story, has fallen in love, has experienced grief. Boiled down to its essence, my work shows unique, queer creatures onstage having universally human experiences.

The creatures that inhabit my work range from burlesque divas to cockroach doppelgängers of myself.[1] They are all expressions of drag, which I define as the use of artifice as a means to expose truth. Drag has been used by queer people throughout history to express something about how they feel—a part of their gender and/or sexuality that may not be apparent without that artifice. I'm thinking about such examples as the revolutionary gender expression of Weimar Berlin, and the drag balls we get a snapshot of in the film *Paris is Burning* (1990). In both examples, queer people use drag to express themselves in innumerably nuanced ways—there is, of course, gender, but also fantasy versions of themselves with qualities from best and most beautiful to ugliest and worst. Weimar and the balls are also two cultures created by and for disenfranchised peoples using drag to parody the social classes and racial stereotypes that oppress them. In a post-*Drag Race* world, when millions of viewers all over the world have become accustomed to safely consuming images of drag performance on their TVs in their living rooms without having to set foot in a gay bar or actually engage with a queer person, I see great value in remembering that "delivering realness" was once political, not just slang for good drag. I am inspired by artists who have used the outrageousness of camp drag to demonstrate universal humanity. Take the scene when John Waters had Divine eat dog shit in *Pink Flamingoes* (1972). It's the most outrageous, un-relatable thing she could do, but the moment always leaves me feeling connected to the patheticness of the character's misguided plight for fame and love.

I developed my signature drag look performing masculinity in a context where most of my colleagues were performing femininity. When I began using drag in my work, the predominant look for contemporary drag kings involved little artifice—not much make-up and off-the-rack men's clothes for costuming. These aesthetic choices can serve as a show of butch-ness, but they can also extend the gender stereotype that men require little grooming so drag kinging should follow suit. I chose to be a drag king using as much

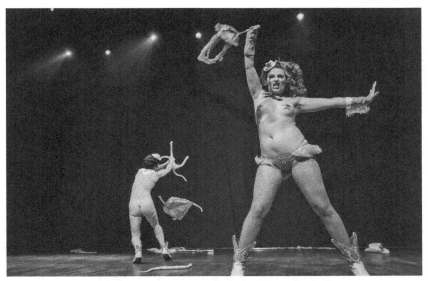

FIGURE 1.2 Lou Henry Hoover and Kitten LaRue. Photo by Alan Hayslip. © 2015
Allan Hayslip Photography.

and aesthetically similar artifice to the drag queens and burlesque performers I work with. I see this as something of a third wave feminist approach to
drag kinging, further queering the paradigm of drag by reclaiming from drag
queens (many of whom are men) the feminine process of putting on make-up
and subverting it to create a masculine result.

Performing as this showboy of a drag king is not only an aesthetic choice,
it is also my way of matching the depth of process and commitment to transformation that my favorite drag queens undertake. I want to use my own
transformation to honor and pay homage to the history of drag. By taking
on a drag persona, I honor the people who bravely expressed their identity
through cross-dressing, even in a period when cross-dressing was a crime.
I honor the fags and butches that rioted with kick lines outside The Stonewall
Inn. I honor all the people whose sacrifices along the battle for gay rights have
allowed me to have the career as a queer artist and the life as a queer human
that I have.

My performance of gender is not limited to masculinity. I also perform
as a drag queen and as a burlesque artist. Sometimes I choose to perform
femininity because a female persona allows me to express the concept, feeling, or idea of a piece more fully. Sometimes there are opportunities that
are only open to me if I perform femininity, instead of masculinity, because
a director is casting women, not men or drag kings. It gives me a personal

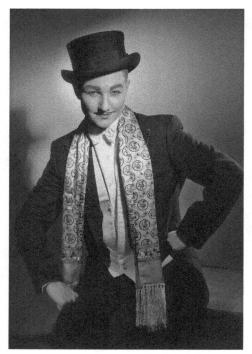

FIGURE I.3 Lou Henry Hoover. Photo by Neil Kendall. © Neil Kendall.

thrill of secret, subversive pleasure that I, a butch-identified lesbian, appear as one of five burlesque dancers in full showgirl regalia onstage in the PBS *Great Performances* special *Tony Bennett and Lady Gaga: Cheek To Cheek Live!* (2014). Our ensemble of neo-burlesuqe dancers pay homage to and reclaim the classic image of a group women identically dressed in rhinestones and feathers, giving this outrageous, glorious, funny, and sexy representation of femininity a new context. I think that most of the TV audience would be surprised to meet me out of that particular drag. I experience those moments as powerful acts of anti-misogyny and feminism, knowing that the gender constructs I present are tools imbued with the brilliant strength of the women who have employed them to their own advantage throughout history. It's always an honor to join the radical women who are performing femininity today.

Using artifice to reveal truth begins with drag and extends into the performative action of my work. I employ highly choreographed and specific movement for Lou onstage, so each moment is opportunity for expression. I am pairing the self-awareness one must cultivate as a choreographer with the persona's—Lou Henry Hoover's—lack of self-awareness in order to

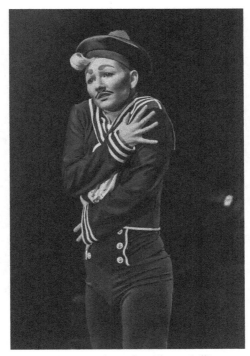

FIGURE 1.4 Lou Henry Hoover. Photo by Olena Sullivan. © Olena Sullivan/
Photolena.

create an experience for the audience. This could be likened to the relationship between many choreographers and their dancers, where the choreographer is constructing a big picture by giving dancers only the information
and motivations they need to execute their piece of the puzzle. I enjoy the
special trick of playing both the choreographer and performer. I can make
studied choices as a choreographer and play the fool as an actor. As choreographer, I stand in a studio and decide that my piece *There Once Was a
Man* (2014) needs a moment for reconciliation between Lou and his wife
before the beer-bottle-jerk-off section so the audience still likes Lou. Then
I get to go onstage as Lou and not worry about if the audience likes me or
not: I can just ride the map of emotions from remorse to contentedness to
lust. The result of this disjuncture is camp, as the term is currently used
by myself and my contemporaries. It's acting with an extra dose of suspension of disbelief. It's having a five-minute-long interaction between Kitten
and Lou onstage with Kitten getting obviously more and more frustrated
with Lou, but Lou not noticing. Onstage in that trajectory I'm holding
onto innocence and obliviousness so the audience can take a ride. This is

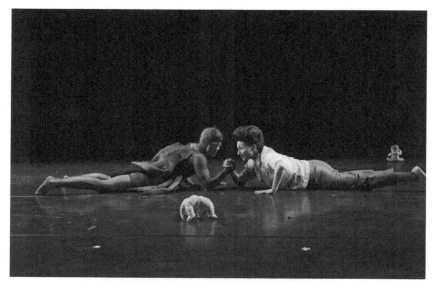

FIGURE 1.5 Elby Brosch and Lou Henry Hoover in "There Once Was a Man." Photo by Sarah Nesbitt.

my way of referencing and invoking the spirit of twentieth-century camp, an aesthetic with many facets. One of my favorite flavors of camp is the gay coding found in the ideals of femininity and masculinity portrayed in twentieth-century film—the result of queer artists, especially choreographers and directors, working in a pre-*Glee* world, when a mainstream audience rejected homosexuality entirely.

I am obsessed with the relationship between comedy and tragedy. Both the moment that something is so pathetically tragic it becomes hilarious and the moment that comedy drops away to reveal a pang to the heart. Louis CK (especially in the TV series *Louie*) is one of my heroes on this front. I often employ a character in a sincere attempt that is failing, which requires both a level of theatrical prowess and choreography that allows performers to be specifically performing the trying-to-get-it-right, as opposed to the failing. I look to great physical comedians of the silent film era like Charlie Chaplin for inspiration here. Finding this quality is the biggest challenge I face when translating my work onto other dancers. I consider my choreography to be based in emotion There is always a specific thought or feeling informing each movement. For multiple dancers to be in unison they must be going through this mental exercise in unison. They must execute the movement as perfectly as they can even if the movement is choreographed to appear somehow "failed."

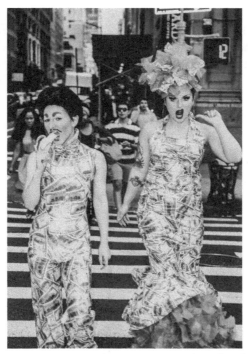

FIGURE 1.6 Lou Henry Hoover and Kitten LaRue. Photo by Eli Schmidt. © Eli Schmidt Photography Inc.

This artifice may look like candy coating, but it is not superficial. This artifice is the drag and theatrical trickery I employ in order to reveal the truth of my own human-ness, and the universality of the experience of being human. This artifice comes from my desire to connect, to be generous with my audience. I create performance work to continually rediscover the simple fact that while we are each our own unique snowflakes of otherness, even that sentiment is deeply common to the human experience.

Note

1. Much of my work and research has and continues to take place in collaborative partnerships. I would like to thank and acknowledge the following artists: Director of The Atomic Bombshells Burlesque, my wife and performance partner Kitten LaRue, whose vast canon of knowledge and aesthetic sensibility regarding the history of camp and music combined with her ability to stay on the pulse of what is popular results in highly entertaining intelligent spectacle;

BenDeLaCreme, a drag queen whose expertise on queer performance art and gender theory is beautifully evident in her hilarious content-driven performance; and modern dancer turned drag queen Cherdonna Shinatra, whose unwavering drive to get at something more unexpected, more original, and more honest results in truly surprising and unforgettable dance-based performance.

2

"Our Love Was Not Enough"

QUEERING GENDER, CULTURAL BELONGING, AND
DESIRE IN CONTEMPORARY *ABHINAYA*

Sandra Chatterjee and Cynthia Ling Lee

▶ *rapture/rupture*
▶ in conversation with Cynthia Ling Lee and Shyamala Moorty

A bejeweled, feminine figure stands upstage with her gaze slightly lowered, as the melancholy sweet strains of a Hindustani stringed *sarangi* fill the stage. Head covered with a sheer golden *dupatta* (scarf), she gestures as if drawing a *ghunghat* or veil delicately across her face. Her traditional costume and movement clearly mark her as a performer of kathak, a classical dance form from the northern part of the Indian subcontinent. She turns slowly toward an imagined presence, walking with longing and hesitation, then runs forward as a female voice says with yearning, "I was drawn to you." The dancer quickly kneels and drinks from her cupped hands, fingers tracing down her throat sensually. Soon afterwards, we hear the poetic line, "I was a foreigner in your world," while the performer gestures *alapadma* upwards in a staccato rhythm, as if eager to speak, only to turn away in disappointment.[1] The mention of foreignness disrupts the Indian classical imagery. This disruption is amplified as the performer slowly pulls the *dupatta* and jeweled *tikka* off her head to reveal her short, boyish hair and East Asian (rather than South Asian) features, punctuated by the plaintive line: "Beloved, our love was not enough."

This is a section of our piece, *rapture/rupture* (2013), a contemporary *abhinaya* work by Cynthia Ling Lee (movement and performance), Shyamala Moorty (direction), and Sandra Chatterjee (theoretical dramaturgy) of the

Post *Natyam* Collective. In this performance excerpt, we see a glimpse of
how multiple modes of *abhinaya* highlight the performer's failure to live up
to a dominant kathak discourse that calls for purist notions of culture, race,
nation, religion, and femininity.[2] These failed identifications point out the
multiple ways in which she is lacking or "not enough." While *rapture/rupture*
choreographs lack, it also produces a dancing subject who should not exist,
whose hybrid body, whose ethnic mismatch, whose gender nonconformity,
and whose same-sex love across cultural difference exceed the boundaries of
dominant kathak discourse. Embracing lack as a mode of exceeding dominant boundaries enables a queer dance-making practice that interweaves the
queering of gender and cultural belonging while opening up the possibility of
queer desire. This essay traces how the piece was developed through a collaborative process, which inextricably entangled choreography and scholarship,
recounting the ways in which the choreographic theorizations of *rapture/rup-
ture* unfolded step-by-step.

rapture/rupture emerged from one of our highly structured online creative processes: the *Subversive Gestures Feedback Loop*.[3] As a transnational,
web-based coalition of dance artists, we use online collaborative processes to
produce dance and media works that reimagine South Asian dance through
feminist-of-color, queer, postcolonial, and diasporic lenses. Trained in different
Indian classical dance forms, we started working together in 2004 to counter
a postmodern aesthetic hegemony that embraced objectivist abstraction over
aesthetic values central to Indian dance such as narrative, facial expression,
and emotion.[4] Critiquing the hegemonic primacy of "Western" aesthetics in
defining contemporary dance globally continues to be important to us as a
decolonizing act. At the same time, we actively work against diasporic-nation-
alist, Orientalist, romanticizing, and exoticizing visions of Indian classical
dance, while creating interdisciplinary politically engaged performance work
embracing hybridity and contemporaneity.

During the *Subversive Gestures Feedback Loop*, we engaged in choreographic
studies, dramaturgical feedback, and theoretical readings on gender and performance from South Asian and Euro-American perspectives. Working in a
feedback loop between theory and practice, we set out to research ways to denaturalize Indian classical kathak's script of idealized femininity to facilitate
more fluid, diverse possibilities for performing gender in South Asian aesthetic
contexts. In this essay, in addition to charting the *Subversive Gestures Feedback
Loop*, we also analyze our process using theoretical insights generated in other
contexts, including our engagements with queer/ing as a performative tactic,
as well as intersecting theorizations of Asian American choreographic practice with critiques of Eurocentric discourses of the "contemporary" in central

and northern European contexts. This essay therefore continues our praxis-based process, bringing to light multiple levels of queering—queering gender, queering cultural belonging, and queer desire—by analyzing key moments in our process.

Transnational Theorizations of Queer and Queering

What do we mean by queer and queering? In our earlier theorizations of queer South Asian performance, we have "[regarded] any embodied performance that opens up possibilities for eroticism, sexuality, and gender outside of heteronormative patriarchal structures as potentially queer."[5] We therefore consider the term "queer" to be not only aligned with non-normative genders and sexualities, but as queer theorist David Halperin states, "queer is by definition *whatever* is at odds with the normal, the legitimate, the dominant."[6] We follow gender studies scholar Ruth Vanita in finding the fluidity of "queer" more productive for South Asian contexts than the identity categories of LGBT, for the "identity categories originating in late 19th century Europe" translate imperfectly into postcolonial contexts and their diasporas.[7] Our use of "queer" is also informed by its etymological resonances with the German word, "quer," which means "transverse," foregrounding its meaning "across."[8] For queer theorist Eve Kosofsky Sedgwick this implies a reading of queer as "multiply transitive," so that queering as "cutting across" can apply beyond the realm of gender and sexuality.[9] For Post *Natyam* Collective member Sandra, who is a native German speaker, this dimension of "queer" holds primary importance and resonates with the phrase "quer denken"—to think outside the box. While there are conflicting opinions in the larger collective regarding expanding queering beyond gender and sexuality, the two of us find the verb "queering," referring to active processes of questioning, challenging normativity, and counteracting naturalization,[10] to be more productive than the fixity of the adjective "queer" and the noun "queerness."[11]

These theoretical transnational dialogues about the term "queer" have led us to expand our notion of queer/ing further through what we think of as queering cultural belonging, or cultural queering. We define queering cultural belonging as a subversive disruption of a dominant naturalized cultural norm that complicates notions of cultural authenticity, appropriation, and identity-based representation, particularly in relation to artistic production. In the context of *rapture/rupture*, queering cultural belonging aims to undo the easy equation between ethnicized and racialized identities, cultural and artistic production, and (post)national imaginaries without ignoring uneven power hierarchies or histories of inequality.[12] Indian classical dance has been extensively theorized in relation to nationalist and diasporic formations that rely on the performance of "authentic Indianness," where performing femininity properly has become entangled with performing Indianness properly. However, little has been said about the fact that non-Indian classical practitioners are also pressured to perform cultural authenticity, even as the conflation between race, nation, and artistic production makes this a logical impossibility. In the United States, the genre of contemporary South Asian dance is typically associated with second-generation South Asian American dancing bodies whose hybrid movement vocabularies and autobiographical explorations are typically read as artistic "attempt[s] to bridge their eternally hyphenated sel[ves]."[13] Meanwhile, postmodern and contemporary dance routinely remain culturally unmarked. We argue that Cynthia's failure to perform idealized Indian femininity in *rapture/rupture* is an example of queering cultural belonging that grapples with and moves beyond the ethnicized essentialism often associated with Indian classical dance, while at the same time troubling the legacy of racialized self-representation that adheres to Asian American dance and questioning the unmarked status of postmodern and contemporary choreographic strategies.

29 Subversive Gestures: Multiplying Queer Critiques

The *Subversive Gestures Feedback Loop* began with a work-in-progress by Shyamala Moorty (director) and Cynthia Ling Lee (performer) titled *29 Subversive Gestures*, conceived as a tribute to American choreographer Joe Goode's solo, *29 Effeminate Gestures* (1987).[14] In his solo, Goode uses postmodern choreographic strategies to trouble identity categories and destabilize gender norms, reclaiming effeminacy from his position as a white gay cisgendered man. We initially sought to straightforwardly translate Goode's critique of white American masculinity to a context of South Asian femininity. However, we came to realize that Goode's dramaturgical approach of critiquing masculinity could not simply be flipped to address femininity and that we needed a more layered compositional approach to address the additional issue of cross-racial performance.

29 Subversive Gestures combined US postmodern, identity-based, and contemporary South Asian choreographic strategies to performatively articulate a critique of idealized femininity in Indian classical dance. As kathak scholar and anthropologist Pallabi Chakravorty explains, the chaste, spiritual, and "respectable" femininity that dominates Indian classical dance is entangled with notions of cultural and religious nationalism:

> During the nationalist phase in the early twentieth century, the revival of Indian classical dance came to be associated intimately with the construction of India's national identity . . . the sole bearers of this spiritual identity, [Indian leaders] proclaimed, were the (upper-middle-class, and upper-caste) Hindu women.[15]

This entanglement of nation, femininity, and classical dance is particularly loaded in an Indian American diasporic context where nostalgic connections to a distant homeland are reproduced through performances of classical dance.[16]

Shyamala invited Cynthia to dance in *29 Subversive Gestures* because of Cynthia's self-avowedly troubled relationship to embodying classical images of Indian femininity and her fluidity of gender presentation in everyday life. A kathak and postmodern dancer, Cynthia is a Taiwanese American, feminist, and cisgendered woman who studied kathak as a young adult in India under a traditional female guru. Cynthia articulated her personal preferences for gender presentation during a *Subversive Gestures Feedback Loop* writing exercise as follows:

> One day I might feel like dressing like a man, another to get all femmed out, another to be androgynous, another to mix gendered fashion codes in unexpected ways. . . . One of my favorite ways of dressing is as an Indian male, or more specifically in a mix of Indian and western clothes, including key items that are gendered male in an Indian context.

Shyamala, a mixed heritage Indian American choreographer trained in ballet, post/modern dance, bharatanatyam, and yoga, was interested in intersecting Goode's queer and postmodern compositional methodologies of "cross-gesturing"[17] and "subversive repetition"[18] with classical *abhinaya*. Dance scholar David Gere defines cross-gesturing in relation to cross-dressing to refer to performing gendered movements and gestures that are "off-limits" within a heteronormative frame.[19] Gender theorist Judith Butler discusses subversive repetition as a strategic repetition of gender codes that facilitates a "subversion of identity" from "within the practices of repetitive signifying."[20]

Goode's postmodern choreographic device of using repetition of gendered movement to accrue multiple meanings in *29 Effeminate Gestures* initially seemed consonant with *abhinaya*, where a dancer brings multiple interpretations to a poetic line through repetition. In *29 Effeminate Gestures*, the hypermasculine image of Goode aggressively wielding a chainsaw to split a wooden chair down the middle is followed by five repetitions of a sequence of twenty-nine effeminate gestures, ranging from the "limp wrist" to "the finger-fluttering wave."[21] The sound changes with each repetition, progressing from silence, to spoken text ("If you feel too much . . . if you gesticulate too much . . ."), to war sounds, to electronica layered with Polynesian drumming, to "gender-modified lyrics to a tune from *Fiddler on the Roof*."[22] With each repetition, the meanings accrue, contradict, proliferate, and implode, revealing a seemingly natural gender's "openness to resignification and recontextualization."[23]

Inspired by Goode's structure, *29 Subversive Gestures* uses as its starting sequence twenty-nine gestures associated with female characters from kathak *abhinaya*. To borrow from Butler's theorizing of how acts become recognized as gender performance, these stylized corporeal gestures have "congeal[ed] over time" to embody a traditional Hindu femininity that mobilizes Indian classical dance to support heteropatriarchal nationalist and diasporic agendas.[24] The work's ensuing variations attempt to critique and complicate the gestures using text, soundings, and hybrid movement vocabulary along a wide gendered spectrum.

In her dramaturgical feedback, Sandra stated that *29 Subversive Gestures* did not have the power of Goode's clear, single-minded critique of the limits of (white) American heteronormative masculinity. The fact that *29 Effeminate Gestures* is situated in a single dance tradition and performed and choreographed by a white gay male allowed Goode to focus on one culturally situated notion of gender. *29 Subversive Gestures*, however, invoked multiple cultural gender codes through its sustained and interlinked use of kathak and postmodern dance performed by a Taiwanese American female, without setting up a singular image of femininity to be "broken" or deconstructed.

In order to incorporate concerns of cross-racial performance, cultural authenticity, and cultural nationalisms into our gender critique, we started reexamining aspects of *29 Subversive Gestures* through a praxis-based process. This process resulted in three choreographic sketches, "Goode-style Deconstruction," "Intersex Nayi/aka," and *rapture/rupture*, which form the case studies for the rest of this essay.[25] Our process raised complex questions in connection with the performance-making methods of postmodern dance, identity-based queer performance, and kathak *abhinaya*: how are gender, cultural belonging, and desire conceptualized through Indian *abhinaya*, US identity politics, and poststructuralist critiques of identity while also being inflected by our individual positionalities as Taiwanese American, Indian

American, and German Indian women who are queer or are allies? How do our critiques of gender intersect with racialized discourses on cultural authenticity? Is it productive to use postmodern dance's tools of self-reflexivity, citationality, and discursive openness (which share a culturally specific aesthetic trajectory with central European contemporary approaches to dance) to choreograph critiques of idealized Indian femininity, when postmodern dance is entangled with whiteness? How might we take advantage of autobiographical performance's ability "to bring into being a self" through the enunciation of queer, female, and Asian American experiences while honoring how *abhinaya* is intended to transcend the performer's individual identity?[26] How might we use the compositional tools of *abhinaya* to critique, disidentify with, and queer the gendered script of Indianness that it is so often used to embody?[27]

Denaturalizing Idealized Indian Femininity: Subversive Repetitions

Our first choreographic sketch, the "Goode-Style Deconstruction," employed subversive repetition to critique and break apart a script of idealized Indian femininity. Modeled after Joe Goode's postmodern compositional approach, our study used six sound-based variations to contrast, undermine, and critically recontextualize a sequence of *angika abhinaya* gestures appropriate for a female character. The study challenged classical kathak's dominant mode of performing femininity in terms of gender and ethno-cultural nationalism: it highlighted the performer's "lack" or failure to conform to an idealized regime of femininity while foregrounding her Taiwanese American identity or "lack" of Indianness.

The base phrase for the "Goode-style Deconstruction" consists of a section from *29 Subversive Gestures* that denotes an idealized female character frequently performed in the classical repertoire—refined, sensual, decorated, and feminine. The phrase utilizes relaxed but clear *hasta mudras* or hand gestures to suggest adorning oneself (braiding hair, gazing into a mirror, putting on earrings) and sensuality (circling her breasts), while employing kathak's seductive glances, known as *nazar*.

The first subversive repetition counterposes these images of femininity with text spoken live by the performer that points out her "lack." Some of the text refers to the inadequacy of Cynthia's physical appearance by Indian standards of feminine beauty, such as her boyishly short hair or smaller East Asian eyes ("not long enough," "not fish-eyed enough"). Other text refers to an inability to live up to feminine ideals of behavior and emotion: "not modest enough, "not vain enough." In a direct reversal of Goode's original piece, which crosses over the acceptable boundaries of dominant masculinity through excess, or the aesthetic of "too much," this text speaks of the inadequacy of failed femininity, the feeling of "not enough."

The second variation evokes the emotional and physical costs of trying to perform this idealized female character using vocalized sounds that communicate displeasure, pain, and violence.[28] The performer repeatedly utters a painful "Oww! ow . . . OWW!!" while braiding her imaginary hair, implying the physical pain of beautification. When tracing her eyes she says melodically, "ching chong, ching chong . . . ," the Orientalist, Chinese racial slur contrasting with a seductive Indian neck movement.

In the third repetition, the dancer performs a critical feminist intervention that troubles kathak's hegemonic history: she speaks academic prose that highlights kathak's Muslim, secular, and female courtesan influences while dancing the original feminine phrase. Her declaration that kathak's official history was rewritten to "ensur[e] a male, patriarchal, and thoroughly Hindu lineage for the form" critically historicizes her performance of an overdetermined idealized Hindu femininity.[29]

Having textually framed kathak as a syncretic form, the fourth repetition of the "Goode-style Deconstruction" physically ruptures the base phrase's performance of embodied feminine Indianness, removing any semblance of cultural "purity" by introducing markedly hybrid movement and language. The dancer performs a speeded up, rhythmic version of the original gestural sequence, physically disrupting the feminine gestures through dynamic changes in direction, speed, falls, lunges, and wide second position stances.

After these four repetitions that denaturalized the performance of idealized femininity, reframed kathak as a syncretic form, and expanded kathak's possibilities for gendered movement, the final repetition evokes queer loss, with the performer mourning her estranged Indian female guru. While dancing the gestures that she learned from her teacher, the dancer poetically laments that their love was not enough to bridge their cultural differences. She says: "Beloved, I brought you into my body . . . I was a foreigner in your world . . . and in the end, *pishi*, our love was not enough."[30] This melancholic section corresponds roughly to Goode's last variation, in which he sings a queer version of the song "Sunrise, Sunset" from *Fiddler on the Roof* in a raw, throat-wrenching tone. While Goode's version invokes the father, "the very model of appropriate gender-specific behavior," our version invokes the performer's estranged female guru, her literal "model [for] appropriate gender-specific behavior" within classical kathak.[31]

Overall, the choreographic sketch, "Goode-Style Deconstruction," revealed how queer failure and lack challenged notions of cultural authenticity as well as gender norms: it constituted a performance of queering cultural belonging. However, we found it insufficient and problematic to use predominantly Western choreographic tools on Indian movement vocabulary, a reiteration of a colonizing methodology that does not give space for the full emotional potential and gendered possibilities of *abhinaya*. Therefore, our second and third sketches explored the critical potential of *abhinaya* techniques as compositional tools rather than using *angika abhinaya* as a signifier of idealized Indian femininity to be broken down using compositional tools from US postmodern and European contemporary dance.

Ekaharya Abhinaya and Gender Fluidity

Our second sketch, "Intersex Nayi/aka," draws on kathak's *ekaharya abhinaya* tradition, a technique whereby one performer shifts between portraying multiple gendered characters without changing costumes. Rather than using *ekaharya abhinaya* to portray known characters in mythological or other culturally familiar stories, Cynthia's performance strives to embody gender fluidity.

Kathak scholar Purnima Shah describes *ekaharya abhinaya* as enabling a spiritual transcendence of one's (gendered) self, which she connects to Hindu philosophical concepts of *advaita*, or non-dualism.[32] One might critique Shah for emphasizing an exclusively Hindu philosophy and thus foreclosing historically significant Muslim contexts and secular functions for kathak *abhinaya*. Nevertheless, given the fact that gendered performances of Indian classical dance are often roped into identity-based discourses of cultural authenticity, Shah's perspective serves as an important reminder that the gendered characters portrayed by a classical dancer are not meant to express one's personal identity. Hari Krishnan, whose scholarship focuses on the secular contexts of South Indian court dance traditions, also emphasizes that the performance of gendered characters are "not about real men and women but rather about reproducing idealized and culturally desired types."[33]

In "Intersex Nayi/aka," Cynthia corporeally shifts between gendered movement without a traditional narrative frame that contains and justifies the character shifts. She braids her imaginary long hair, strokes her imaginary beard, boldly throws dice, gazes coyly, and changes her carriage and the size of her kinesphere while traveling and sitting. She uses *ekaharya abhinaya* as a corporeal technique that facilitates performing outside the "normal" boundaries of one's gender identity and sexed body.[34] In line with a poststructuralist critique of identity, *ekaharya abhinaya* contradicts the "organicist conception of the link between body and identity," challenging essentialist notions of identity.[35]

Because *ekaharya abhinaya* goes beyond the affirmation of a personal identity as embedded in the sexed body, "Intersex Nayi/aka" becomes an abstracted performance of gender fluidity based on a stylized technique. "Intersex Nayi/aka" also differs from classical *ekaharya abhinaya* in how it brings a queer ambiguity to the traditional clear switch between gendered characters, which is often marked by a *palta* or spin.

Wearing a long-sleeved orange kurta with a *dupatta* tied around her waist, akin to a male kathak dancer, Cynthia at times gradually morphs from "feminine" to "masculine" movement: she shyly shakes an imaginary pair of dice with her legs folded demurely underneath her, the shaking growing more energetic as her legs gradually move into a wide masculine sitting position until she boldly tosses the dice on the ground, hands spread wide in victory. At other times, she shifts erratically between gendered embodiments, moving between braiding her hair and stroking her beard like a broken, repetitive record. To a viewer enculturated in kathak, this creates confusion about whether the performer is switching between characters, or if she is performing one gender nonconforming character moving through a range of gendered expression.

We also found that the "Intersex Nayi/aka" introduced questions of sexual desire into our choreographic process. Cynthia's performance, as is traditional in *abhinaya*, is addressed to an imagined other—a beloved with whom she flirts and plays dice. The love stories of classical Indian *abhinaya* typically function within a heteronormative frame: when an insider audience sees a familiar *nayika* (heroine or female character type), they will imagine a corresponding *nayaka* (hero or male lover) to whom the performance is addressed. However, the gender ambiguity of Cynthia's character(s) calls this heteronormative framework into question: when a protagonist character defies gender binaries, then what might the audience imagine the gender identity of the invisible beloved to be? What kind of potential does this open up for performing queer desire through Indian dance? These questions informed our third and final choreographic experiment, *rapture/rupture*, which became a fully realized work that is performed publicly.

rapture/rupture: Queering Love Poetry

rapture/rupture repurposed *abhinaya*'s tradition of love poetry to bring together multiple threads of queering: queering gender, queering cultural belonging, and queer female desire. *rapture/rupture* intersects identity politics and classical Indian aesthetics through poeticized autobiography, cross-dressing *aharya abhinaya*, and physical eruptions on a broad gendered spectrum. Intersecting culturally idealized gender types from classical Indian dance with the performer's ethnically and gender "mismatched" body, the work reconfigures *viraha* (love-in-separation) as queer female desire infused by an intense lack. Here, *viraha* becomes the (im)possibility of love to transcend difference when cultural purity and rigid gender roles are at play.[36]

This piece begins with the dancer, Cynthia, coyly sitting on the ground with her eyes downcast, a shimmering image of Indian femininity. She wears an iridescent deep orange *anarkali kurta* (dress) over dark pink *churidar* pants, a magenta brocade vest accentuating her breasts, and a long, sheer golden *dupatta* draped over her head, shoulders, and chest. Bejeweled, she wears a *tikka*, bangles, necklace, and earrings. Sitting in the downstage corner watching the dancer, Shyamala recites in a soft female voice: "Beloved, our love was not enough." As she repeats the opening *sthyai*, or poetic refrain, Cynthia uses hand gestures, torso movements, and subtle facial expressions to color this refrain in different ways—shy, self-conscious, angry, resigned— the dancer and vocalist playing off each other to create emotional variations.[37] The music shifts melodically to the *antara* as Shyamala says, "You were my mirror / when you moved I moved / me an imperfect copy." Cynthia bows deeply, placing her forehead reverentially on the ground, then sits up, looking into an imaginary mirror in her right hand, smiling in admiration. She boldly circles her breast with her right hand in a sensual movement, then uncertainly echoes the movement with her left hand, looking up for approval.

rapture/rupture is based on a *viraha* (love-in-separation) poem addressed to a female beloved. In part, *rapture/rupture* builds on Cynthia's earlier theorizations, which consider gendered identification, guru–disciple relationships, and *abhinaya* in relation to psychoanalytical theory.[38] Cynthia noted a strong resemblance between Lacan's mirror stage and learning kathak *abhinaya* as a form of gendered identification with one's guru. As illustrated in this opening section of *rapture/rupture*, the text and movement ("you were my mirror") reference the process of learning to embody a culturally specific, idealized form of femininity from one's kathak guru through repeatedly imitating and internalizing her movement. The choreographic assignment that gave rise to *rapture/rupture* extended this use of psychoanalytic theory beyond mirror stage identification: it was inspired by Butler's theorization of hyperfemininity as a consequence of heterosexuals' melancholic incorporation of same-sex attachments from early childhood:

> If a woman has disavowed her early homosexual attachments and lost those objects, those other women, those other girls, as possible objects

of love, cannot even acknowledge that she has lost them, or cannot even acknowledge that she has loved them; she incorporates them as parts of herself, modes of identification and this means that they come to survive for her as her own character traits. She incorporates them—makes them, in a way, into her own body, her own bodily sense and comportment, and this incorporation is precisely the opposite of—and the consequence of—unacknowledged loss.[39]

What choreography of queer desire might result if we framed a female disciple's performance of idealized femininity as the result of residual same-sex attachment to her female guru? We formulated the following assignment to explore this idea:

Create a melancholic *padam* about a lost love, in which the beloved is an Indian woman.[40] Start the *padam* in hyperfeminine Indian garb and physicality. As the lost love is increasingly acknowledged through po-etic mourning, have your body language and physicality shift towards being more androgynous and incorporating the physicality of cultures outside of India.[41]

The resulting poetic text for *rapture/rupture*, written by Cynthia, was steeped in *sringara rasa*, the aesthetic flavor of love that dominates kathak *abhinaya*, overlaying romantic love onto aspects of her actual relationship with her guru.[42] Traditionally, guru and *shisya* (disciple) are bonded through a lifelong love, a love that softens the disciple's body and makes the *shishya* open to incorporating her or his guru's dance.

The assignment also specified that the refrain of the poem should include the words "not enough," connecting to earlier studies and making queer lack central to the emotional import and compositional structure of the work. Classically, the refrain of a poetic *abhinaya* song is regarded as containing the song's dominant emotion—its *sthyai bhava*—out of which spring emo-tional variations and narrative developments. Here, the main *sthyai* or re-frain of *rapture/rupture* is "beloved, our love was not enough," speaking to a failed love. Each section of the poem also contains a textual variation on the refrain that fleshes out and reveals its multiple facets of meaning. These variations articulate personal interpretations in relation to larger social sys-tems with impossible ideals ("as much as I tried, I was not enough," "beloved, I was not Bengali enough"), eventually critiquing these systems ("kathak was not enough," "and perhaps, beloved teacher, you were not enough"). In this opening section, the inability of the student to adequately imitate her beloved/teacher—"as much as I tried, I was not enough"—points to a failed or incomplete culturally specific gender identification.

As the piece continues, the classical imagery gradually begins to unravel on textual, physical, and costume levels: the performer proves to be neither feminine enough nor Indian enough, embodying a culturally queer defiance to kathak's idealized Indian femininity. Textually, the poem starts to intersperse seemingly autobiographical references with the stock imagery, many of which refer to the dancer's cultural and ethnic difference: "I was a foreigner in your world," "I was not Bengali enough." In the third section, the dancer sits demurely during the words, "but I could not be you [the female guru]," only to have her legs unexpectedly open into a wide masculine position. Unable to contain her body—"my body would erupt with otherness"—she falls onto her left side, her right leg wildly swinging and kicking sideways and outwards multiple times in sync with her audible breath, while Shyamala violently fragments the lines: "my stride too large/my eyes too small: Erupt? body Other! Other erupting with, with not enough Not ENOUGH ERUPTING my stride STRIDE too large Eyes eyes too small. . . ." The dancer comes to a halt, sitting in a wide, frontally oriented position with a confrontational look on her face, her *dupatta* tangled and her skirt messily flung over her shoulder.

rapture/rupture's multiple poetic and physical references to the performer's non-Indianness are a form of queering cultural belonging that undermines nationalist-diasporic constructions of Indian classical dance as a symbol of cultural purity. Cynthia notes that "there has always been a friction between my ethnic identity as a Taiwanese American . . . and my artistic identity as a kathak dancer, primarily because I don't look Indian . . . [but am still asked to] perform 'Indianness.'"[43] *rapture/rupture* further undoes this notion of cultural purity through hybrid movement as exemplified by Cynthia's wildly careening, full-bodied expansion of kathak gestures, her mixture of Indian and Western clothing, and the sound, which combines Hindustani music with English language poetry modeled on South Asian literary form. Through these different performative tools she hails multiple audiences with different bases of cultural and artistic knowledge. As a more subtle contradiction of Hinduized Indian kathak's investment in cultural and religious purity, *rapture/rupture* includes Muslim elements such as *ghazal* poetic imagery and the Mughal-style costume. For Cynthia, the inclusion of Muslim material reclaims a syncretic version of kathak's history that gives more space for her own ethnic and cultural difference.

In addition to queering cultural belonging and choreographing queer desire, *rapture/rupture* queers gender through a combination of

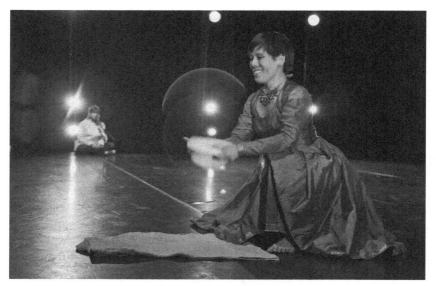

FIGURE 2.1 Cynthia Ling Lee (*foreground*) and Shyamala Moorty (*background*) in Post *Natyam* Collective's *rapture/rupture*. Photo by Sarah Nesbitt.

cross-gesturing physical movement and cross-dressing *aharya abhinaya*. Halfway through the piece, the performer rips off her *dupatta* and her *churidar* pants, which she boldly replaces with a pair of carpenter jeans and a fedora hat, fearlessly running full-tilt backwards with large strides. These costume changes are intended to mobilize the power of drag by denaturalizing the relationship between "anatomical sex, gender identity, and gender performance" upon which "heterosexual coherence" rests.[44] The costumes, which mix masculine, feminine, and androgynous Western and Indian clothing in unexpected configurations, correspond to Cynthia's preferred range of gender presentation while also constituting a cultural cross-dressing.[45]

Queering *Viraha*: Longing, Lack, and Queer Potentiality

rapture/rupture combines the strategies of the "Goode-style Deconstruction," which critiques gender norms in relation to personal identity, and the "Intersex Nayi/aka," which references ideal gender types separate from the performer's identity. As such, *rapture/rupture* reveals productive intersections between using identity-based autobiography and *abhinaya* to perform queerness in a South Asian aesthetic context. Looking at *rapture/rupture* through the lens of US identity politics, the work can be read as using autobiography to create critical distance from nationalist constructions of kathak's idealized Indian femininity. After all, its textual content (relationship with guru), movement vocabulary (kathak and postmodern vocabulary), and gendered costumes (mixture of masculine and feminine) reflect various aspects of Cynthia's personal history and identity. One possible reading of *rapture/rupture* is as a chronological "life story" that follows the trajectory of coming out stories, where the performer's initial performance of idealized Indian femininity leads to growing resistance and ends with the emergence of her "true" androgynous self. Another autobiographical reading might foreground the conflict that arises because of Cynthia's ethnic mismatch with a culturally marked dance form.

Yet *rapture/rupture* also resists being read as a straightforward autobiographical expression of the performer's identity through its poetic ambiguity and abstraction, which are rooted in South Asian aesthetics. Rather than use (white) postmodern aesthetic tools to unsettle the performance of a coherent self and fixed identity, the work does so using Indian compositional tools. As Cynthia commented during the feedback process:

> The stylization, repetition, and abstraction provided by the *abhinaya* . . . as well as the poetic structure with its strategy of a repeated refrain that accrues new meaning and thus moves away from narrative literalness, displace the confessional contract and performance of an "authentic" self that often adheres to autobiographical performance.[46]

Black queer interdisciplinary performance artist Anna Martine Whitehead, a fellow artist who performed alongside us in *Confetti Sunrise: An Evening of Queer Dance* curated by Clare Croft at the University of Michigan, noted that the structure of Shyamala speaking in the first person and Cynthia physically interpreting the text creates a dual subject that unsettles the singular "I."[47] If viewed through an Indian lens of gender roles rather than an identity-based autobiographical lens privileging a "personal code of gender," *rapture/rupture* might be understood as trying to make space for alternative gendered roles and multiple cultural identifications outside of those normally performed by Indian classical dance.[48] As Cynthia wrote during one of her theoretical feedback responses, "Can we make space for the butch, the genderqueer, the androgyne, the masculine woman, the effeminate man within Indian classical *abhinaya*?"

rapture/rupture ends with the performer contemplatively taking off her pink vest and traditional kathak *kurta*, revealing her vulnerable body in sports bra and jeans, before putting on a simple, unisex cross-tied *kurta* that can also read as a Chinese style jacket. With soft, subtle movement, stationary in space but expansive through wide, almost floating arm movements, her gestures reference a utopic space where queer desire can be realized:

> i imagine us in a room together
> . . .
> an open channel between two hearts
> two women dancing and reciting bols
> like and unlike each other

The above lines' expression of queer togetherness-in-difference recall José Esteban Muñoz's ideas of queerness as utopia and potentiality. He writes:

> Queerness is not yet here. . . . We may never touch queerness, but we can feel it as the warm illumination of a horizon imbued with potentiality. . . . Queerness is a longing that propels us onward. . . . Queerness is that thing that lets us feel that this world is not enough, that indeed something is missing. . . . Queerness is essentially about the rejection of a here and now and an insistence on potentiality or concrete possibility for another world.[49]

Viraha's unique, bittersweet quality of yearning, in which the sweetness of possible union with a divine or human beloved is tinged with the bitterness of inevitable separation, animates countless works within South Asian poetic, dance, and music traditions. *rapture/rupture* reconfigures this unique quality of *viraha* for a queer agenda, imagining union with a same-sex beloved, a guru, and, perhaps, a more whole self. The piece uses "lack" to indict systems that foreclose cultural queering and gender fluidity while using queer desire—the ability of love to connect us across seemingly insurmountable difference—to imagine, with sweet bitterness, the possibility of another way of being in the world, in which one's "lack" ceases to be failure and instead becomes a source of power, love, and connection. In the performance of its failure to conform to norms, *rapture/rupture* gestures toward a culturally queer, gender non-conforming, and queer desirous character type/subject who chooses fluidity, multiplicity, and contradiction over narrow notions of purist authenticity.

Yet in the end, *rapture/rupture* finds this togetherness-in-difference impossible, underlining how the pressures of "the world outside" suffuse queer desire and longing:

> but there is never just a room
> there is always the world outside
> and in the end, beloved,
> our love was not enough

Interlacing her hands to signify love-in-union, the performer slowly travels backwards, her hands quietly straining to stay together before separating, cradling loss and emptiness as the lights fade.

While *rapture/rupture* ends without the consummation of queer togetherness-in-difference, the work's queer utopian potential lies in its hope that it may move and be witnessed by "forward-dawning" *rasikas*, or ideal sympathetic spectators.[50] These *rasikas* live at the edge of more easily identifiable existing communities and may resonate with *rapture/rupture* in different ways.[51] We choreograph for an emergent, intersectional audience of *rasikas* who may not exist yet; who may share our deep emotional investment in Indian aesthetics, as well as postmodern or contemporary approaches, and an equally urgent political need to critique how any of these aesthetics can be used to perpetuate exclusionary systems; who may live between cultural worlds; whose dreams for a future include multiple fluid possibilities for gendered and cultural embodiment and decolonized queer desire.

Acknowledgments

Sandra Chatterjee worked on this article in the context of the research project *Traversing the Contemporary (pl)*. Austrian Science Fund (FWF): P_24190-G15.

Notes

1. *Alapadma* is a mudra or a hand gesture in which the fingers fan open. The word *alapadma* means opening like a flower.
2. *Abhinaya* refers to stylized performative communication of emotional intent in Indian classical dance. Most typically associated with the use of gesture and facial expression to interpret love poetry and tell stories, *abhinaya* actually has four aspects: *vachika*, or communication through voice; *aharya*, or costume; *angika*, or body; and *sattvika*, which is difficult to translate into English but refers to state of mind/involvement.

3. The collective engaged in the *Subversive Gestures Feedback Loop* from November 2012 to February 2013.

4. Our collaborations started during graduate school in Los Angeles in the first decade of the twenty-first century, before a new interest in emotion and affect emerged in postmodern dance and contemporary dance in our home contexts, to which we have dispersed since.

5. Sandra Chatterjee and Cynthia Ling Lee, "Solidarity—*Rasa*/Autobiography—*Abhinaya*: South Asian Tactics for Performing Queerness," *Studies in South Asian Film and Media*, The Body: Indian Theatre Special Issue, 5, no. 1 (2013): 130.

6. David M. Halperin, *Saint = Foucault: Towards a Gay Hagiography* (New York: Oxford University Press, 1997), 62

7. Vanita qtd. in Chatterjee and Lee, "Solidarity—*Rasa*/Autobiography—*Abhinaya*," 130.

8. Eve Kosofsky Sedgwick, *Tendencies* (Durham: Duke University Press, 1993), xii.

9. Sedgwick, *Tendencies*, xii.

10. See Donald E. Hall, *Queer Theories* (New York: Palgrave Macmillan, 2003), 22 and 56.

11. Sandra Chatterjee, Cynthia Ling Lee, Shyamala Moorty, and Meena Murugesan, Skype Conversation about Queer/ing, July 14, 2015.

12. Our articulation of queering cultural belonging, discussed here in the context of the *Subversive Gestures Feedback Loop* and *rapture/rupture*, is crucially informed by how "othering" works in the postnational context of the European Union, particularly Sandra's research and personal experience with contemporary Indian dance in Germany and Central Europe. The term "culturally queer" emerged from a dialogue discussing contemporary Indian dance case studies from Germany and the United States alongside each other, in relation to the frameworks of (classical) Indian dance, cultural nationalism, and US and German multiculturalisms. The term initially opened the possibility to discuss cultural difference and hybridity within Europeanness and European choreographic production as exceeding existing categories. See also Fatima El Tayeb, *European Others: Queering Ethnicity in Postnational Europe* (Minneapolis: University of Minnesota Press, 2011).

13. Yutian Wong, *Choreographing Asian America* (Middletown, CT: Wesleyan University Press, 2010), 52.

14. *29 Subversive Gestures* was created in August 2012 for BEHOLD!, a queer performance festival curated by Leo Garcia at the Highways Performance Space in Santa Monica, California. According to Meiling Cheng, Highways was founded by Tim Miller and Linda Frye Burnham to promote "boundary-breaking, issue-oriented, and identity-centered performances [that] reflected Burnham's preference for multidisciplinary experimentation and socially relevant art and Miller's commitment to queer cultural definitions and intercultural collaboration." As such, Highways has been central for the development of queer performance art

in Southern California as well as being an important space for politicized artists of color to show new work. *In Other Los Angeleses: Multicentric Performance Art* (Berkeley: University of California Press, 2002), 186.

15. Pallabi Chakravorty, "From Interculturalism to Historicism: Reflections on Classical Indian Dance," *Dance Research Journal* 32 no. 2 (Winter 2000–2001): 111. Kathak historically has both Muslim and Hindu influences. The Hinduization of kathak due to processes of religious and cultural nationalism is specific to kathak as practiced in India and its diaspora and manifests differently in Pakistan and Bangladesh. Cynthia received the bulk of her kathak training in India, and Chakravorty was her first kathak teacher. For more on how secular Islamic elements are sidelined in normative, India-centric versions of kathak history, see Margaret Walker, *India's Kathak Dance in Historical Perspective* (Farnham: Ashgate, 2014) and Pallabi Chakravorty, *Bells of Change: Kathak Dance, Women and Modernity In India* (Kolkata: Seagull Books, 2008).

16. Sandra Chatterjee, "Undomesticated Bodies: South Asian Women Perform the Impossible" (PhD diss., University of California, Los Angeles, 2005).

17. David Gere, "*29 Effeminate Gestures*: Choreographer Joe Goode and the Heroism of Effeminacy," in *Dancing Desires: Choreographing Sexualities On and Off the Stage*, ed. Jane C. Desmond (Madison: University of Wisconsin Press, 2001), 376.

18. Judith Butler, *Gender Trouble* (New York: Routledge, 1999), 42.

19. Gere, "*29 Effeminate Gestures*: Choreographer Joe Goode and the Heroism of Effeminacy," 376.

20. Butler, *Gender Trouble*, 185.

21. Gere, "*29 Effeminate Gestures*: Choreographer Joe Goode and the Heroism of Effeminacy," 357 and 367.

22. Gere, "*29 Effeminate Gestures*: Choreographer Joe Goode and the Heroism of Effeminacy," 372.

23. Butler, *Gender Trouble*, 176.

24. Butler, *Gender Trouble*, 43.

25. A *nayika* refers to a female heroine, while a *nayaka* refers to a male protagonist.

26. Deirdre Heddon, *Autobiography and Performance* (New York: Palgrave Macmillan, 2008), 3.

27. José Esteban Muñoz, *Disidentifications: Queers of Colors and the Performance of Politics* (Minneapolis: University of Minnesota Press, 1999).

28. This compositional approach is inspired by Goode's vocalization of warlike sounds such as machine-guns and explosions in *29 Effeminate Gestures*, which Ramsay Burt, in his writing about Goode's solo, interprets as the violent consequences for performing effeminacy. "The Performance of Unmarked Masculinity," in *When Men Dance*, ed. Jennifer Fischer and Anthony Shay (New York: Oxford University Press, 2009), 157.

29. Cynthia Ling Lee and Shyamala Moorty. "29 Loop 6 Variations," Vimeo video, 6:23, February 16, 2013, https://vimeo.com/59816332. See also http://post-natyam.blogspot.com/2013/02/29-subversive-gestures-final-loop.html.

30. *Pishi* refers to father's sister in Bengali and is commonly used to connote intimate social relation beyond the realm of blood relatives. Disciples of Cynthia's kathak guru affectionately refer to her as *pishi*.

31. Gere, "*29 Effeminate Gestures*: Choreographer Joe Goode and the Heroism of Effeminacy," 373.

32. Purnima Shah, "Transcending Gender in the Performance of Kathak," *Dance Research Journal* 30 no. 2 (Fall 1998): 3.

33. Hari Krishnan, "From Gynemimesis to Hypermasculinity: The Shifting Orientations of Male Performers of South Indian Court Dance," in *When Men Dance*, ed. Jennifer Fischer and Anthony Shay (New York: Oxford University Press, 2009), 379–91. Projesh Banerji explains how these character types are codified in terms of types of heroes (*nayakas*) and heroines (*nayikas*) in various writings pertaining to poetry, performing arts, and visual arts, as well as in the *Kama Sutra*. Various texts classify the *nayikas* with different emphases and subdivisions. For example, classification occurs in terms of social status (divine women, high-class women, maids, and courtesans); social relationship (married or public); age; numerous subdivisions characterizing her social relationship (experienced, well versed in love, sarcastic, happy, longing, proud, and vain); temperament (a well-wisher for her husband, temperamental with changing moods, with feelings for someone other than the husband, and angry); and appearance. *Dance in Thumri* (New Delhi: Abhinav Publications, 1986), 9–13.

34. Gere, "*29 Effeminate Gestures*: Choreographer Joe Goode and the Heroism of Effeminacy," 375.

35. Susan Foster, "Choreographies of Gender," *Signs* 24, no. 1 (Autumn 1998): 2.

36. *Viraha* is typified by a longing for union that is not realized. The reasons for the separation between the protagonist and beloved can be multiple: because one's beloved is with another person or away from home, because there has been a quarrel, etc. One important expression of *viraha* is the spiritual *bhakti* dimension of the human soul longing to be united with the Divine, who is imagined as lover.

37. Avanthi Meduri describes how vocalist, dancer, and drummer engage in simultaneous improvised emotional variations on a shared poetic text in traditional Bharatanatyam *abhinaya*. "Multiple Pleasures: Improvisation in Bharatanatyam," in *Taken by Surprise: A Dance Improvisation Reader*, ed. Ann Cooper Albright and David Gere (Middletown, CT: Wesleyan University Press, 2003), 141–50.

38. Cynthia Ling Lee, "The Bhakta and the Feminist: Gender and Identity-Formation in Kathak Abhinaya," MFA research paper, University of California, Los Angeles, 2006.

39. Judith Butler and Vasu Reddy, "Troubling Genders, Subverting Identities: Interview with Judith Butler," *Agenda: Empowering Women for Gender Equity*, Special Issue: Sexuality in Africa, 18, no. 62 (2004): 121.

40. A *padam* is a love song rendered in *abhinaya* from the South Indian classical repertoire. *Padams* are not a part of kathak repertoire, but given Shyamala's and Sandra's training in South Indian classical dance, the collective often uses the term.

41. Cynthia Ling Lee and Shyamala Moorty, "29 Subversive Gestures Choreography Assignment 3: Not Enough Padam," The Post *Natyam* Collective (blog), January 11, 2013, http://postnatyam.blogspot.com/2013/01/29-subversive-gestures-choreography.html.

42. *Sringara rasa*, or love and its corresponding *bhavas* in *abhinaya* is conceptualized in terms of multiple kinds of love: in addition to romantic and erotic love, it can be motherly, sisterly, platonic, etc. *Rasa* describes the aesthetic flavor ideally received by the audience. The *bhava*, or emotional intent performed by the dancer is conceptualized as distinct from *rasa* but with an ideal correspondence: *sringara rasa* generally corresponds to *rati bhava* (*bhava* of love), or as in our example, specifically *viraha* (love-in-separation).

43. Email interview with Cynthia Ling Lee, November 9, 2013.

44. Butler, *Gender Trouble*, 175.

45. In the case of India, the fact that women are more commonly expected to wear traditional clothing than men affirms their status as the bearers of tradition, illustrating the entanglement of performing Indianness and femininity.

46. "29 Subversive Gestures Loop, Padam complete Draft," The Post *Natyam* Collective, http://www.postnatyam.blogspot.com/2013/02/29-subversive-gestures-loop-padam.html#comment-form.

47. Anna Martine Whitehead in discussion with Cynthia Ling Lee and Shyamala Moorty, February 18, 2015.

48. Krishnan, "From Gynemimesis to Hypermasculinity," 383.

49. José Esteban Muñoz, *Cruising Utopia: The Then and There of Queer Futurity* (New York: New York University Press, 2009), 1.

50. Muñoz, *Cruising Utopia: The Then and There of Queer Futurity*, 1.

51. Thus far, *rapture/rupture* has been performed at the following venues: *Braiding Rivers Festival of Indian Dance* at Links Hall in Chicago, *Rapture and Rupture: Love and Emotion in Contemporary Dance* at the University of Salzburg, *Dance Conversations II* at the University of California at Irvine, the *Los Angeles Women's Theatre Festival* at The Electric Lodge in Los Angeles, University of North Carolina at Greensboro, Congress on Research in Dance/Society for Dance History Scholars' *Writing Dancing/Dancing Writing* Conference at the University of Iowa, *Confetti Sunrise: An Evening of Queer Dance* at the University of Michigan at Ann Arbor, *Erasing Borders: Festival of Indian Dance* in New York, and *Making Change for Better Communities Through Dance* at Swarthmore College.

3

Women Dancing Otherwise

THE QUEER FEMINISM OF GU JIANI'S
RIGHT & LEFT

Emily E. Wilcox

▶ *Right & Left*
▶ in conversation with Gu Jiani and Emily Wilcox

Despite the fact that one of China's most prominent contemporary choreographers is a publically transsexual woman,[1] and that indigenous theater in China has a long and well-known history of homoerotic spectatorship and patronage,[2] the idea of "queer dance"—or public reflection on queer identities and experiences more generally—is almost nonexistent in twenty-first-century urban Chinese professional dance circles.[3] Out queer choreographers are few and far between in major domestic dance festivals in China, as are dance productions or academic works that explicitly draw attention to non-normative genders and sexualities through dance. For women, this is even more pronounced, due to a more circumscribed set of possibilities of what constitutes "normal" and "appropriate" for women's performed subjectivities and dancing bodies.[4]

The fifty-minute contemporary dance duet *Right & Left* 右一左一 (2014) by Beijing-based female choreographer Gu Jiani,[5] danced by Gu and Li Nan with projections by media artist Li Ah Ping, presents an important and unusual departure from this larger trend. When approached for inclusion in this anthology, Gu said that she does not consider *Right & Left* a work of queer dance. Thus, the following reading represents my interpretation of the work

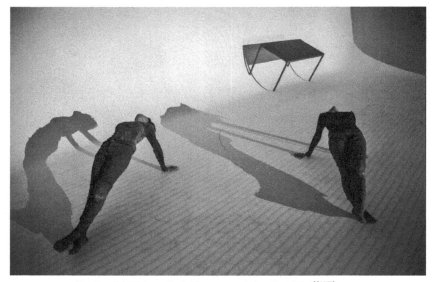

FIGURE 3.1 Gu Jiani's *Right & Left*. Photograph by Fan Xi (范西).

and not Gu's overt intention in creating it.[6] For me, the exploration of human relationships and embodiments enacted in *Right & Left* challenges normative conceptions of women, feminine gender, and female sexuality as typically presented in dance works by Chinese choreographers in twenty-first-century urban China. The term "queer feminism" best describes this intervention because it engages a complex nexus of social norms that engender women's dance movement, including heteronormativity, patriarchy, and gendered constructs of ethno-national identity.[7]

In this essay, I focus primarily on choreography—the ways in which bodies move, on their own, in relation to one another, and in relation to theater space and stage properties. Through this analysis of choreography, I examine two areas in which *Right & Left* draws attention to and in some cases successfully disrupts typical portrayals of women in past works by twenty-first-century urban Chinese choreographers. First, through a comparison with the highly acclaimed contemporary dance piece *Thunder and Rain* 雷和雨 (2002) by Beijing-based female choreographer Wang Mei, I argue that *Right & Left* challenges a common pattern in which female subjectivity and relationships between women are depicted as a product of women's unequal, even abusive, heterosexual relationships with men. I argue that *Right & Left* challenges these portrayals by exploring alternative modes of female subjectivity produced through relationships between women—including homoerotic ones—and by drawing attention to the violence against women perpetuated through works such as *Thunder and Rain*. Second, through an analysis of the presence and absence of culturally marked movement vocabulary in *Right & Left*, I examine Gu's choreographic choices around movement form in relation to her prior training in Chinese classical dance. Proposing the phrase "queer tai chi remix" to describe Gu's use of Chinese classical dance movement in this work, I suggest that while expanding the space for queer female subjectivity within ethno-national politics, Gu nevertheless avoids the issue of gender normativity as it relates to technique conventions and ethno-national identity in dance styles marked as ethnically "Chinese."

Apart from choreography, choices in costuming, hair, sound, lighting, and stage design also contribute to the queer feminism of Gu Jiani's *Right & Left*. While I will not address all of these elements here, two details should be mentioned, as they are important to the development of the choreographic meanings discussed below. *Right & Left* takes place in a white stage space set with one rectangular table and two stools. This choice is significant in relation to the history of Chinese theater, since "a table and two chairs" comprised the traditional stage set for Peking opera and other forms of indigenous theater in China. Here, the use of the table and stools places the dancers and their activities within a social frame, identifying them as dramatic figures rather than abstract bodies in space. In terms of costuming, it is also significant that the two female performers wear nearly identical costumes (long-sleeved knit shirts and gray leggings) yet have very different hairstyles. One of the dancers wears her hair in a short cut that would be recognized as "boyish" to Chinese audiences.[8] In contrast, the other dancer wears her hair in bangs and a medium-length braid, a conventionally "feminine" hairstyle common for young women in Chinese dance works. This difference in hairstyle sets up a situation in which one dancer can be read as gender conforming and the other as gender non-conforming, or the two together as a butch-femme/ T-P couple.[9] To avoid imposing a single interpretation on this hairstyle choice, while also marking the important differences it connotes at certain places in the choreography, I use the names "Short-hair" and "Braid" to refer to the two performers.

Young women living in contemporary China face significant pressure to conform to the intersecting social expectations of heterosexuality, patriarchy, and gender normativity—pressures that are reflected in the predominant modes of representing women in dance works by twenty-first-century urban Chinese choreographers. By drawing attention to these practices and providing alternatives to them, Gu Jiani's *Right & Left* makes an important contribution to a new field of queer feminist dance in China.

Sexuality, Subjectivity, and Women

Wang Mei 王玫 (b. 1958), a prolific choreographer and professor at the Beijing Dance Academy (BDA), is one of the leading figures in twenty-first-century Chinese contemporary dance. Wang began her career as a performer and later choreographer of Chinese ethnic, folk, and classical dance.[10] Then, in the late 1980s, she was part of the inaugural group of students in an experimental modern dance program led by Yang Meiqi at the Guangdong Dance Academy, what led to the formation of the Guangdong Modern Dance Company.[11] Since 1990, Wang has taught modern dance and choreography at BDA, serving as the most important promoter of modern dance within China's conservatory system. When I studied at BDA in 2008–2009, Wang's classes were regularly over-enrolled, and choreographers trained in what many then called the "Wang Mei style" populated nearly every major dance ensemble in China.

Among Chinese dance scholars, Wang's 2002 contemporary dance drama *Thunder and Rain* is considered one of the most canonical works of twenty-first-century Chinese dance, and it is viewed by many as a breakthrough in portrayals of women's subjectivity, sexuality, and feminist perspectives.[12] The authors of a recent study argue that in *Thunder and Rain* Wang Mei "takes woman as her subject . . . works from a feminist viewpoint . . . [and] makes visible a complete woman's psychology."[13] *Thunder and Rain* is an adaptation of one of China's most famous modern plays, Cao Yu's *Thunderstorm* (1934), which recounts the demise of a Chinese family plagued by incest, jealousy, and an autocratic patriarch. Wang's version focuses on the story's three female characters, in particular, the middle-aged second wife, Fanyi.[14] In the play Fanyi's husband forces her to take "medicine" for what he calls her "mental illness." Meanwhile, Fanyi is involved in a failing love affair with Ping, her husband's son from a previous marriage.[15] Like *Right & Left*, *Thunder and Rain* uses minimalistic stage sets and everyday clothing (except in one group scene), and the movement vocabulary is a blend of vernacular movement and contemporary dance.

Although *Thunder and Rain* makes an important contribution to feminist choreography by foregrounding female experiences and emotions, it does so in a way that pits women against one another and portrays their agency and self-value as dependent upon heterosexual relationships to men. A sequence of interconnected duets reveals the relationships between the three female characters. In the first segment, Fanyi has just been rejected by Ping and is intensely upset. She meets Sifeng, the younger woman with whom Ping is now romantically involved, and Sifeng at first comforts her with a moving embrace. This act of care is revealed to be insincere, however, when Sifeng suddenly pushes Fanyi away, lets out a ridiculing laugh, and then removes her coat to taunt Fanyi with her younger, presumably more sexually appealing, body. A group of young women dressed similarly to Sifeng swarms onto the stage and chases Fanyi, a manifestation of the latter's inner anguish. Then, an older woman—the former lover of Fanyi's husband—appears. Like Sifeng, she laughs condescendingly, then performs a long soliloquy in which she criticizes Fanyi for believing she can still compete with younger women for the attention of men. "Think about it, who would want a woman like you?" she shouts. The key to everlasting beauty and youth, the older woman counsels, is learning to give up: "If you go away now, you will remain in his heart forever." The scene ends with the three women dancing side-by-side to tango music, basked in red light with expressions of ecstasy, enjoying what appears to be a shared fantasy of everlasting appeal achieved through self-sacrifice.[16]

In *Thunder and Rain*, the audience gets to know Fanyi through her violent subjugation to the various male characters, and her subjectivity seems to be produced by these encounters. In one sequence, she stands inclined on her tiptoes, her body making a forty-five degree angle to the floor, as her husband grips her head under one arm and appears to drag her along the stage by her neck. Immediately following this, she repeatedly runs after and throws herself at her husband, grasping and clinging onto him. A similar dynamic emerges in Fanyi's relationship to Ping—the romantic affair around which the plot largely centers—even to the extent that Fanyi's sexual enjoyment appears to be a product of, or least compatible with, Ping's mistreatment of her. The long duet that characterizes the pair's relationship begins with Fanyi attempting to back away from Ping, suggesting that she does not want a romantic encounter. Ping nevertheless grabs her tightly by the wrist and does not let her go. He pulls her toward him and twists her arms around her body until she cannot move. Then, Ping's manipulation of Fanyi's body increases in intensity: he thrusts her head back and forth, grips her by the waist, and rubs his hand along her face, neck, and chest. At this point, Fanyi's resistance fades. As Ping grabs her breast with his hand, she thrusts her head back in apparent enjoyment. Then, she turns and embraces Ping tenderly. A long sequence ensues that seems to portray mutually consenting sex, including a "flying" pose with Fanyi outstretched and suspending in the air atop Ping's extended legs. This scene suggests that Fanyi derives extreme pleasure from her encounter with Ping, so much so that his rejection of her for a younger woman becomes the primary defining feature of her character in the remainder of the production.

While there is, of course, great variation in how women are depicted in twenty-first-century urban Chinese concert dance, and it is impossible to generalize based on one work alone, the rejected heterosexual woman is an extremely common trope. Moreover, women's sexuality is often portrayed as being linked to this experience of rejection, and this produces a kind of gendered violence in which men are expected and permitted to determine women's fates, including what they can and cannot enjoy. A variety of processes lead to the reproduction of this vision in new choreography. For example, a female contemporary dance choreographer I knew while living in Beijing told me that she had entered a duet into a local dance competition, but, after the first round of judging, was advised to make changes because of what was described as the "inappropriateness" of the work's theme: an amicable heterosexual one-night stand. The work was changed to instead portray a man and woman who sleep together, after which the man rejects the woman, and the remainder focuses on the woman's sadness. This was seen as more "appropriate" than a couple enjoying a sexual encounter on equal and mutually unattached terms.

In contrast to the older and more established Wang Mei, Gu Jiani 古佳妮 (b. 1988) is a young, independent choreographer in the early stages of her career. Like Wang, Gu works primarily in the medium of contemporary dance. In 2008–2012, Gu was a dancer with the Beijing Modern Dance Company, and in 2013, she and Li Nan 李楠 set up their own Beijing-based arts collective, N SPACE, which became the creative platform for *Right & Left*.[17] Gu and Li devised *Right & Left* between April and August, 2014, at the Jiaotang 焦堂/ Sofun gallery space in Beijing.[18] It was then presented in the Guangdong Dance Festival, China's most important international contemporary dance festival, that November.[19] In 2015–16, *Right & Left* toured abroad to the United States, Australia, and Hong Kong, and in 2016 Gu was commissioned by the Shanghai International Arts Festival to create a new work.[20] Although *Right & Left* has not yet received the attention of major Chinese dance critics, Gu's work has generally been well received in China's contemporary dance community. In 2011 and 2013, Gu won "Best Young Choreographer" and Bronze Medal in Choreography awards at the Beijing International Ballet and Choreography Competition. The 2013 work, a short duet titled "By My Side" 身边 performed by Gu and Li, could also be read as a work of queer dance.[21]

Gu's work *Right & Left* departs from portrayals of women found in *Thunder and Rain*. First, not only are men not physically present, but the relationship that develops between the two female dancers appears in no way to depend upon male desire. Instead, a form of intimacy and care emerges between the two women. When the work begins, the dancers move in unison, performing a relationship of equality that lacks obvious signs of competition or self-comparison like those found in *Thunder and Rain*. Next, the dancers interact in a way that suggests romantic intimacy, while also maintaining parity in the relative power of each over the other. Playing with two stools, the women exchange roles sharing weight, lowering to the floor with their bodies in parallel, and allowing their feet and legs to brush against one another. The most explicit sequence occurs when a tangled set of inversions brings Braid's face between Short-hair's thighs, then her body seated backward on Short-hair's lap, legs wrapping around in a reverse embrace. As they roll to the floor, their torsos press against one another and their faces nearly meet. Although there is little overtly sexual contact, a sense of queer intimacy develops. This happens in part from the use of the stools, which suggest a domestic space, and in part because of the clothing and haircuts, which suggest a blurring between gender sameness and gender complementarity.

While the sequence described in *Right & Left* presents an alternative to the unequal, competitive, and abusive relationships presented in *Thunder and Rain*, the one that immediately follows mimics them in order to generate critique. A change in music signals a break between the two scenes: a playful piano melody is replaced by a heavy electronic static. Short-hair turns toward the audience, staring intensely, as she slowly takes a seat on one of the stools. Throughout the next scene, Short-hair is completely passive, while Braid manipulates her body, evoking the way that Ping engaged with Fanyi in *Thunder and Rain*. The difference, however, is that Short-hair does not resist. With her palm on the side of Short-hair's head, Braid gives a hard push and sends Short-hair's torso bobbing back and forth like a metronome. Then, Braid rolls Short-hair's head between her hands and presses her hand along Short-hair's face. Short-hair's neck and arms are limp, allowing her body to flail with each push or pull. Then, the flurry of motion is interrupted by a sudden stillness, as Short-Hair's body falls limp and motionless over the top of the stool. A direct comparison can be made between this scene and Fanyi and Ping's duet, with the difference that, here, Short-hair does not respond to Braid's manipulations. Throughout the interaction, Short-hair's sustained inertness acts as a foil to Fanyi's initial resistance and then enjoyment, both of which had implied that Fanyi's subjectivity emerged in response to, or was sustained by, Ping's actions. By portraying Short-hair as completely without subjectivity in this sequence, *Right & Left* challenges the broader idea perpetuated in *Thunder and Rain*, namely, that the woman is an equal participant in, and even complicit in or welcoming of, abusive treatment by her male partner.

In the next sequence, Gu pushes this theme further, questioning whether such violent interactions are so commonplace as to engender the perception of femininity. At this point Short-hair is sitting upright on the stool and facing the audience, while Braid's arm is wrapped around her neck like a stranglehold. This resembles the position of Fanyi when her husband dragged her in *Thunder and Rain*. Braid's arm squeezes around Short-hair's face, guiding it into a forward tilt into the audience. Short-hair's eyes suddenly appear enlarged, her chin narrowed, and her face white against Braid's dark gray shirt, all while her eyes look forward and slightly upward. The position eerily resembles the familiar pose of so many "cute" selfies, and she suddenly appears conventionally feminine for the first time. The neck of her shirt hangs loose from the previous actions and falls to expose her shoulders and upper chest. The viewer suddenly wonders: is it the changes to her clothing and how the lighting is landing on her face that has shifted her gendered appearance—or is it how her body is being moved?

If the sequences above offer a critical intervention into *Thunder and Rain's* portrayal of heterosexual relationships, then the following one speaks to that among the three females. Performing the alteration of one woman's appearance by another, it suggests adornment or "beautification" in the form of a gesture that could simultaneously be read as violent. First, Short-hair stands caught with her arms twisted around her waist, as Braid proceeds to hang the two stools from Short-hair's body, one from the back like a backpack and the other from the front like an oversized belt. As if Short-hair were a paper doll and the stools a set of push-pins, Braid presses the legs of the stools into convenient crevices: over the shoulders, under the armpits, under the crotch, around the hips. In a scene as absurd as it is poignant, Braid then guides Short-hair's arms to hold the two stools in place on her own body. Finally, holding onto the legs of the stools, Braid leads Short-hair into a series of twirls, as if the two were social dancing. Darkness slowly closes in on the stage, causing Short-hair's silhouette to be cast in shadow against the back wall. With the stools still hanging on her, their round tops add curves to Short-hair's hips and chest, while the eight stool legs appear in the shadow image like so many rods or spines sticking out of her torso. Finally, Braid steps away and, as if controlled by the momentum, Short-hair continues to twirl.

When read alongside Wang Mei's *Thunder and Rain*, Gu Jiani's *Right & Left* presents a new set of possibilities for performing women in Chinese contemporary dance. On the one hand, by presenting two women in a non-antagonistic, even intimate, relationship that is not mediated by male desire, *Right & Left* dislocates women's psychological and sexual subjectivity from its dependence upon and subordination to male desire. On the other hand, by embodying gendered violence through a female couple, in which the Tomboy appears to be subjected to the manipulations and adornments by her Femme partner—and made somehow strangely more "feminine" in the process—this invites the audience to reflect on multiple issues related to gender normativity and the ways in which women are typically portrayed in intimate relationships. In *Right & Left* queer and feminist critique intersect to rethink (or re-perform) representations of women on multiple levels.

"Queer Tai Chi Remix," or De-gendering the Nation

Since the early twentieth century, the image of the suffering woman has often been an allegory for the ailing nation in Chinese performance culture; yet while woman's bodies and experiences stand in for the nation metaphorically, women are rarely depicted as the primary agents of national salvation or development.[22] With this in mind, the next section of *Right & Left* is interesting for the way it challenges conventional understandings of women's relationship to national culture, first by staging these conventions and then by undoing and complicating them.

If, following the manipulation sequence, Braid plays a social role marked as "masculine" and Short-hair one marked as "feminine," the next scene can be read as a clear enactment, followed by critique, of conventional ideas about the respective roles of men and women in the national political sphere. After Short-hair's spinning is engulfed by shadow, the lights come on again to reveal Braid standing tall at the front of the stage and staring into the audience, while Short-hair, the two stools still encumbering her body, stands at the back, hunched forward with her eyes cast toward her own feet. As if in separate worlds, the two perform different actions simultaneously. Braid performs a manic sequence in which she repeatedly brushes the top of her head with both hands while staring into the audience, causing her hair to become increasingly disheveled. Meanwhile, Short-hair, still hunched over, carefully and quietly balances one stool atop the other's feet, constructing a small rectangular space between them. As Braid's head-brushing motions intensify in speed and range, Short-hair crouches down and shrinks her body to fit into the space between the two chairs. This scene is abstract and minimalistic, and it would be a mistake to read it too literally. However, the image of Short-hair, as "woman/feminine," contorting herself to fit a metaphorically domestic space, while Braid, as "man/masculine," admonishes herself in an act that could be read as public, even intellectual, self-reflection provokes clear resonances with habits of modern Chinese nationalist discourse, in which gender difference is mapped onto a constructed distinction between private and public spheres.[23]

Evidence that this scene references the theme of the gendered nation becomes clearer as it unfolds. After Short-hair quietly disappears from the stage, taking the stools with her, Braid is left alone on the space of the white surface and table with which the work began. Staring into the audience, Braid takes a wide step to the side and sinks into a lowered stance with weight distributed evenly between both feet. Her hand slowly floats to one side, and she begins a sequence of movements clearly based on the Chinese martial arts form *taijiquan*, also known as "tai chi." The link between this movement sequence and Chinese national and cultural identity is unmistakable—it appears in multiple forms of globalized popular culture associated with China, from martial arts films to wushu performance to a variety of contemporary dance styles that aim in different ways to embody "Chinese" (or in some cases "Taiwanese") culture, such as the Cloud Gate Dance Theater of Taiwan and the Beijing Dance Academy's Chinese classical dance curriculum. As Braid performs the movement, her body shows visible marks of the relationships and experiences that have already transpired on stage over the course of the performance—her hair is disheveled, her shirt stretched and loosened, and marks from contact with the white dusted floor still hang on her knees and shoulders. Thus, in her performance of the tai chi movements, Braid inserts an already established queer female subjectivity into the national or cultural imaginary of "China."

Placing a queer female subject at the center of the national imaginary is not the extent of this sequence's intervention. What happens next does something potentially even more drastic to normative discourses about how gender constructs and is constructed through national space: after performing several movements in a standard tai chi mode, Braid then seamlessly intertwines these actions with movements that break from it, which are unrecognizable as part of any established "Chinese" movement aesthetic. Allowing her left hand to drop and then rise up across her body like a clock hand, then arching her upper body and head back into a reverse arc, she is no longer performing tai chi. However, just as smoothly, she then drops back down to the low sinking stance, lowers her hands to waist level, and continues the previous sequence. With this intermingling of movement vocabulary, some marked as Chinese and some not, Braid does more than place a new body within the existing national form; she constructs her own version of the form, thereby redefining what is meant by "China" through her inhabiting of it. Here, play is central to Gu's intervention. Much as the two women played with the stools as a way of rethinking sexual intimacy, in this scene Braid plays with national form as a way of rethinking national space.

When Short-hair rejoins Braid, performing her same movements in a different orientation, this suggests the replicability, and thus inheritability, of a queered national culture. Drawing on the literature of postcolonial gender and sexuality studies, cultural critic Gayatri Gopinath has argued that queer sexuality tends to be excluded from national imaginaries because it is presumed to endanger the possibility of genealogical lineage at the center of biological and patrilineal notions of national identity.[24] Thus, when Short-hair doubles Braid's altered version of the national movement form, this suggests a queering of the conventional nation, in at least two ways: first, it proposes a model of reproduction based on a pairing of two women, in which patrilineal relations are unnecessary and irrelevant; and, second, it suggests that national culture is open to remolding and proliferation through the unrestrained bodily agency of women, something usually thought to endanger it.[25] The entire next duet is carried out in this hybrid movement style, a kind of queer tai chi remix. Pulsing rhythms add syncopation to the familiar floating hands; tilted torsos and angular arm lines break up the quintessential roundness of the movements. Here, nationalized form is no longer a guide for how a Chinese woman "should" move. Instead, it becomes a resource to be mined and transformed through her productive creativity.

Despite the fact that modern Chinese movement vocabularies like PRC Chinese classical dance were formed through processes of constant change and reformulation, many dance practitioners in China today find them highly restrictive when it comes to developing individual expressive styles.[26] Over years of conducting ethnographic fieldwork among professional dancers in China, I found that most dancers who rejected dance styles coded as "Chinese" did so because of what they described as the perceived lack of stylistic freedom these forms imposed. Gu Jiani's professional bio narrates a similar process of her own artistic development. After being trained in both ballet and Chinese classical dance, it states, Gu was "dissatisfied with the monotony of conventional training, [and] she embarked on a path of meditative self-discovery."[27] Such a story suggests, following what has become a standard narrative for modern and contemporary dancers and choreographers around the world, that conventional or classical technique and self-discovery are somehow mutually exclusive.[28]

Gu's creative use of movement marked as conventionally "Chinese" in *Right & Left* troubles this notion. By staging a reinvention and appropriation, rather than a complete rejection, of conventional forms, Gu performs something similar to what Gopinath identifies in her work as a queering of the nation from within, one that does not rely on a flight to an imagined "elsewhere." Gopinath writes,

> Given that leaving, escaping, and traveling to a presumably freer 'elsewhere' is not an option or even necessarily desirable for many subaltern subjects, we must take seriously the myriad strategies through

which those who remain (out of choice or necessity) conspire to rework the oppressive structures in which they find themselves.[29]

In Gu's case, fleeing to an "elsewhere" is certainly possible: the entire rest of the production is composed using movement languages that do not use movement forms marked as "Chinese." Thus, by inserting the tai chi movements in this sequence, Gu suggests a concerted effort to find ways of performing as a queer female within the space of the nation, rather than outside it. Like the women in Gopinath's texts, Gu suggests through this sequence that the rejection of conventional or culturally coded spaces is not a prerequisite for queer existence or self-expression.

What Gu does not engage with directly in this scene, however, is the aesthetic definition of gendered bodies that is also a strong component of many "Chinese"-coded movement forms. Chinese classical dance, one of the forms Gu studied in her conservatory training, is composed of "male" and "female" movement vocabularies that differ from one another. These movement styles grew out of the history of Chinese indigenous theater, in which male and female characters traditionally moved differently.[30] Since cross-gender performance was a central component of Chinese indigenous theater from at least the late eighteenth century, gender difference became something separated from the sex of the actor—something to be created and performed through artistic skill.[31] While this denaturalized the connection between gender performance and the actor's sex, it also led to a firm codification of normative gendered embodiment, as actors (until the 1920s primarily men) were trained to play characters recognizable as "men" or "women" on stage.[32] Within the PRC Chinese classical dance curriculum, tai chi movement is one of the few forms conventionally performed by both men and women. In the entirety of *Right & Left*, there is no use of movements from the Chinese classical dance vocabulary coded specifically as "female" or "male." Thus, by avoiding gender-specific movement actions in her citation of the Chinese classical dance repertoire, Gu avoids engaging fully with the problem of how gender-queer expression can exist or be explored within the national form as it is defined in PRC dance.

The Risks of Dancing Queer

What does it mean to talk about queer dance in a context in which "queer dance" as a concept does not exist? For Chinese citizens in twenty-first-century urban China, identifying publically as homosexual can bring serious negative social consequences, such as being fired from one's job, being harassed by police, lacking access to regular medical care, and being shunned by friends and family.[33] Even though homosexuality was formally decriminalized and depathologized in China in 1997 and 2001, respectively, there continue to be no legal protections for homosexuals, and in 2008 representations of homosexuality were banned from public media.[34] Thus, when I asked Gu Jiani whether she considered *Right & Left* a work of queer dance, her first answer was "no," but then she asked, "What is queer dance?" Part of writing about queer dance is thus starting these conversations, opening up the possibility for dance-making and dance-viewing to become a hearth for queer activism and community building.

Speaking openly about sexuality is not easy in China. While conducting fieldwork among Chinese dancers in 2008–2014, I audiotaped over two hundred interviews that dealt with sensitive topics ranging from political violence during the Cultural Revolution to corruption and bribe-taking in today's dance schools. There was only one time, however, that an interviewee asked me to stop a recording midway so that something could be shared off record. When I turned off the tape, the twenty-year-old male contemporary dancer who sat across from me in the corner of a nearly empty restaurant in Beijing said in a hushed voice, "Actually, I'm gay." If expressing one individual's private identity in this context was so sensitive, how can queer identities be performed publically on a stage, in dance performances that require the collaborative support (and thus risk-taking) of many entities, institutions, and bodies?

In twenty-first-century urban China, as in many places around the world, people who do not conform to social expectations about gender—whether because they are homosexual or simply do not embody social norms about how "women" or "men" should behave—face discrimination and, often, violence. Queer dance is about challenging such social expectations about gender in all their forms. It is only by challenging these expectations and showing alternative possibilities that damaging and discriminating habits can ultimately be made visible and overturned.

Acknowledgments

I am grateful to Clare Croft for inviting me to participate in this anthology and for her insightful and supportive feedback throughout the writing and revision process. I am also grateful to Gu Jiani for sharing a complete video of her performance in Beijing, which served as the subject of this analysis. Tremendous thanks go to Alison Friedman of Ping-Pong Productions for introducing me to Gu Jiani's work and for facilitating Gu's 2015 visit to the University of

Michigan. This project benefited from generous funding and support from the American Council of Learned Societies, the Kenneth G. Lieberthal and Richard H. Rogel Center for Chinese Studies, and the Confucius Institute at the University of Michigan.

Notes

1. Andrew Kimbrough and Jin Xing, "Jin Xing in the New China: Redefining the Mainstream," *Drama Review* 48, no. 1 (T181) (Spring 2004): 106–23.
2. Andrea S. Goldman, *Opera and the City: The Politics of Culture in Beijing, 1770–1900* (Stanford, CA: Stanford University Press, 2012).
3. My use of "China" here designates the People's Republic of China. It does not include Taiwan or diasporic communities.
4. These observations are based on ten years of experience as an ethnographer and historian of Chinese dance, a former student at the Beijing Dance Academy, and a producer of dance exchanges between China and the United States.
5. Family names come first in China. Gu (rhymes with "you" with a hard "g") is her family name and Jiani (pronounced "jeeah-nee") is her given name.
6. More on Gu's thoughts about the work can be found in the video interview that accompanies this book.
7. By using the terms "queer" and "feminist" together, I am drawing on a tradition of scholarship that recognizes the potential for shared concerns and intersections between queer and feminist critique. I follow Mimi Marinucci, one proponent of a specifically "queer feminist" analytic, when she writes, "this solidarity [between queer and feminist critique] seems born of a deep understanding that the oppression of women and the suppression of lesbian, gay, bisexual, and transgender existence are deeply intertwined." Mimi Marinucci, *Feminism is Queer: The Intimate Connection between Queer and Feminism* (London: Zed, 2010), 106. While I would add that this is not always the case, and that LGBTQ individuals often experience different and/or greater forms of oppression even than women do in highly patriarchal societies, I contend that the alliance is a useful one in this case and for dealing in general with situations in which heteronormativity, gender normativity, and patriarchy operate as intersecting forms of social violence.
8. The 2005 controversy over the "tomboy" aesthetic of Li Yuchun, the short-haired female performer who won first place in a Chinese television singing contest *Supergirl*, suggests that this type of gender performance would be read as nonconforming among popular Chinese audiences. See Xin Huang, "From 'Hyperfeminine' to Androgyny: Changing Notions of Femininity in Contemporary China," in *Asian Popular Culture In Transition*, ed. Lorna Fitzsimmons and John Lent (London: Routledge, 2013), 133–55.

9. "T-P" refers to the concept of "Tomboy-Po" (Po refers here to the Mandarin word *"laopo,"* a colloquial term for "wife"), used among many lesbians in urban twenty-first-century China. It is sometimes compared to the butch-femme concept, though it is not entirely the same. See Elisabeth L. Engebretsen, *Queer Women in Urban China: An Ethnography* (New York: Routledge, 2014). On the contested, variable, and changing meanings of "butch-femme" among queer females in North America, see Esther D. Rothblum, "The Complexity of Butch and Femme among Sexual Minority Women in the 21st Century," *Psychology of Sexualities Review* 1, no. 1 (2010): 29–42.

10. Feng Shuangbai 冯双白 et al., *Zhongguo wudaojia da cidian* 中国舞蹈家大词典 (Dictionary of Chinese dance artists) (Beijing: Zhongguo wenlian chuban she, 2006), 18–19.

11. For more on this program and Wang's role in it, see Ruth Solomon and John Solomon, eds., *East Meets West in Dance: Voices in a Cross-Cultural Dialogue* (New York: Routledge, [1995] 2011).

12. Jin Hao 金浩, *Xin shiji Zhongguo wudao wenhua de liubian* 新世纪中国舞蹈文化的流变 (New century Chinese dance culture and transformation) (Shanghai: Shanghai yinyue chubanshe, 2007).

13. Dong Yinghao 董英豪 and Wang Jing 王婧, "Wudao zhong de nüxing biaoshu" 舞蹈中的女性表述 (Women's expression in dance), *Minzu Tribune* 民族论坛 8 (2012): 108–9.

14. For a comparative analysis, see Tang Xumei 汤旭梅, "Wuju 'Lei he yu' dui 'Leiyu' de jiegou yu chuangsheng" 舞剧'雷和雨'对'雷雨'的解构与创生 (Dance drama *Thunder and Rain*'s deconstruction and recreation of *Thunderstorm*), *Journal of the Beijing Dance Academy* 北京舞蹈学院学报 (2007/3): 107–12.

15. For a complete English translation of the play and a discussion of it in historical context, see Xiaomei Chen, *The Columbia Anthology of Modern Chinese Drama* (New York: Columbia University Press, 2010).

16. *Thunder and Rain* video recording, performed by the 2002 Modern Dance graduating class of the Beijing Dance Academy's Choreography Department, author's collection.

17. "*Right & Left* promotional materials," Jiumai Cultural Promotion Corporation, http://cama.cc/goods/show-417.html.

18. For social media documentation of the creative process, see "GO_NSPACE 身体计划," Beijing Weibo Internet Technology Corporation, http://www.x-weibo.net/u/5032902718/p_4.html. The analysis provided in this essay is based on a video recording of the work taken in this space in 2014. The same recording is included in the video database that accompanies this book.

19. "Eleventh Guangdong Dance Festival Online Program, 2014," Guangdong Dance Festival, http://www.gdfestival.com/en/programme.php.

20. "Choreographer Gu Jiani," Ping Pong Productions, http://www.pingpongarts.org/projects/56/.

21. "By My Side" 身边, Wudao.com, http://q.dance365.com/topic/10032004? ordertype=desc.

22. Xiaomei Chen, *Acting the Right Part: Political Theater and Popular Drama in Contemporary China* (Honolulu: University of Hawai'i Press, 2002); Shuqin Cui, *Women through the Lens: Gender and Nation in a Century of Chinese Cinema* (Honolulu: University of Hawai'i Press, 2003); Rosemary Roberts, *Maoist Model Theater: The Semiotics of Gender and Sexuality in the Chinese Cultural Revolution (1966–1976)* (Leiden: Brill, 2010).

23. Wendy Larson, *Women and Writing in Modern China* (Stanford, CA: Stanford University Press, 1998).

24. Gayatri Gopinath, *Impossible Desires: Queer Diasporas and South Asian Public Cultures* (Durham, NC: Duke University Press, 2005).

25. Doris Croissant et al., eds., *Performing "Nation": Gender Politics in Literature, Theater, and the Visual Arts of China And Japan, 1880–1940* (Leiden: Brill, 2008).

26. On the history of change and individual voice in PRC Chinese classical dance, see Emily Wilcox, "Han-Tang *Zhongguo Gudianwu* and the Problem of Chineseness in Contemporary Chinese Dance: Sixty Years of Controversy," *Asian Theater Journal* 29, no. 1 (2012): 206–32.

27. Gu Jiani promotional materials. Supplied by Gu Jiani and Ping Pong Productions, March 2015.

28. For a critique of this narrative, see Ananya Chatterjea, "On the Value of Mistranslations and Contaminations: The Category of 'Contemporary Choreography' in Asian Dance," *Dance Research Journal* 45, no. 1 (2013): 4–21.

29. Gopinath, *Impossible Desires*, 91.

30. Li Zhengyi 李正一 et al., *Zhongguo gudianwu jiaoxue tixi chuangjian fazhan shi* 中国古典舞教学体系创建发展史 (History of the development of the teaching system of Chinese classical dance) (Shanghai: Shanghai yinyue chubanshe, 2004).

31. Joshua Goldstein, *Drama Kings: Players and Publics in the Re-creation of Peking Opera, 1870–1937* (Berkeley: University of California Press, 2007).

32. The ban on women in Peking opera lasted from the late eighteenth century to the early twentieth century. On the reintegration of female actors into Chinese theater and their impact on gender performance, see Siyuan Liu, *Performing Hybridity in Colonial-Modern China* (New York: Palgrave Macmillan, 2013). On a genre of Chinese theater in which women traditionally play the roles of both male and female characters, see Jin Jiang, *Women Playing Men: Yue Opera and Social Change in Twentieth-Century Shanghai* (Seattle: University of Washington Press, 2009).

33. Lisa Rofel, "Grassroots Activism: Non-Normative Sexual Politics in Post-Socialist China," in *Unequal China: The Political Economy and Cultural Politics of Inequality*, ed. Wanning Sun and Yingjie Guo (New York: Routledge, 2013), 154–66.

34. Rofel, "Grassroots Activism," 155.

4

The Hysterical Spectator

DANCING WITH FEMINISTS, NELLIES, ANDRO-DYKES, AND DRAG QUEENS

Doran George

Setting the Stage

I'm in the Betty Pease Studio Theatre at the University of Michigan at a 2012 queer dance conference. We are viewing Jennifer Monson and DD Dorvillier's diptych *RMW(a) & RMW* (1993/2004). The dancers, a bitch-mother and daughter, menace the edges of a sparse stage. Sporting a satin mini-dress with a black-on-white print pattern suggesting overgenerous zebra-like cuts, Monson's body is all big-cat-drag-queen-top. Her sleek wig ups the ante of the natural redhead beneath while Marlene Dietrich's pencil-thin eyebrows battle for facial territory with Baby Jane Hudson's greedy lipstick. I'm a deer in Monson's carnivorous headlights, but she's focused on returning Dorvillier's intense and piercing gaze. Trimmed with gold piping, Dorvillier's emerald green short-sports-shorts scream 1980s, thereby cohabiting happily with a long, and ostentatious, loosely curled black mullet-wig. Dark as dried blood, her Morticia lips sparkle with cheap glitter, undergirding the clichéd green eye shadow through which Dorvillier meets and incites the delicious nasty gaze of her street-queen mother. Only the tinkling of overheated fresnels breaks the silence. Then high-pitched guttural machine-gun laughter spills from my lungs; *RMW(a)*, the first part of the diptych, has rendered me hysterical.

Fueled by the destabilizing impact upon me of *RMW(a) & RMW*, this essay considers gender critique in select dances from Monson and Dorvillier's Manhattan Lower East Side dance scene. I identify in East Village dance distinct strategies for staging femininity that elicit feminist, queer, and transgender viewers. Yet by collapsing the distinctions between these different viewing positions, *RMW(a) & RMW* disturbs the clear sense of inside and outside upon which discrete and stable sexual and gender identities depend. The diptych thus plunges me into hysteria, where I reclaim the condition from psychoanalytic diagnosis that was used to circumscribe proper femininity. Beyond identity's boundaries, I navigate territorial tensions between feminist, queer, and transgender theories and activism, exposing their respective limitations upon embodiment.

Some feminist and queer theorists position femininity and femaleness as legitimate or critical only for particular sexed and desiring bodies. This territorialism overlaps with Western concert dance's privileging of the female body as its proper vehicle of expression. As a result, dancing men find their masculinity and heterosexuality brought into question even while gay subjects have, until recently, rarely been staged. Yet concert dance's conventional femininity also circumscribes the institutional and representational possibilities for women. Since its early twentieth-century beginnings, American modern dance resisted and compounded such conventions, both reconstructing and recapitulating gender norms. Likewise, the examples I analyze sometimes resolve tensions between feminism, queer, and transgender, and sometimes reaffirm patriarchal gender asymmetry and exclusionary normative identity.

To understand my hysterical spectatorship, this chapter identifies conflicting agendas in the staging of femininity in others of Monson's works, as well as pieces by her East Village colleagues Neil Greenberg and John Jasperse. I equate the feminist viewer with the contesting of gender-asymmetry, the queer viewer with establishing lesbian and gay visibility, and the transgender viewer with claiming legitimacy for occupying a sex/gender in conflict with that assigned at birth. In a journey through the different dances, I ricochet between the different viewing positions, failing to identify coherently with any one, and thereby foregrounding my inability to stabilize the dynamics of desire (Freud's basis for coherent identification). *RMW(a) & RMW* initiates this trajectory by exposing my assimilation of multiple Others and preventing me from crystallizing a stable self, which, in psychoanalysis, characterizes Hysteria.[1]

To define the viewing positions, I get on the psychoanalyst's couch and disclose childhood experiences, autobiographically establishing my hysteria. My aim is transparency about the essay's limits because to marshal feminism, queer, and transgender into single, distinct viewing positions erases their myriad historical and theoretical interdependencies and antagonisms, while also glossing over their internal complexities.[2] By disclosing my body history, I also foreground a problem with coherent identity. Some feminist readings reveal how, in establishing a stable self, psychoanalysis historically places white, heterosexual masculinity at its apex, and that coherent identity thus inherits a dependence on categorizing and stratifying various Others.[3] Embracing the tensions between feminist, queer, and transgender identities coursing through my body, I mobilize what is lost in the territorializing of a coherent sex-sexuality-gender identity.

East Village dance lends itself to thinking through feminist, queer, and transgender viewing positions because, since its early 1980s consolidation, the milieu has dealt explicitly with gender and sexual politics. Rather than define an artistic movement, this essay considers a few examples in detail, focusing on the territorializing of access to gender critique; but I offer here some contextual information to frame my discussion. Responding to political, economic, and social exigencies ushered in by Reagan, a group of East Village artists wrangled with rabid marginalization as attacks were made on reproductive rights, and people dying of AIDS were denied proper medical attention. With irony and anger, they staged gender and sexual identities as they were being defined in the culture wars.[4] In line with the era's leftist protocols, they focused on marginalization to which they could lay claim. The dances on which I focus contest heterosexual gender by intervening into the presumed association of dance theater with conventional femininity, without reflecting explicitly upon other axes of identity. African American dancer-choreographer Ishmael Houston-Jones drew attention to black artists' underrepresentation in the East Village with special showcases.[5] But, although his white colleagues probably saw the value of such projects, they rarely reflected on their own racial specificity. To avoid giving the impression that the critiques presented by Monson, Dorvillier, Greenberg, and Jasperse account universally for gender or sexuality oppression, I suggest a number of times how race changes the argument. I thereby hope to open my methods to research that I have not achieved within the scope of this project.[6]

East Village artists often survived with little funding, and the dissemination of their choreography was limited. They worked in spaces equivalent to off-off Broadway, like the converted, disused public school that became Performance Space 122; and also relied on sympathetic organizations donating time in buildings that already served another purpose, like St. Marks Church, which still doubles as a house of worship and Danspace Project's theater. Sheltered from large theater protocols by its small-scale economy, the East Village scene supported experimentation in motile embodiments of political exigencies, which often impacted dance theater more broadly. Despite the role of identity politics, however, rather than proselytizing, the small and well-informed audiences preferred playful, risky, implicit and veiled references that resisted transparent meaning. My familiarity with the milieu generally, and Monson specifically, contributed to my hysterical viewing of *RMW(a)* & *RMW*. My direct dialogue with the artists informs my theorization of their work.

Let's Get Hysterical

A prime example of choreographic experimentation, *RMW(a)* & *RMW* contests heterosexual gender by refusing to separate feminist, queer, and transgender viewership. Through its compositional structure the dance erodes the exclusionary logic of coherent identities, situating me in the frenzy of hysteria. The "(a)" following the first titular utterance of "RMW" connotes that this half of the dance is a revisiting of work first staged in 1993. *RMW(a)* was created a decade later. Since then the duo have performed their archival dance once a year. As Monson and Dorvillier dance their original work *RMW*, which is now the latter half of the diptych, the cause of my disorientation becomes clear. It reminds the audience of the radical departure that *RMW(a)*'s drag queen catwalk constitutes for Monson in particular. In *RMW*, the dancers lose their wigs and don denims, white T-shirts, and bomber jackets; the only thing separating them from 1990s andro-dyke street fashion is the hangover of heavy make-up from the night of cross-dressed prowling in which they were engaged only theatrical moments before. *RMW* thus reveals a shimmering late twentieth-century lesbian as behind *RMW(a)*'s foray into male to female performance. However, the remnants of thickly applied drag-queen make-up thwart any coherence or stability of familiar female homosexuality. In the diptych's chronology, *RMW*'s denim-clad dancers (the andro-dykes who displace the drag queens) represent the pre-existing work, symbolizing the historical precursor for the diptych, and foretelling in reverse the drag queens they will become. The remaining make-up refuses to belie the theatrical progression currently on view, obscuring access to authentic Sapphism as dykes emerge in the shadows of drag's spectacle. Monson and Dorvillier thus entangle a 1990s metro-lesbian and a contemporary retro gay spectacle of 1980s drag, removing viewers' certainty about where to direct their desire. This robs the spectator of the way that they would normally know and locate themselves in a coherent identity.

With sartorial, movement, and structural choices, the diptych denies singular viewing positions; it prohibits reassuring coherent identification, or an appropriate trajectory of desire. The choreography thus parallels the queer critique of naturalized male and female identity for which feminist theorist Judith Butler has become iconic.[7] *RMW(a)* & *RMW*'s andro-dykes and drag queens also expand upon Sue-Ellen Case's flouting of distinct embodied territories, which she achieved coevally with Butler. A queer performance theorist, Case tore gendered semiotics from heterosexual convention, evacuating the biological referent of the penis from the scene of desire. In "Towards a Butch-Femme Aesthetic" (1988), by masquerading heterosexual categories in their lust for each other, lesbians unseat the naturalized fantasy that reproductive sex, sutured to a supposed opposition of male and female, is the foundation of sexuality. A femme directs her desirability toward a butch, who performs and undermines the masculine(ist) power to desire. Case thus delights that "the female body, the male gaze and the structures of realism are only sex toys for the butch femme couple."[8] The bodies and desirability that Monson and Dorvillier display toward multiple and conflicting Others, not only destabilize a heteronormative male spectator, but set feminist, queer, and transgender viewer-positions in motion. Through a deviant use of history, the dance disintegrates coherent identity, confusing and luxuriating in multiple trajectories of desire.

By insisting that the significance of the female body in Western concert dance is central to any staging of gender critique, this essay uses East Village dance to reconsider methodological differences in some theories of gender and its critique. My feminist viewer identifies with dances by Monson that contest gender asymmetry (other than *RMW(a) & RMW*), but my queer spectator insists that the choreography leaves troubling sexual difference in place. I understand this deficit through queer theory, which claimed to rectify a tendency, in its precursor of feminism, to naturalize the category of sex. Meanwhile, Greenberg and Jasperse seem to critique the category of sex, arousing my queer viewer, but they jettison feminism by staging gay-male femininity that affirms femaleness as its origin. Read in this way, Greenberg's and Jasperse' queer strategies neglect to account for gender asymmetry, and thereby still fail to contest heterosexual gender. While their work is queer, the inattention to feminism limits queer possibility. *RMW(a) & RMW* is central to my argument because it exposes an underlying heterosexual logic in some queer performance. Monson and Dorvillier cleave conventional femininity from their femaleness by embodying drag-queen femininity for which a male body appears to be the origin. They thus reveal sanctions about the gender to which women have access in queer strategy, and demonstrate that, unless received notions of sex and gender are challenged in both sexes, heterosexuality recapitulates its omnipotence, robbing female dancers of critical agency. By uncovering limits in queer gender transgression, *RMW(a) & RMW* opens possibilities for my transgender viewer.

Defying Asymmetry

To discover the roots of my feminist viewing, I invite you into my child-hood home. By age 5, I was aware that, due to our shared femininity, my mother and I had less say than the men in the family. Long before discover-ing 1980s feminism in my teens, I secretly rooted for the women in weekly family viewings of a comedy game show, called *It's a Knockout* (a creation by Guy Lux initially aired in 1966), which involved feats of strength, ingenuity, and teamwork. Fast forward to the early 1990s, and my desire to see the women match the men finds satisfaction in Monson's *Finn's Shed* (1991), a dance that avoids explicit signs of masculinity or femininity. With vocabulary that appears functional, *Finn's Shed* betrays Monson's history of dancing for Pooh Kaye's company that staged an exciting and disturbing displacement of conventional femininity. For example, in *Bring Home the Bacon* (1984) Kaye, Monson, Claire Bernard, Ginger Gillespie, and Yvonne Meier slammed into walls, the floor, and each other, eschewing illusion and recognizable codes of gender through sheer endurance. Having met Kaye in the East Village scene, Monson achieved prominence there dancing for and choreographing work on her colleagues. She also gained recognition in similar scenes around and beyond the United States. A duet for Monson and Jasperse, *Finn's Shed* pre-miered at St. Mark's.

In the duet Monson transformed Kaye's crash-and-burn aesthetic with an androgynous childlike quality, seeming to avoid the adult sexual drama entailed in gendered display. There is nothing girly about the lack of hesitation with which she and Jasperse give weight fully and generously to each action, but neither are the dancers aggressive or ambitious enough to be nursery-rhyme boys. On a starkly untheatrical stage, wearing overalls that obscure bodily contours and represent practicality, Monson and Jasperse embody a "neither/nor" of gender, directing any athleticism back inward or toward each other by cushioning their play with mutually soft landings. Zeena Parkins's discordant and zany soundtrack bounces bizarrely from one organ-like note to another, propelling the dancers with no other purpose than the playful ex-change of weight. Kinesthetic pleasure underpins the unostentatious delight with which they run at each other, leap, knock each other over, spin, or sus-pend momentarily in a precarious balance. Their limbs never appear decora-tive, but facilitate easy landings, mutual support, and efficient balances. When arms or legs move with excited complexity, they catch the toppling, off-balance body; or amplify momentum and extend propulsion. Meanwhile, with a placid regard, Monson's and Jasperse's eyes follow the direction of their movement, focusing the audience on the mechanics of dancing.

By subduing sexual difference in a heterosexually cast pas de deux, *Finn's Shed* achieves greater gender equivalence than was hoped for but denied by Monson's predecessors. For example, internationally renowned Merce Cunningham, choreographing since the 1950s, and Trisha Brown, who gained prominence two decades later, both rebuffed classical ballet's and early modern dance's polarizations of gender. Like these artists, Monson avoids obvious signs of femininity, which, along with them, she configures as theatrical artifice. With formalism, Cunningham rejected modernist and classical lexicons, which *Finn's Shed* and several of Brown's works extended in task-like vocabulary that built on early 1960s innovation.[9] Yet along with Brown, Cunningham naturalized the idea that men are stronger than women by choreographing distinct embodiments of an equivalent vocabulary such as having the male dancers do most of the lifting.[10] In strong contrast, Monson denaturalizes such gender asymmetry in *Finn's Shed* by standing her own ground in relation to Jasperse; she takes her turn lifting him and aiding his suspensions. Moreover, with a functional sensibility in ongoing gamboling motion, the duo also desexualizes their liberal use of indiscriminate physical contact. With a sober gaze the dancers seal out heterosexuality as Monson's head rests on Jasperse's ass, and their faces fall into each other's crotches.

My feminist viewer identifies with Monson as she exceeds the lesser physical capacity often equated with women's social inferiority. Iris Marion Young, a political theorist, argues that "typically 'feminine' styles of movement and comportment" correlate with diminished access to what philosophers call "transcendence."[11] Young thus affirms the urgency of my rooting for women in the TV game show of my childhood, and the relief I find in Monson's gender equivalent vocabulary. Yet law scholar Kimberlé Crenshaw reveals the whiteness of such politics, pointing out that "society ... creates sex-based norms ... which racism operates simultaneously to deny; Black men are not viewed as powerful, nor are Black women seen as passive."[12] While patriarchy might broadly misrepresent women as dependent and passive, Crenshaw insists that black women struggle with their "failure to live up to such norms," a problem that also affects working-class women, who are denied the "privilege" of frailty not least because of the manual work they often perform. Contesting asymmetry by willing the women in *It's a Knockout* to win, perhaps then betrays my household's racial specificity and class aspirations as much as Monson's approach to establishing equivalence does of her whiteness.

Because whiteness tends to naturalize itself, my feminist viewer begins bumping up against her critical limits.[13] To the degree that gender asymmetry claims a biological basis, some feminism, often associated with the 1970s, asserts the pre-cultural female body as a means to resist patriarchy.[14]

These theories configure the constraints of femininity as artificially imposed upon women's natural potential, but they thus universalize themselves, erasing their cultural specificity and proffering immutable sexual difference. As Crenshaw points out, when it is assumed that all women are configured as frail or passive in contrast with their true nature, some women's struggles get marginalized. With its aesthetic interventions that seem to configure femininity as theatrically superficial, contemporary dance exhibits the problems of naturalized whiteness. Contact improvisation, for example, which emerged in the 1970s, entails weight-sharing techniques that, by enabling women and men to lift and support each other, as Monson and Jasperse do in *Finn's Shed*, seems to cut through gender differences.[15] Contact improvisers differed from much 1970s feminism by underplaying rather than emphasizing gender difference in the construction of nature, but the emphasis on mechanical bodily capacity seemed to displace theatrical artifice by staging an authentic self in a style that dance scholar Cynthia Novack calls "the dancer is just a person."[16] By drawing attention to the means of kinetic execution, dancers highlighted function, staging a kind of "bodily authenticity" that seemed to displace culturally imposed power relations. This is how Monson's equivalent physical capacity to Jasperse reads, and it is what my feminist viewer identifies with. Yet, as well as erasing the differences in gender asymmetry's impact that Crenshaw asserts, as an emancipation strategy, "natural equality" also jettisons the critical use to which conventional femininity can be put.

Signifying Male Homosexuality

My hysteria first refuses a singular identity by insisting on the queer potential of the conventional femininity rejected by my feminist viewer. To understand this tension, let us briefly return to my childhood machinations over gender. To those around me, I was a feminine "boy," and therefore gay, long before I felt erotic urges for anyone. By my hormonally volatile pre-pubescent teens, I had also ascribed to this belief, and, fueled by gay identity's irreverence in the 1980s political struggles against Margaret Thatcher's homophobic legislation, I left my rural English village for an urban gay ghetto at age seventeen. Signs of femininity such as my pronounced assibilation of "S" and my motile "delicacy," earned me queer conspicuousness, whereas performing contact improvisation's anti-theatrical gender equivalence would configure me as merely male. As a strategy for emancipation, androgyny fails women without Monson's dynamic ability to assert their equivalence to men, while male embodied queer and transgender difference disappears.

We find the problem of evacuating feminine conspicuousness in what Trisha Brown calls her "one phrase fits all genders" approach. The choreographer avoided "undignified" movement for the male body, and "clichéd images of . . . muscular male movement" in modern dance.[17] Against hypermasculinity at one end of the gender spectrum, lack of dignity at the other reveals itself as male femininity. To secure her male dancers' virility while discarding modern and classical gender roles, Brown demonized conspicuous gender transgression, jettisoning gay-male visibility. Gender equivalent "authentic" dancing thus risks foreclosing access to the concert stage for bodies that identify with explicit femininity, be that as queer conspicuousness on male bodies, or what seems like more a conventional version on women.

Monson does not repudiate male femininity in *Finn's Shed*, in fact there is a delightfully swishy flavor to Jasperse's dancing. But neither does she exploit the queer potential of such nellie-ness in the way that Greenberg and Jasperse do in their choreography.[18] Capitalizing on dance theater's historical association with femininity, the men stage emasculated dancing male bodies as queer subjects. Repurposing vocabularies that foreground rather than sublimate femininity's exceptionality, they achieve gay-male visibility by denaturalizing the relationship between sex and the performance of gender. Male dancers delight in their embodiment of femininities that, for them, have historically been taboo. Yet by ironically foregrounding theater's artifice, they convey cynicism about the movement language's integrity, and consciousness of how dance constructs its bodies. Greenberg and Jasperse therefore insist that, like heterosexually sexed dancing, 1970s authenticity is culturally contingent rather than natural.

Greenberg's *Really Queer Dance with Harps* (2008) exemplifies this approach. The piece was half of an evening-length program seen in art-houses in major American cities such as the Los Angeles REDCAT where I saw the work in 2010. Like Monson, Greenberg is a prominent East Village figure, but Greenberg also danced for Cunningham, an influence that is visible in Greenberg's focus on kinetics and repudiation of narrative. Greenberg nevertheless stages political themes, having got his first significant recognition for *Not-About-AIDS-Dance* (1994), which etched the havoc that the virus wrought across his personal life, and New York's artistic community, onto formal movement investigation.[19] Yet as much as gender critique, what Greenberg calls "non-normative phrasing" also contributes to the titular indication that our expectations about dance have been screwed with in *Really Queer Dance with Harps*. He thus extends Cunningham's infusion of eccentricity into formality, staging male femininity as quirkiness in queer dancing that avoids narrative references to homosexual identity.[20]

Greenberg queerly deploys conventional femininity in a way that Butler describes using the metaphor of figure and ground. She insists that when "'feminine' identity [as figure is] ... juxtaposed on the 'male body' as ground ... both terms ... lose their internal stability and their distinctness from each other."[21] Her thesis that heterosexuality depends on an apparent congruence of sexed bodies and gendered performances concurs with the perspective of those around me who took my childhood femininity as a sign for homosexuality. The final section of *Really Queer Dance with Harps*, "Coda," exhibits the critical use of figure and ground, contrasting sharply with *Finn's Shed*'s androgynous practicality. Small groups of dancers flounce back and forth in a childlike display that fails to take them anywhere. Jumps and steps flounder in their execution with a lack of purposeful direction, highlighting the dancers' self-consciousness. Unlike Monson and Jasperse, Young would say Greenberg's dancers are "throwing like girls"; taking pleasure in the feminine motility that for Young engenders diminished access to transcendence. Yet they push out nonchalant chins, daring anyone to question their lack of athletic commitment, and heads drop coyly from side to side. Greenberg juxtaposes corporeal maleness with kinetic white femininity. Soft-wristed

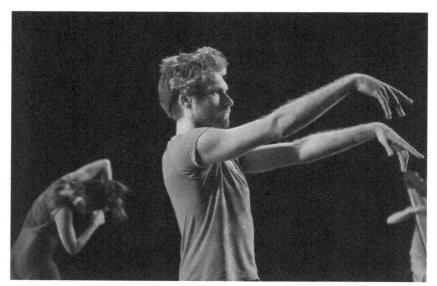

FIGURE 4.1 In Greenberg's *Queer Dance with Harps*, Colin Stilwell complicates a clichéd "gay limp wrist" by dancing it with both extended arms, while adding to the gender confusion of gesture with his masculine beard and feminine flower. In the background Christine Elmo avoids explicit social references in what would be broadly understood as an abstract gesture. Photo by Frank Mullaney.

superfluous arms throw into the air as ostentatious punctuation to each significant shift of weight; they serve no purpose for balance or propulsion, framing the movement as a childlike attempt to be a ballerina, a hyper-feminine vocabulary that is synecdoche for theatrical dancing itself. Flowers in the dancers' hair, a red curtain dressing a usually sparse stage, and a fanciful refrain strummed out by an onstage harpist, all enhance the overall girly-ness.

My queer viewer identifies with Greenberg's irreverent staging of male femininity because, despite modern dance having been one of the most open closets for gay men, heterosexual masculinity historically dominates the concert stage.[22] At age six, I declined my mother's invitation to join my best friend in ballet class, terrified that my secret gender "problem" would be revealed. *Really Queer Dance with Harps* gives the finger to heterosexual dance establishments, and a broader cultural concern about the sexuality that male femininity supposedly indicates. Yet the dance also represents an alternative to the denial, within gay subculture, of social or sexual subjectivity for the effete. Writing in a Western metropolitan context, Alex Robertson Textor argues that girly boys represent levity or humor for gay men by signifying queer visibility in a fraught conjunction of pride and shame. Serving as projections for the shame of failed masculinity and pride in the queer significance thereof, drag queens, nellies, and sissies manifest the resulting battle over meaning in their often-ironic embodiment femininity.[23] Martin Manalansan's ethnography of New York gay Filipino pageantry highlights the cultural specificity of the ironic embodiment of femininity. He found that "most Filipino cross dressers described their [drag] . . . in opposition to the parodic, scandalous and comedic forms of cross-dressing that they saw as a white or Western practice."[24] Greenberg references parody, yet more than laughter, he procures interest in his male femme by emphasizing quirkiness, and fondness with the amorous harp's refrain. *Really Queer Dance with Harps* thereby resists the femme-phobia encumbering white American gay-male culture since the 1950s.[25]

The Necessity of Feminism

Despite my queer viewer's delight in the gay-male visibility achieved in *Really Queer Dance with Harps*, my feminist spectator insists that although, like Monson and Jasperse in *Finn's Shed*, male and female dancers share a vocabulary, they access critical agency asymmetrically. To the degree that Monson's rambunctious flouting of femininity overshadows Jasperse nellie-ness, whatever else is queer in Greenberg's dance, within its representational structure, the women cannot resist heterosexuality to the same degree as the men. The hyperbolic femininity on which the queer dancing depends is too close to what has historically been compulsory for dancing women. This is because the metaphor of figure and ground does not move in both directions in contemporary dance to the degree that it does in queer subculture. Although Butler gives examples of lesbians critically embodying masculinity, like Case's butch, modern dance's association with femininity hinders a concert-stage corollary for dancing women. Greenberg's girls could be boys being girls, which is perhaps terribly queer. Yet they draw attention back to the men's contravention of masculinity, so even if they escape being old-fashioned ladies displaying hyper-femininity, it is merely as a chorus for the boys. In this dance with harps, the "really queer" body is thus male, overshadowing dancing female critical agency.

Greenberg intended to investigate slippage between identity and ambiguity, staging clichéd gay gesture as both queer sexuality on the men and movement quirkiness on the women.[26] His approach exemplifies the broader East Village idiom of tackling political exigencies while resisting representational transparency. But like the shortfalls of Cunningham's attempts to neutralize race and gender through formalism,[27] Greenberg still naturalized sexual difference. Although men and women perform an equivalent rather than overlapping vocabulary in the coda section of *Really Queer Dances with Harps*, the choreography fails to address the specific ways in which femininity signifies on differently sexed bodies in contemporary dance. Dances such as Tere O'Connor's *Rammed Earth* (2008),[28] and Jasperse's *Truth, Revised Histories, Wishful Thinking, and Flat Out Lies* (2009),[29] stage comparable disparities of gender critique across sexed bodies. Such privileging of male bodies both draws attention to the power of familiar kinetic codes in dance, and feminism's indispensable role in queer choreography.

By drawing a parallel between the change in gender critique (from *Finn's Shed* in the early 1990s to *Really Queer Dance with Harps* in the next century), and the development of theories of gender, I wish to reveal the intellectual context in which women dancers seem to lose critical agency. In order to exit from a hetero-oppositional construction of the female body, Monson resisted the obvious gendered codes that Greenberg actively deployed. This difference mirrors the change in strategy for which queer theory became symbolic. Butler, for example, argues that exiting heterosexual gender is impossible, taking to task the idea that an authentic body-self offers refuge away from the oppressive theater of patriarchy. Both Butler and Case also point out that when it aims to extinguish heterosexual genders, feminism forfeits resistance achieved through the redeployment of categories of sex within queer subculture.[30] To rhetorically denaturalize heterosexual sexual difference, queer theory mobilizes the hyperbolic embodiment of heterosexual gender, like that of Greenberg's girly boys.[31] Sexual difference consequently loses its enshrined natural status and is instead relegated to the socially constructed status of gender. For Butler, corporeality achieves its pre-cultural illusion through the sedimentation of performative (gendered) acts that obsessively reiterate the immutable truth of sexual difference.[32] She famously states: "Indeed, sex by definition will be shown to have been gender all along."[33] Theatrical exhibitionism in *Really Queer Dance with Harps*, in comparison with the anti-theatrical androgyny of *Finn's Shed*, seems to embody the shift toward contesting natural sexual difference.

Queer theory's ascendance attended a broader politicization of theatricality in lesbian and gay activism. ACT UP (AIDS Coalition to Unleash Power) is perhaps most famous for its use of hyperbole in nonviolent direct action and civil disobedience to protest against the US government's lack of effective response to the AIDS crisis. Beginning in the 1980s, ACT UP staged what Butler calls "the hyperbolic 'performance' of 'die-ins'" which she connects to "the theatrical 'outness' by which queer activism has disrupted closeting distinctions between public and private."[34] To the degree that their gender performance signifies homosexuality, girly boys and butch girls exemplify this outness. For Butler then, critique and activism are launched with the transvaluation of extant gender categories, not in a fictional "authentic" space beyond their discursive power. Political intervention takes place within layers of reflective meaning as a self-referential hyperbolic theatricality. Yet theoretically, this leaves women in contemporary dance, for whom feminine flamboyance is politically impotent, without critical resources.

Dancing that reflects on rather than claiming to transcend existing vocabulary politicizes theatricality in a comparable way to queer activism. Greenberg choreographs the lesbian and gay subcultural strategy of simultaneously exhibiting apparently oppositional categories of sex: girl-boy. Yet to the degree that male femininity is read as homosexuality, it tends to overshadow the misogyny within gay-male culture toward cissexual and trans women, as well as effeminate men, as is evident with the long-standing use of the phrase "no fats no fems" in singles ads and on dating sites.[35] Similarly those who configured my childhood femininity as a sign of male homosexuality, obscured my experience of gender asymmetry (my early awareness that feminine-identified family members enjoyed less say). Gender transgression likewise often trumps feminist viewership in queer dance because nonconforming bodies seem to be beyond heterosexual dynamics. So my feminist viewer asks: How can dance prosper from queer subcultural strategies, while also resisting heterosexuality's gender asymmetry?[36]

Performing Lesbian Androgyny

Seen through a queer lens, Monson's androgyny reveals itself as a crucial site of lesbian identification. Recalling the andro-dykes in *RMW*, the dance that initiated the diptych with which I opened this essay, lesbians may avoid familiar oppositional gender codes precisely because of the associations of more explicit femininity. Femme dykes, for example, often complain that heterosexuality's omnipotence renders their lesbianism invisible;[37] this is one reason why Case finds traction in the visibility butch gains in relation to femme. Arguing that they resignify heterosexuality, Case, along with Butler and others, also responded to the demonizing of dykey genders in the 1970s women's movement. Lesbians' predilection for androgyny in the late twentieth century attests to battles over gender. Sociologist Mignon Moore notes that "in their efforts to assimilate into the larger women's movement, 1970s lesbian-feminists [were] . . . disparaging of feminine and masculine gender display . . . and encouraged . . . androgynous gender presentations." Her insight frames a study of New York African American dyke culture, which she argues was "less influenced by efforts to replace butch and femme identities" because of limited participation of these women in 1970s feminism.[38] Moore's scholarship underscores the racial specificity of Monson's dancing androgyny but also highlights how it connects with a lesbian subcultural strategy of rejecting, rather than hyperbolically embodying, heterosexual genders.[39]

In the "reality" beyond theater's artifice, initially manifested in 1970s androgynous dancing, Monson found a means to move the relationship between theatricality and politics in the opposite direction to that which I associate with Greenberg's dance. While *Really Queer Dance with Harps* mirrored how ACT UP amped up theatricality, to cultivate her "real female body," Monson referenced an androgynous sensibility of street protest, bringing queer activism to the theater. In 1993, for example, she had New York's activists, The Lesbian Avengers, lay face down on the stage at St. Marks Church, pounding their fists, and building up to a roar. Part of a full evening of Monson's work, *The Lesbian Avengers Pounding Dance* began with the women entering the dance-floor from the audience, underscoring their ordinariness compared with dancers who appear from the wings. The choreography therefore repudiated both theatricality and conventional femininity by referencing street protest.

Although *Really Queer Dance with Harps* premiered a decade later than *Pounding Dance*, the contrast between them exemplifies dykes' unique struggle. The Avengers formed coevally with ACT UP to fight for queer women's visibility precisely because the US AIDS crisis compounded the representation of male homosexuality as synonymous with all non-canonical sexualities, erasing lesbianism. Sex between women carries a lower risk of contracting the virus than sex between men, recapitulating the myth that caused Queen Victoria to refuse to criminalize lesbianism: the threat of queer sexuality depends on a penis, lesbian sex is no sex at all. So the prolific and destructive representation of gay-male sex during the 1990s actually contributed to the erasure of dykes. Phallocentric ideas about sexuality often collapse female homosexuality into homosociality, or a heterosexual male fantasy. The appropriation of heterosexual femininity, by which men achieve queer visibility, can thus contribute to the erasure of lesbianism; a duet of flamboyant girly girls too easily evokes a high school slumber party or straight male porn. Notably there was a lot of crossover in membership between the Lesbian Avengers and ACT UP New York, indicating dykes felt that the government's ignoring of the AIDS crisis was their struggle. But it is fair to assume that the emphasis on gay men was problematic in ACT UP's internal politics, which added to wider cultural invisibility, necessitating the formation of a separate women's organization.

The Avengers contested social erasure, such as protesting when the press ignored the firebombing of a queer Oregonian home. Yet, in her *Pounding Dance*, Monson staged an embodied practice rather than represent explicit political rhetoric or characterize lesbian identity. She thus shared Greenberg's East Village tendency toward opacity of message, rejecting the transparent truths often proffered in queer solo performance. Referring to the personal story telling with which 1990s queer folk affirmed their struggle, performance scholar David Román insists, "autobiography fits into the model of identity on which lesbian and gay politics is founded."[40] By contrast, *Pounding Dance* avoided explicit references to identity by staging a contradictory performer-experience: lying face down on the floor might suggest defeat, and yet the gradual increase of the ground-thumping sound and vocal charge staged human-sonic resistance. Monson's street-protest aesthetic was not unlike the task-like approach in 1970s contact improvisation. Yet the choreographed chagrin disbanded with the naïve pleasure of her duet with Jasperse, even while *Pounding Dance*, like *Finn's Shed*, repudiated feminine flamboyance and avoided masculine heroism by creating its collective power from the sum of individual minimal actions. Affirming a shared bond and common purpose, the Lesbian Avengers, of which Monson was a member, dramatically transgressed the familiar staging of the female body.

Monson avoided the solo performance strategy of defining lesbian identity because of sharp differences she observed between women. She recalls local Florida separatists who refused to house the gay men with whom the Avengers arrived when a trailer was burned to the ground; and the difference between the working-class butch who experienced the attack and Monson's largely middle-class New York activist colleagues. Her training practice similarly reflects a desire to hold her gender identity open; she explains that in the 1980s, she "wanted to be as powerful as a man but there was a rawness and a vulnerability that I really valued."[41] Monson hints at how raw vulnerability is seen as oppositional to male strength, perhaps connoting femaleness. Blending masculinity and femininity in her dancing, she insisted on an existential range for female corporeality, resisting marginalization, but recognizing the limits of a stable identification.

Tackle Rock (1993), a dance that shared *Pounding Dance's* bill, capitalized on androgyny to resist the construction of female upper body nudity as sexual availability. By claiming the contemporary dancing stage for her bare chest, a privilege usually reserved for men, Monson did in theaters what 1990s Lesbian Strength marchers did on the street when they exposed their breasts as an act of defiance. Despite all dancing half naked with Jasperse, who also stripped above the waist, Monson, Dorvillier, and Jennifer Lacey averted lascivious associations. Their playful sharing of weight, not unlike in *Finn's Shed*, as well as mutual carrying and walking while in a squat, all conveyed an infant-like-task-like quality; so while the bare flesh was striking, the dancers deflected lewd associations by refusing to acknowledge any bodily dimension as more significant than moving weight. Yet defiance laced the innocence and functionality, such as when a woman periodically stood atop a co-dancer, gazing monumentally at a distant horizon, with indifference to the way her state of undress might be read.

To assert the advantage of androgyny over theatrical reflexivity, my feminist spectator compares Monson's use of female upper body nudity with that of Jasperse in his *Truth, Revised Histories, Wishful Thinking, and Flat Out Lies*. Steeped in theatrical irony, Jasperse's full evening work toured similar venues to *Really Queer Dance with Harps*. Unlike either Greenberg's or Monson's work, however, the choreography engages in self-conscious explicit cultural referencing. In line with queer theory, Jasperse seeks to reflect upon the constructed nature of sexuality; and with two male dancers wearing only athletic supports, grinding their butts at the audience, he achieves social critique by exposing body parts that are normally concealed in concert dance. Eroticizing the male body, the fleshy rear ends delight in their homosexualizing of the male gaze. However, the booty dance's critical agency relies on two bare breasted women, whose gyrating reminds the audience of the hackneyed female sexual availability that the asses are replacing. Representing transgression in a culture that historically constructs women as either chaste or available, tits become ass cheeks and boys get to be bad-girls after a fashion; but the women remain frozen in signification even while they move with the same commitment as the men.

Jasperse insists that his reconstruction of male and female stripper-dances stages conventions of which none are more or less transgressive or traditional.[42] Yet the movement semiotics procure a male viewer, and the marginal status of homosexuality means that the lads' butts disrupt the heterosexual power dynamics that the ladies' exposed flesh seems to reinforce. Jasperse's fag-centric specter is more disturbing than the asymmetry weighing on *Really Queer Dance with Harps*, but they both rob women of agency. While Greenberg's girly choreography forecloses women's critical embodiment of femininity and claims queerness for girly boys, Jasperse's gay-male pleasure relies on a hetero-sexually available female. The contestation of conventional gender in dancing women is crucial precisely because asymmetry persists in queer dance.

Returning to *RMW* we find a queerly female choreographic strategy that integrates feminist critique. Originally made for a "Sexual ID" series, Dorvillier and Monson embodied and introduced to each other the woman rescued from heterosexual dynamics in works like *Finn's Shed* and *Tackle Rock*. In *RMW*, the two dancers remain in the throes of a kiss as they swing each other around, launch each other over their respective shoulders, and crash each other onto the floor. The intimate connection of the facial orifice burns lust into the otherwise perfunctory sensibility, and the dancers also infuse their utilitarian vocabulary with violent fervor, recalling *Pounding Dance*'s angry community. Yet with interpersonal tenderness, the duo also embody the rawness and vulnerability with which Monson complicated her desire to be as strong as any man.[43] On the one hand, they resist the hyperbolic performance of masculinity and femininity, yet by ricocheting between motile vigor and subtlety, they blur heterosexual polarities. Monson and Dorvillier engage in what dancer-scholar Emilyn Claid calls "the ambiguous play of gender performance [which] androgyny [can] offer . . . from a queer perspective."[44] My feminist and queer spectators comingle as *RMW* contests asymmetry with rambunctious female bodies performing desire for each other. Monson's dancing subject who extracted femaleness from the clutches of canonical male desire, hankers for another version of herself, creates space for lesbianism on a dancing stage historically hostile to all things Sapphic.

Not the Marrying Kind

With her androgyny, Monson slipped an authentic and stable dancing dyke identity under the queer radar. By eschewing artificiality with a protest sensibility, *RMW* made a union between two women look natural, a crucial maneuver in the 1990s fight for visibility, and no mean feat considering contemporary dance lacks the equivalent for lesbians to the

conspicuousness of dancing masculinity upon which gay men have capitalized. While boys can fag-a-liciously parade their artifice, feminine frolick-
ing between two women risks recapitulating the erasure of lesbianism as
homosociality or a heterosexual male fantasy. But although my feminist
and queer viewer both find some peace in lesbian-realness, neither girly
boys nor dynamic dykes satisfy my transgender spectator. As a child I hid
my cheering for the women when our family viewed *It's a Knockout* on TV
because I was cognizant of phenotype differences between my mother and
I that are linked to gender identity. My parents allowed me to play with
dolls as a small child, and when it was decided that the men should use
the outside loo in my pre-pubescent teens, nobody batted an eyelid when
I refused. Yet I believed that their failure to acknowledge my contravention
of gender norms concealed a plot to have me taken away; I spent hours
behind the living room curtains, scanning the street for doctors in a white
van. Not until my involvement with transgender communities at end of the
1990s did I accept the contradictions of my body and identity. From this
perspective, if male femininity points to a gay man, and female androgyny
to a lesbian, gender difference stands in for stable sexual identities founded
upon cissexual bodies. Natural sexual difference has crept back in, leaving
my transgender spectator betwixt and between.

It is perhaps, however, only by viewing *RMW* from 2015 that dancing dyke
identity gets stabilized. The duet seems to symbolically stage a queer wedding
at St. Marks—the East Village religious institution cum home of dance. The
American marriage equality movement depends on naturalized representations of stable lesbian sexuality in its state-by-state battles for matrimonial
parity between heteros and homos. "Till death us do part" implies life-long
lesbianism, mutual desire between two unequivocally female bodies. With its
task-like androgyny conveying bodily authenticity, infused with girl-on-girl
passion, Monson and Dorvillier's motile Sapphism seems to have foretold
of a lesbian model of the conventional nuptial relationship. The happy coincidence of their ecclesiastical dance venue referenced the sanctity entailed
in the hetero-religious consecration of sexual relations. A bride and bride
were unthinkable then, but now lesbianism regularly achieves the representational coherence and consistency on which the claim for marriage rights
rest. However, *RMW* loses its critical edge if it is reduced to a forerunner of
contemporary social legitimacy. Framing the dance as a precursor to normative lesbianism limits the dance's role to an artifact of East Village political experimentation, superseded by girly boys who insist upon gender's artificiality.
Furthermore, naturalized lesbianism concurs with the denial of my legitimate
access to femaleness; my experience of asymmetry as a feminine-appearing

body is erased in the attribution of girly-boy-gay identity achieved within cis-sexual boundaries of sex in homosexual desire.

To prevent their achievement of lesbian visibility from becoming a mere relic of a bygone century, Monson and Dorvillier rob audiences who continue to encounter *RMW* of any simple experience of nostalgia. The diptych they created on revisiting the duet, and which opened this essay, uses historical reflexivity to reframe the dancing dykes as theatrical constructions in a similar manner to Greenberg's deployment of a feminine coded lexicon as quirkiness. The two-act work *RMW(a) & RMW* puts theatrical parenthesis around *RMW's* Mrs. & Mrs. dyke by setting the stage for the reappearance of 1990s lesbianism with a performance of twenty-first-century hyper-theatrical 1980s-retro-chic street queens. Monson and Dorvillier resisted the teleology of marriage rights that might retrospectively fall on *RMW* by demonstrating that the dance's lesbianism is no less constructed than *RMW(a)'s* drag, which they first stage and then peel away. Ostentatious gender and androgyny both reveal themselves as second skins, suggesting that the memory of street-dykes-gone-by is no more or less artificial than the petrochemical hair they wear as street queens in the present. The dancers stage the lesbians of an earlier era as a flaming recollection that can only be accessed through the mantel of drag. *RMW(a) & RMW* draws attention to identity's constructed nature by embracing femininity's connotation of theatrical artifice.

By establishing the contingency of lesbian identity, Monson and Dorvillier open space for my transgender viewer by demonstrating that queer genders, like their heterosexual corollaries, have been based upon presumptions about which sexed body has access to which gender. In a striking similarity with Greenberg, they deconstruct gender with Butler's metaphor of figure and ground through a virtuoso performance of queer femininity normally associated with male bodies: the deliciously menacing walks, clad in street-queen garb and gesture, which first rendered me hysterical. The incongruence of sex categories arises because, watching the women self-consciously strut, grind joints, and accent gesture, it becomes clear that to the degree that male bodies have been locked out of conventional femininity, women have been denied access to the drag-queen-queer-equivalent. Monson and Dorvillier thus break the contract of queer gender in which subcultural lesbian and gay semiotics are always viewed as transgressive. To ensure that, as Butler puts it, "the term 'queer' is a site collective contestation," *RMW(a) & RMW* secures queer as "never fully owned, but . . . redeployed, twisted and queered from a prior usage."[45] By revealing how drag queen femininity is tied to cissexual masculinity, the dance redeploys queer performance, precisely "queering" it from a prior usage.

When viewed in light of this revelation, Greenberg's girly boys appear to depend for their infraction of heterosexuality on the myth that the female body is the origin of their femininity. As much as Greenberg and Jasperse lock women out of queer critique, they erase a history of queer performance because for the dancing boys' girly-ness to appear transgressive, it must owe a debt to heterosexuality's originality; a pink cookie that's been stolen. Like Jasperse's and Greenberg's dancers, Monson and Dorvillier embody a historically recognizable motile language of femininity. Yet *RMW(a)* insists on queer femininity's historical provenance by staging gender codes that are familiar as those of drag queens. Monson and Dorvillier, like Greenberg, rely on hyperbole to distinguish queer from conventional femininity. However, by foregrounding their female bodies as vehicles for queerness, they evacuate from the scene the naturalized myth of heterosexual genders on which the girly boys feed. When Greenberg's dancers do their swishy thing, it's the fleshy stand-in for the phallus that we assume defines their bodies, and thus determines their contravention of masculinity. But with their female bodies, Monson and Dorvillier, like the butch to the femme, masquerade a queer male economy, as Case says "penis, penis, who's got the penis."[46] The women thus challenge the apparent originality of the heterosexual nexus, cleaving a version of femininity from their own female bodies and mobilizing the critical potential of women's corporeality. The diptych consequently also questions queer gender's presumption of being a foil to the mainstream, insisting that the margins do not always have to be described in relation to a center.

Trespassing into drag, Monson and Dorvillier retrieve critical tools for bodies, other than just gay-male ones, to deconstruct conventional femininity. Bringing to their dance the queer ambiguity they cultivated in *RMW*, the duo reveal that *RMW(a)*'s street-queens' survival depends upon a blending aggression and vulnerability. Censorship and the omnipresent threat of violence meted out against effeminate men demands resoluteness in public displays of femininity. Yet the receptivity to, or seduction of, masculinity, with which such codes are conventionally associated, entails emotional susceptibility. This contrary concoction of *RMW(a)* reads so clearly because, as referred to above, gay-male culture tends to represent drag queens, nellies, and sissies with the same oppositional qualities as sources of pride and shame, bringing adoration and the derision indicated by the phrase "no fats no femmes." Patriarchy calls forth a similar contradiction in conventional femininity, insisting women be receptive, while shoring up the masculine Other with the more aggressive act of seduction, which brings with it susceptibility to violence. However, naturalized heterosexuality overshadows such ambiguity in the logic of equivalence between female and feminine. As street queens, Monson and Dorvillier replace the naturalized femininity that their femaleness usually accrues with one that seems delightfully infected with perverted testosterone because its origin is generally thought of as the queer male body. They thus suture drag's gender ambiguity to their womanhood, insisting upon an existential range in equating femaleness and femininity, much like Monson did by training to be as strong as a man while remaining raw and vulnerable.

Regardless of how convincingly they perform male femininity, however, by suffusing their flamboyance with ambiguity, Monson and Dorvillier remain deliciously dykey. They parse out notes of butch and femme just like Case's couple. Monson imbues theatrical display with a beefy execution of decorative dance by refraining from extending as a ballet dancer would. She thus recalibrates virtuoso elevation by emphasizing her mass; rather than ethereal illusion, her leaps throw weight, and she lands with feet sinking into the ground as large legs fold revealing Monson's substantial architecture growing away from the floor. Meanwhile Dorvillier's childlike rendering of feline aggression is high femme, playfully wallowing in theatrical artifice as she snarls and claws the hand left free in her crawl. But the Dorvillier's conviction introduces a serious potential of assault; any allure of her tiger-princess is laced with the reminder of the damage she can do. Mobilizing femininity in two directions, Dorvillier deflects any attempt to anchor the performance as natural to her female body by executing her intervention behind the veil of drag. By resignifying queer genders, the dancers open new readings of the feminine, articulating drag's complexity across their female fleshy selves. To critically mobilize the equation of feminine and female, *RMW(a) & RMW* thus views drag-queeniness through the lens of lesbian subcultural aesthetics.

In their deviant use of the archive, Monson and Dorvillier manipulate theater's apparent artifice to screw with the supposed factual quality of history, revealing the hysteria that lurks beneath stable identity. In this sense, the diptych brings together critical approaches to dance reconstruction with queer theories of gender. Dance scholar Mark Franko argues that restaging old choreography necessitates metamorphosis. Even while concealing the use of the "new" to reproduce the "old," a performance that claims to simulate an original work relies on contemporary aesthetics and technique. He complains that "the historicist tendency to see the old in the new is characteristic of reconstruction. Its master conceit is to evoke what no longer is, with the means of what is present."[47] For example, although Martha Graham rejected ballet in the early twentieth century, she ultimately integrated the classical technique, transforming the look and aptitudes of her visions of femininity.[48] Yet the Graham company doesn't reference this change in their performances of her repertory. By contrast, Monson and Dorvillier laugh at the reliance of historical verisimilitude upon contemporary paradigms and narrative consistency; with the conspicuous lens of male-to-female drag, they foreground their looking back. In a cocktail of andro-dykes and drag queens who refuse to remain within distinct embodied territories, *RMW(a)* & *RMW* tears gender's historicity apart in the disparity and connection it stages between the original and revised versions of *RMW* from 1993.

By openly screwing with the older work, Monson and Dorvillier acknowledge the rapid change that took place in the conception of queer femininity and femaleness between the 1990s and the twenty-first century. In its onstage evolution, the diptych reverses its historical genesis disintegrating identity coherence. The thickly applied drag make-up of *RMW(a)* smears across the kissing lesbian faces of *RMW*, so the denim-clad women retroactively foretell the queens they will become. By staging *RMW* in the shadow of drag's spectacle, the duo obscures access to any authentic lesbian from the past, and so through gender ambiguity, 1990s lesbianism becomes a memory of the street queens bouncing back and forth. *RMW* consequently appears not as the document of a bygone era, but a living testament to identity's dependence upon the sedimentation of performative acts. We learn about the common source for lesbian and male-to-female drag identity. Juxtaposing conflicting codes of gender signification that puncture the dance piece and their bodies with the conventions of the then and now, Monson and Dorvillier ricochet backward and forward between 1993 and 2012. *RMW(a)* & *RMW* thus disassembles the generally concealed workings of performatively constituted sex and gender, and scatters stable identity across the stage along with historical teleology. The capricious chronicling of historical shift shatters the mirror of coherent identity, and its handmaiden of corporeal truth, upon which theatre is conventionally based. These hidden props of performance are broken for me by my machine-gun laughter as I am drawn by Monson and Dorvillier into labyrinthine hysteria.

Notes

1. For a good overview of Freud's theory of identification, including the role of hysteria, see Kaja Silverman, *The Subject of Semiotics* (New York: Oxford University Press, 1983).
2. Jay Prosser, "Transgender," in *Lesbian and Gay Studies: A Critical Introduction*, ed. Andy Medhurst and Sally Munt (London: Cassell, 1997).
3. Judith Butler addresses this point, arguing that "the construction of the human is a differential operation that produces the more and the less 'human,' the inhuman, the humanly unthinkable." Judith Butler, *Bodies that Matter: On the Discursive Limits of 'Sex'* (New York: Routledge, 1993), 8.

4. Duncan Gilbert, "A Conceit of the Natural Body: The Universal Individual in Somatic Dance Training" (PhD diss., University of California Los Angeles, 2014).

5. For example, Houston-Jones curated "Parallels in Black" at Dance Theatre Workshop in 1987. Interview with author, June 6, 2012.

6. I am influenced here by law scholar Kimberlé Crenshaw's framework on "intersectionality": Kimberlé Crenshaw, *Demarginalizing the Intersection of Race and Sex: A Black Feminist Critique of Antidiscrimination Doctrine, Feminist Theory and Antiracist Politics* (London: Routledge, 2009).

7. Judith Butler, *Gender Trouble: Feminism and the Subversion of Identity,* (New York: Routledge, 1990).

8. Sue-Ellen Case, "Towards a Butch-Femme Aesthetic," *Discourse* 11, no. 1 (1988): 70.

9. For example, in *Slant Board*, part of the 1960s *Dance Constructions* by experimental dance luminary Simone Forti, performers pulled themselves up angled boxes with rope, replacing apparently artificial presentational modern and classical vocabulary with natural incidental movement, see Gilbert, "A Conceit of the Natural Body," 280. Trisha Brown references Forti's influence, Klaus Kertess, Rebecca Davis, Carolyn Davis, Maryvonne Neptune, Michele Thompson, Trisha Brown Company, ARTPIX (Firm) Brown, *Trisha Brown Early Works 1966–1979, Artpix Notebooks* (Houston, TX: ARTPIX, 2004), videorecording, 2 videodiscs (ca. 239 min.): sd., b&w and col.; 4 3/4 in.; as does Kaye, who Monson danced for (interview with the author, August 15, 2011); and the East Village scene identifies with Forti's milieu of the 1960s and 1970s, see Gilbert, "A Conceit of the Natural Body."

10. Dance scholar Susan Foster points out that "Cunningham neutralized all masculine, feminine and sexual connotations by focusing on space, time and motion," but also "articulated gender difference ... [with] overlapping yet distinctive vocabularies ... in which men partnered and lifted women." Susan Leigh Foster, "Closets Full of Dances: Modern Dance's Performance of Masculinity and Sexuality," in *Dancing Desires: Choreographing Sexualities On and Off the Stage*, ed. Jane Desmond (Madison: University of Wisconsin Press, 2001), 174–77. From within the same academic field, Ramsay Burt argues that in Brown's first large concert stage work for a mixed company, *Set and Reset* (1983), when "dancers caught others who jumped or dived into their arms ... [t]he men ... did more than their fair share," even though he insists Brown used "a decentralized structure ... to relocate the excitement of masculine strength and dynamism." Ramsay Burt, *The Male Dancer: Bodies, Spectacle, Sexualities*, 2d ed. (Milton Park, UK: Routledge, 2006), 157–58.

11. Iris Marion Young, *On Female Body Experience: "Throwing Like a Girl" and Other Essays*, Studies in Feminist Philosophy (New York: Oxford University Press, 2005), 138.

12. Crenshaw, *Demarginalizing the Intersection of Race and Sex*, 155.

13. For a comprehensive discussion on the way whiteness erases its specificity, see Richard Dyer, *White* (London: Routledge, 1997).

14. Feminist theorist Julia Kristeva, for example, insists that maternally bequeathed feminine "poetic semiosis" disrupts patriarchal linguistic logic. Kristeva in Butler, *Gender Trouble*, 101.

15. Foster, "Closets Full of Dances," 182.

16. Cynthia Jean Novack, *Sharing the Dance: Contact Improvisation and American Culture* (Madison: University of Wisconsin Press, 1990), 122.

17. Burt, *The Male Dancer*, 157.

18. Sally Banes refers to Jasperse undertaking this approach already in the 1980s. Sally Banes, "Spontaneous Combustion: Notes on Improvisation from the Sixties to the Nineties," in *Taken by Surprise: A Dance Improvisation Reader*, ed. Ann Cooper Albright and David Gere (Middletown, CT: Wesleyan University Press, 2003), 81.

19. Jennifer Dunning, "Immortality and Horror with Aids, Review of Not-about-Aids-Dance by Neil Greenberg," *New York Times*, May 7, 1994.

20. Foster insists that Cunningham "fashioned himself as a maverick"; queerly conspicuous in his own dances, yet not explicitly homosexual. Foster, "Closets Full of Dances," 178.

21. Butler, *Gender Trouble*, 123.

22. Foster discusses the various way in which modern dance has closeted male homosexuality, Foster, "Closets Full of Dances." As late at as 1960s Judson Dance Theatre, Freddie Herko found himself marginalized because his performance was too flaming, which is just one example of casualties from an ongoing struggle to contest the idea that dancing men are inevitably effeminate and homosexual. Foster cited in José Esteban Muñoz, *Cruising Utopia: The Then and There of Queer Futurity*, (New York: New York University Press, 2009), 159.

23. Alex Robertson Textor, "Marilyn Mayhem and the Mantrap: Some Peculiarities of the Male Femme," in *Femme: Feminists, Lesbians, and Bad Girls*, ed. Laura Harris and Elizabeth Crocker (New York: Routledge, 1997), 202.

24. Martin F. Manalansan, *Global Divas: Filipino Gay Men in the Diaspora*, Perverse Modernities (Durham, NC: Duke University Press, 2003), 139.

25. George Chauncey discusses how a largely white middle-class "homophile" movement navigated the extremely difficult social terrain of mid-century America by instituting conformity to heterosexual gender norms: George Chauncey, *Why Marriage?: The History Shaping Today's Debate over Gay Equality* (New York: Basic Books, 2004).

26. Email from Greenberg to the author, July 28, 2012.

27. Foster, "Closets Full of Dances."

28. Seen by the author at the Los Angeles Skirball Center, June 28, 2008.

29. Seen by the author at the Los Angeles REDCAT, April 15, 2010.

30. Butler, for example, argues that Julia Kristeva reified gender categories by theorizing feminine semiosis with the "maternal" body and stabilized the dominance of masculinity by positioning femininity as only ever disruptive relative to logical patriarchal language. Butler, *Gender Trouble*. Meanwhile, Case argues against the idea that butch and femme lesbians conform to patriarchal heterosexuality. Case, "Towards a Butch-Femme Aesthetic."

31. Butler is often at pains to distinguish between theatrical performance and her theory that gender is performatively constituted. She argues that "regulatory norms of 'sex' work in a performative fashion to constitute the materiality of bodies," yet insists that the "theatricality of gender . . . need not be conflated with self-display." Butler, *Bodies That Matter*, 2 and 158.

32. Butler, *Bodies That Matter*, 15.

33. Butler, *Gender Trouble*, 8.

34. "Critically Queer," *GLQ: A Journal of Lesbian and Gay Studies* 1 (1993): 158.

35. Nick Artrip, "College Feminisms: No Fat, No Femme: The Politics of Grindr," *The Feminist Wire*, November 8, 2013.

36. In asking this question, I am building on the groudbreaking work of feminists like Biddy Martin, who argues queer theory often seems to position itself as displacing outmoded feminist ideas about gender, see for example: Biddy Martin, "Sexualities without Genders and Other Queer Utopias," *Diacritics* 24, nos. 2/3 (1994).

37. Laura Harris and Elizabeth Crocker, "Bad Girls: Sex, Class and Feminist Agency," in *Femme: Feminists, Lesbians, and Bad Girls*, ed. Laura Harris and Elizabeth Crocker (New York: Routledge, 1997), 95.

38. Mignon R. Moore, "Lipstick or Timberlands? Meanings of Gender Presentation in Black Lesbian Communities," *Signs: Journal of Women in Culture and Society* 32, no. 1 (2006): 116.

39. I am influenced here by the work of dancer and scholar Emilyn Claid, who recalls repurposing feminist representational strategies from the 1970s for queer performance in later decades, see Emilyn Claid, *Yes? No! Maybe—: Seductive Ambiguity in Dance* (London: Routledge, 2006).

40. Holly Hughes and David Román, *O Solo Homo: The New Queer Performance*, 1st ed. (New York: Grove Press, 1998), 4.

41. Jennifer Monson, phone interview with the author, January 13, 2010.

42. Jasperse email to the author, November 7, 2012.

43. Ann Cooper Albright refers to this kind of ambiguity in *Finn's Shed*. Ann Cooper Albright, *Choreographing Difference: The Body and Identity in Contemporary Dance* (Middletown, CT, and Hanover, NH: Wesleyan University Press and University Press of New England, 1997), 54.

44. Claid, *Yes? No! Maybe*, 70.

45. Butler, "Critically Queer," 154.

46. Case, "Towards a Butch-Femme Aesthetic," 64.

47. Mark Franko, "Repeatability, Reconstruction and Beyond," *Theatre Journal* 41, no. 1 (1989): 58.

48. Mark Franko, *Dancing Modernism/Performing Politics* (Bloomington: Indiana University Press, 1995).

5

Chasing Feathers

JÉRÔME BEL, *SWAN LAKE*, AND THE ALTERNATIVE
FUTURES OF RE-ENACTED DANCE

Julian B. Carter

This essay follows the fleeting trace of swans across time and choreographic
tradition. Airborne, feathers materialize atmospheric currents felt more than
seen; pursuing them carries me again and again away from the dances of the
here and now and into a magic room in the back of my head, a room flutter-
ing with generations of bird-women repeating the rituals of their becoming.
I am grasping at feathers, trying to articulate what swans make manifest as
they flit through contemporary performance, rather than situating a whole
ballet in its larger tradition. And yet each pinion dropped into a contemporary
dance seems to materialize and transmit the cultural DNA that shapes ballet's entire elaborate system of technique, its affective aesthetic, and its shared
imaginative forms. Each feather evokes the sensory appeal of accumulation,
pattern, and geometric triangulation. Each quivers with pride in elite status;
with the dangerous romance of submission to power; and with the legacies of
misogyny, elitism, and imperialism that inform classical dance in the West.
Inherently compound and repetitive structures, feathers do not lend themselves to conventional argumentative trajectories.[1] They make me want to re-
enact in text the cygnine idiom's tendency to curve back on itself, and with it
the power and the limit of queer temporality theory to describe these floating
fluffs of down.

Re-enactment and Repetition

This text is not an attempt at the literal reconstruction of the dance that is its
subject. Instead the following pages consider Jérôme Bel's 2004 *Veronique*

Doisneau in relation to recent discussions of re-enactment in performance art, the better to follow the fleeting trace of swans in/to contemporary choreography.[2] Bel is a French avant-garde conceptual choreographer whose work interrogates conventional understandings of what constitutes "dance." In *Veronique Doisneau* Bel merges spoken word with movement (and stillness) to re-present both past and future aspects of one individual's career as a dancer. The resulting complex temporality allows Bel to launch a (characteristically critical) exploration of classical ballet's aesthetic and institutional intersections with contemporary dance. As part of this project Bel draws on Rudolph Nureyev's 1984 staging of *Swan Lake*, opening questions about how the queerness of Nureyev's characters informs the different works into which they travel, remnants of their previous contextual connotations clinging to their feathers as they fly into new stories.

I do not mean only that we can look back at *Swan Lake* and reinterpret it from a queer perspective, nor that its history informs its present usages, though both these things are also true.[3] Rather, I am thinking of the specific narrative construction of queerness in Nureyev's ballet, where it expresses a morbid and irresponsible attachment to juvenile subordination. In this pathologizing analysis the essence of queerness lies in the prolongation and repetition of an outmoded dependency: childhood goes on too long and goes over the same ground again and again. *Veronique Doisneau*'s extensive movement passages from *Swan Lake* and *Giselle* seem to express just such a reiterative, drawn-out relation to time.

This temporality initiates a peculiar multiplication effect. Balletic quotations in the context of a specifically retrospective biographical dance are little re-enactments folded into larger (re)creative projects; even at this level of generality *Veronique Doisneau* is not one but several dances, which can be understood as belonging to several possible times. Such choreographic and temporal pleating brings different historical cultures into intimate proximity. Thus in *Veronique Doisneau* feudal peasants' vulnerability to aristocratic predation is performed through the same gestural sequences that meditate on strict occupational hierarchies and mandatory retirement for twenty-first-century French government workers (but here I'm getting ahead of myself. More on this later).

Much critical work on re-enactment engages its queer temporal effect, what Rebecca Schneider describes as the "warp and draw of one time in another time" and Elizabeth Freeman calls "the mutually disruptive energy of moments that are not yet past and yet are not entirely present either."[4] Such work suggests that both past and present can change as the interface between them is altered by re-enactment's capacity to revivify the past outside of what we usually understand as its proper moment. Indeed, Schneider's brilliant book *Performing Remains* argues that the pursuit of an embodied experience of authenticity (such as takes place among Civil War battle re-enactors) can bring different historical moments and historical actors into powerful juxtaposition, such that "the bygone is not entirely gone by and the dead not completely disappeared [... while] the living are not entirely (or not only) live."[5] These descriptions resonate powerfully with *Veronique Doisneau* in that no choreography can make biographical claims without folding and compressing time, if only because any given dance is shorter than (most) lives. Different historical moments can, however paradoxically, coexist in the bodies of dancers who are simultaneously present in performance as themselves and as the (past and future) persons they re/present.[6]

The intimacy between temporal multiplicity and the proliferation of the subject onstage suggests that re-enactment theory's temporal address needs to be expanded so that it can attend to the way that bodies multiply in the folds of time. Yet dance, like theater and music, has been neglected in discussions of re-enactment.[7] Performance scholar Amelia Jones suggests that this may be in part because these arts are based in a script or score and so are inherently and intentionally repeatable.[8] In sharp contrast, performance art is widely believed to derive its force from a kind of 'real-life' corporeal and affective presence that has been imagined as allowing for a powerfully unmediated, unique, and ephemeral moment of contact between performers and audience members.[9] Concert dances are less likely to generate this kind of force as an event because they are composed in the shelter of the studio and are designed to be repeated; their basic form does not usually rely on or respond to live interaction with an audience. Even when a dance work is improvised in performance it is backed up by the process of rehearsal, and behind rehearsal, the classes or other practice sessions that build technique. As a result it is not immediately obvious that anything conceptually significant can emerge from an intentional re-performance of something that is always a re-performance anyway.

Nevertheless, the distinction between dance and performance art has been questioned and undone for decades, both choreographically and critically.[10] Concert dance's very reliance on repetition can be imagined as a kind of ontological intimacy with re-enactment, and so construed as an incitement rather than a barrier to interpretations that focus on re-enactment's temporal fold. On the one hand, both choreography and embodied technique change over time. So do the myriad aesthetic/social conventions and material/technological resources that shape programming, orchestration, lighting, and audience participation and response, with the result that even the most carefully

reconstructed dance can never be an exact replica of its previous materializa-
tions.[11] On the other hand, the repetition across time of particular choreographies (construed broadly to include narratives, characters, motion pathways,
gestural sequences, dynamic impulses and associated costuming) also may
have the effect of bringing those movements from the past into the present
and with them material echoes of the social worlds in which they took shape.
Re-enactment is an artistic strategy for engaging repetition's interface with
temporal change. As André Lepecki has proposed, re-enactment facilitates
understanding, at once retroactive and anticipatory, of the creative and critical
potential in an original that was not materialized in its previous forms and yet
was in a sense already there as an alternative expression of its inventiveness.[12]
Thinking of dance through re-enactment theory's attention to the mutual
"warp and draw" of past and present highlights the charged and contradictory
relation between the choreography of a work—its abstract formal existence—
and an actual physical instantiation of that work in a body that can never be
only itself.

Proliferating Subjects Dreaming Alternative Futures

Veronique Doisneau was a dancer who was beginning her final season when
Bel received a commission to make a dance for her company's repertory. He
responded with what he describes as a "documentary" in which "the dancer,
close to the retirement age, alone on stage, retrospectively and subjectively
considers her own career as ballerina inside this institution."[13] But the work
positions Doisneau as a hyperbolically plural subject in relation to the material
she performs, with the effect that "her own career" appears to be neither hers
alone nor entirely about her subjectivity. Neither is the time of this retrospective performance simply past. On the contrary, Doisneau's career is a vehicle
for a temporally complex and socially objective account of "this institution."

The institution in question is the time-drenched Ballet de l'Opera National
de Paris (Paris Opera Ballet, or POB). POB's global prestige reflects its status
as the oldest national ballet in the world, whose broad and deep repertory
includes both glorious staging of the classics and avant-garde contemporary work. As a contemporary account of a venerable institution, *Veronique
Doisneau* necessarily takes place in several times at once: it draws on and represents the classical tradition of Western theater dance, but does so "retrospectively," within the dramaturgical frame of a moment in the future of
the nineteenth- and twentieth-century works it presents on stage. The folded
time of re-enactment thus shapes Bel's basic concept. It is also reflected in

his repetitive choreographic structure, which cycles from speech about dance to illustrative movement and back again. This structural folding initiates the multiplication of Doisneau's physical presence onstage, a multiplication underscored by the content of both narrative and choreography.

Almost half of *Veronique Doisneau* consists of Doisneau standing down-stage center, in rehearsal clothes and a wireless mic, talking to the audience about her experience of dancing at POB. She begins with the kind of data that appears in her Human Resources dossier—her name, her age and marital status, her salary and her place in the institutional hierarchy—and so we learn that Doisneau holds the status of *sújet*, a mid-level dancer who works with the corps de ballet and is also eligible for casting in some soloist roles. *Sújets* are talented and seasoned performers but they are not feted and idolized: they do not conventionally have dances named for them, nor is their retirement usually treated as an occasion of any significance for the institution or the public. As the subject of Bel's dance, however, Doisneau acquires an institutional prominence usually reserved for *étoiles*, the most celebrated dancers in the company. Doisneau thus appears as a paradoxically plural subject/*sújet*, at once the subject of Bel's institutional documentary, a lowly member of the corps, and the solitary star glowing on Paris Opera's deep and historic stage.

A further multiplication: all of the movement Bel quotes from other choreographers was composed for more than one dancer. Doisneau performs a pas de trois from *La Bayadere*, an ensemble passage from a Merce Cunningham piece called *Points in Space* (1987), and a pas de deux from *Giselle* before taking on a full-corps sequence from *Swan Lake*. These dances are simultaneously referential fragments of larger works and complete re-enactments of the single *sújet*'s movements; as such they draw attention to the gap between their choreography and their actual materialization, the gap in which time folds and the subject proliferates. This is what I mean when I say that the body re-enacting a dance is never only itself. When Doisneau performs these bits of dances, she materializes them in the bodily present she shares with her live audience. She simultaneously indexes her previous experience of executing these steps, as well as her physical ability to dance roles she tells us she has not previously performed. Finally, she directs our attention to the absent bodies of additional dancers who were integral to Doisneau's experience of ballet and yet who do not appear before us in Bel's re-creation of that experience.

When we see Doisneau as one among many, even though she is alone onstage, we are witnessing the institutional hierarchy that mediates relations between the individual performer and the larger collective: Doisneau stands before us as a soloist who embodies and is embedded in the *corps de ballet*, the inherently plural body of ballet. Classical corps work consists of many dancers moving in perfect time, their individual expression subordinated to the theatrical effect of the flock. Achieving such unison requires strong technique acquired through years of repetitive practice that mirror in the individual dancer's body the larger history of ballet, each performance of the classical repertoire repeating and referring to its predecessors. Every member of the corps, then, manifests many bodies striving to resemble one another both synchronically and diachronically. This striving for physical resemblance stretches time like a bird's wing, extending to enfold the dancers in a present experience of the past. In so doing it constitutes their collective movement as specifically classical ballet.

Like the classical body politic whose structure it repeats, the body of ballet is organized into strictly segregated ranks, each with its own functions and duties. The maintenance and replication of hierarchical social order is a persistent theme in the dances Bel quotes in *Veronique Doisneau*.[14] After Doisneau has explained that there was never really any question of her promotion to starring roles, she tells us that she dreamed of dancing the title role in *Giselle*, one of the most prestigious roles in classical ballet. Then she steps into a practice tutu and walks calmly offstage, the better to enter again as Giselle.

This moment is a retirement gift that Bel makes to Doisneau, who gets to realize some measure of her dream, albeit on a bare stage and humming the music over her headset as she dances. In a larger frame, however, this dance is not only about Doisneau and her dreams but is also about Paris Opera Ballet's institutional hierarchy and the way that it materializes and aestheticizes a deep cultural tradition of social inequality. Bel uses Doisneau's miniature re-enactment of *Giselle* as a vehicle for putting POB's caste system onstage, and so opening it to critical review.[15]

Bel's critique works in large part through re-enactment's effects on time. Re-enactment tends to produce futural effects while looking backward—that is, it draws awareness to the present as the past's future, while it simultaneously opens possibilities for an alternative future that may follow from its present alternative version of the past. Choreography, too, speaks to the traditions from which it emerges while it anticipates its own performance as well as the re-performance that provides the measure of its success. Dances live to the extent that dancers embody them in ever-changing present moments. Thus *Giselle*'s world premiere was at POB in 1841 and again in *Veronique Doisneau* in 2004. This latter performance contains the ballet's multiform past while it also materializes that past's future, both linked to and different from its origins.[16] But while the dance itself can inhabit multiple temporalities with ease, the dancer is rendered less nimble by the institutional constraints on her movement: Doisneau stumbles over the future tense.

When Bel has Doisneau re-enact her career, she seems simultaneously to narrate and redress her unfulfilled desire to embody Giselle: the alternative present of re-enactment moves toward an alternative future, one in which Doisneau will have danced Giselle at POB. Put another way, her performance of the dance that bears her name is a moment of emergence into a future that is physically different from and socially more celebrated than the one her previous career trajectory supports: it is the future to a past other than the one she has actually lived. Giselle as re-presented in the context of *Veronique Doisneau* would then seem to be a breakthrough role, taking place in an opening in time that also opens the occupational hierarchy. Act I of *Giselle*, in which the eponymous peasant girl thinks she's going to marry the Duke, echoes this opening to an alternate fairy-tale future. But just as Giselle's infatuation is fatally dashed by the revelation that her Duke is about to wed a woman of his own rank, Doisneau's new future as a Paris Opera Ballet star runs smack into institutional limits. This performance will be followed by her state-mandated retirement, so that her first appearance in the position of an *étoile* is also necessarily her last. Besides, her execution of this choreography does not effectively compensate for her previous failure to achieve the promotion necessary to legitimate her adoption of the role. Danced without costuming, music, or Duke Albrecht, the steps of the pas de deux themselves lack the performative authority retroactively to change her occupational rank. Thus Doisneau's performance does at least three things: it presents Doisneau as Giselle; it re-enacts Giselle's class predicament; and it represents Doisneau's failure to dance Giselle. Doisneau's position at Paris Opera Ballet cannot be changed to allow her emergence into stardom because POB's caste structure is not flexible enough to accommodate the temporal opening that promises a different future than the one the past predicts.

Complicity in Hierarchical Time: *Swan Lake*

There is another reason that Doisneau cannot be said to dance Giselle: her excerpt from the ballet is only three minutes long, a compression of time extraordinary even in the already-squeezed temporal frame of biographical dance. At the climax of *Veronique Doisneau*, Bel develops duration in the opposite direction, toward gesture that is sustained too long. He does this with the grand pas de deux from *Swan Lake*. Conventionally *Swan Lake*, like *Giselle*, deploys dozens of identical corps dancers to support its female star; but while Bel allows Doisneau to embody the title character in *Giselle* for a moment,

Bel's version of *Swan Lake* keeps her firmly in her place in the corps. This segment begins when Doisneau tells us "One of the most beautiful things in classical ballet is the scene from *Swan Lake* where thirty-two female dancers of the corps de ballet dance together but in this scene there are long moments of immobility, the 'poses.' We become a human decor to highlight the stars. And for us it is the most horrible thing we do." Then she calls for music and begins to dance; but the dancing in question is almost entirely still.

Doisneau's plural pronouns prepare us to be alert to the immaterial presence of the swans that have surrounded her in previous performances of this dance, their feathers trembling just at the edge of perception; at the same time our eyes register Doisneau's solitary stillness because there is nothing else to look at. We have time to reflect on the importance of still presence in contemporary choreography, and on the fold in time that lets us see such stillness as something that has been present in classical dance for a century and a half. And we have time to contemplate how dancing collective dances as solos simultaneously magnifies and diminishes Doisneau's importance. She is the focus of all eyes, unaccompanied and uncostumed, executing movement choreographed as a contribution to a collective effect. As we wait and watch we may waver between seeing the dance as a showcase for Doisneau's effort and accomplishment, and as a mocking exposure of her inadequacy to the impossible task of representing thirty-two swans and a pair of principal dancers all by herself. Nothing in the choreography itself supports or refutes either interpretation, so that the opposites co-exist in a perfect balanced tension much like that exhibited by Doisneau's slender muscled arms.

Then again we may get bored, or tense. The audience begins to rustle and cough after only ten seconds. Even as we witness the labor Doisneau is performing, we experience the force of the evaluative schema that would interpret her as "doing nothing," or nothing significant, because she slows down time to the point that we can't see anything happening. Her performance of suspended time is simultaneously a dramatization of her impressive self-discipline and of its failure to propel her career further up the ladder of rank. A few steps provide beautiful relief. Doisneau is suddenly a swan, wings beating as she extends her neck parallel to the floor—but these few steps lead only to another sustained pose. Seven full minutes later, the music swells. Doisneau inclines her head toward center stage and ripples her elbows slightly, and the audience bursts into applause. Doisneau, however, reacts neither to the music nor the applause, maintains her position for several more seconds, then steps to a new position as a new musical theme begins. The applause dies unevenly, as though the audience is developing that uncomfortable sensation of having clapped at the wrong time. Or for the wrong reason.

We have been applauding for the principal dancers who would have concluded their grand pas de deux at that moment, had they been onstage at all.

In this awkward moment audiences are asked to recognize our complicity with the hierarchical structures of value that make Doisneau's dancing body appear to be worth less than those of the principal couple who are not actually present on the stage before us. Those structures of value refer not only to rank within the POB but also to the monarchies in which the national ballet of France took shape. Paris Opera Ballet was founded in 1661 by Louis XIV; the Palais Garnier, in which *Veronique Doisneau* was staged, was built for the Opera in the 1860s by Napoleon III and includes an architectural tribute to the Hall of Mirrors at Versailles. When Bel sets us up to applaud for the invisible principals in *Swan Lake*, we are given the opportunity to consider extended duration and suspended time in terms of the stubbornly persistent aesthetic legacies of absolutism as these are re-enacted in every performance of the great classical ballets. In the world of Paris Opera Ballet, princes must marry for dynastic reasons while peasants must keep their place; princesses are political pawns; and everybody wears magnificently embroidered velvets and silks, sewn by invisible hands. On one level this means only that POB is in the business of staging fairy tales. On another level, this stage, in this palace, is where the kings and queens of France still command adoration for their superior grace and poise.

When we applaud for Prince Siegfried and the Swan Queen despite their absence, we are experiencing the pull of an absolutist aesthetic, caught up in admiration for power expressed as and through physical control: ballet's beauty manifests the triumph of the rational will (Louis XIV is still known as the Sun King for his character in a court ballet that glorified his rule as a model of Apollonian order).[17] But our admiration does not simply transport us backward in time or carry the politically laden posturing of the *ballet de cours* into the present unchanged. Complicity means "folded together"— in Bel's quotation from *Swan Lake* the temporality of postmodern dance, its interest in stillness and bodily presence, mingles across four centuries with the temporality of court dance at Versailles. Past and present tug on one another. For a moment we seem to be living in an alternative future in which the Revolution isn't quite complete, so that the civil servant standing center stage both replaces France's toppled royalty and manifests its continued potency.

Arrested Development and Alternative Futures

The swansdown wafting through Bel's dance carries a history that remains stubbornly present after its moment has passed, so that we see the persistent influence of political forms long after their original governmental supports are overturned. *Veronique Doisneau* is a critical call for an alternative future for French dance, one in which affective and aesthetic attachments to ballet (figured as an archaic art reflecting relations of domination) are left behind more decisively. This critical logic is so familiar. Inappropriate attachments, archaic forms, illegitimate exercises of power: Bel's call for a new approach to choreography sounds eerily like an argument for reparative therapy, the psychic and social reorganization of desire around a more proper object. In this logic ballet occupies the position of a gayness that needs maturational development, both personal and political, into a potentially (re)productive relational form.

The flurry of feathers thickens: from behind the swan corps, enter the Prince who doesn't want to grow up. The *Swan Lake* performed by POB is based on the usual nineteenth-century Petipa/Ivanov choreography but was restaged by Rudolph Nureyev in 1984 so that the story focuses on Prince Siegfried and his inner turmoil.[18] Earlier versions of the story depict Siegfried as a party boy who would rather go hunting with his friends than marry and take up the mantle of kingship. His attitude threatens dynastic stability and must be corrected, but the stereotypical masculinity of its expression seems to promise that this Prince will straighten out when he finds the right woman. In Nureyev's version, however, the situation is much more dire. His Siegfried is a sensitive, solitary youth indifferent to women and awkward in the company of men. His father is dead and his mother is distant; his sole intimacy takes the form of dependence on and submission to his handsome, domineering tutor. It is therefore no surprise that the only woman he can imagine loving is not a woman at all, but a bird—and even then he finds it challenging to distinguish his beloved from other waterfowl. Siegfried personifies a classic mid-twentieth-century psychoanalytic description of gay men as castrated, narcissistic, deluded, prone to valuing inappropriate objects, and vulnerable to domination by more powerful people.

Although this reading of POB's *Swan Lake* is rarely articulated, Siegfried's queerness is something the dance can be said to know about itself. Even the Nureyev Foundation acknowledges that one might choose to read this *Swan Lake* as referring to "latent homosexuality."[19] The adjective works as a rhetorical strategy for maintaining the open secret of Nureyev's own gayness, but it is no more accurate as a descriptor for the dance than for the life. In one extended exchange in Act I, the tutor lifts, spins, and manipulates the entranced Prince until the boy is on his knees at his feet, one pale sculpted leg extended behind him in a mirror reversal of the White Swan's famous bowing pose; at that moment, the tutor hands the Prince the crossbow his mother gave him when he came of age and ordered him to marry. The symbolism is not subtle, nor is the gestural placement of the bow's central shaft. In this scene of instruction the lesson seems to be that access to virile power requires submitting to an older man's authority.[20] Then there is the striking way that the tutor mediates Siegfried's introduction to the Black Swan in Act 3, offering his daughter not only as a replacement for the White Swan but also as a female substitute for himself in a crystalline triangle of homoerotic displacement. My point is not that this *Swan Lake* is an unambiguously gay text, but rather that its ambiguities are drawn from a conventional menu of strategies for avoiding direct discussion of sexual variance. Most pertinent for my purposes here is that Nureyev figures Prince Siegfried as problematically immature.[21]

Queer analyses of heteronormative time emphasize the conventional life trajectory from birth through childhood and adolescence to reproductive adulthood, punctuated with milestones that certify our progressive development through these predictable stages or that identify our failures to move forward at the expected time. Prince Siegfried's birthday party opens the action of *Swan Lake* because his coming of age marks the moment when he must take his father's crown and find a queen. The narrative arc of the ballet traces the tragic consequences of Siegfried's lack of interest in these adult projects in favor of sustaining a boyish dreaminess that he expresses through his dependence upon his tutor. The homoeroticism of Nureyev's *Swan Lake* converges with its pathologization to produce a vision of Prince Siegfried as tragically suspended in an androgynous youth whose extension past its acceptable temporal limit renders him inadequate to the royal mantle of manhood.

Veronique Doisneau's re-enactment of *Swan Lake* uses a similar temporal suspension to represent the limit of Doisneau's development as a dancer at Paris Opera Ballet. Queer cultural theorist Jack Halberstam notes that many gay cultural practices—such as nightclubbing—are not deviant for their content so much as for their temporality, specifically their persistence past the age at which we are supposed to grow out of them. He makes the case that not growing out of going out allows queer people to invest in collective social experience, sharing a kind of perpetual adolescence oriented toward the group, long after their straight age peers "normally" pair off into isolated family units.[22] Halberstam's insight can be laminated onto *Veronique Doisneau* to suggest that Doisneau's career as *sûjet* approximates the same kind of developmental arrest that is manifest in Prince Siegfried's queer failure to marry and to rule. Spending decades with the corps means maintaining a permanent adolescence in relation to the expected trajectory of maturation as a classical ballet dancer, in which each promotion means less stage time embedded in groups of women or dancing alone, and another step closer to starring as half of a featured heterosexual couple. Bel literalizes this arrest in

Doisneau's physical stillness in her excerpt from *Swan Lake*, where the corps dancer's role is shown to be one of endless deferential support for a romance that does not address her directly. Always a bridesmaid, never a bride: where Halberstam imagines a thriving queer nightlife, Doisneau's suspension in the corps paradoxically leaves her as isolated in her *Swan Lake* as the Prince who, surrounded by eligible young ladies, wishes he could marry a bird.

Entr'acte

It is tempting to conclude that Bel sees POB's institutional hierarchy as in need of a revolution as decisive as the one that undid dynastic rule in France, and that he is using Doisneau to question a problematic affective attachment to an archaic art that aestheticizes relations of domination. Shouldn't Mme. Doisneau have grown out of her little-girl ballerina dream? Shouldn't dance in general have moved on to more current, more democratic forms?

Certainly there is something both pathetic and poignant about Doisneau's effort to fill the stage, alone and without support from the dramatic technologies of costumery, lighting, sets, and music. But the very absence of theatrical magic and the emphasis on her simple physical presence suggest that if Bel is staging the inevitable failure of an outmoded art form, he is simultaneously staging something we can recognize as successful according to present aesthetic standards and needs. The rejection of the arts of illusion in order to allow a less mediated contact with the artist's presence is a hallmark both of performance art and of the tradition of critically engaged dance-making out of which Bel's work emerges.[23] Bel offers thoroughly contemporary dance that re-enacts past choreographies in and for the now.

Re-enactment complicates the present, making us feel how we are always folded in time, always in physical relationship to a past that can take new forms through and in our bodies. As Doisneau's re-enactments fold time, they bring the forms of beauty enabled by France's monarchical past into its republican present and vice versa; that is to say, Bel has his dancer materialize the unexpected aesthetic convergence of classical and postmodern choreographic devices. Thus, in its extended stillness Doisneau's performance of *Swan Lake* echoes a contemporary strategy for pushing at the boundaries defining what dance is and can be, creating a moment of slippage between postmodern work and the multiple traditions it both mobilizes and critiques. What alternative forms can emerge in that temporal slide?

Following feathers through folded time has led me from absolutist aesthetics to a pathologizing vision of homosexuality as a fundamentally antisocial manifestation of arrested development. Still I want to emphasize that Bel does not simply use Doisneau to indict ballet as an artistic reflection of entrenched systems of power and oppression. While his re-enactments of the classics demonstrate how aesthetics and politics dovetail in a cultural legacy that works to keep people, including Doisneau, in their allotted places, he simultaneously has his *sujet* perform an alternative future. Again and again Bel offers us oppositions that turn out to be leaning on one another for support. While he exposes the cultural logic through which Doisneau's career at Paris Opera Ballet can be narrated as a failure to leave the corps, he also creates a starring role for her at POB. When he stages her inevitable inability fully to represent multiple dancers in her own small frame, he also stages the importance of the collective to which she is integral. When he has her dance the scene of Giselle's first appearance in her afterlife, he shows us Doisneau's emergence into the character at the same moment we witness the death of her career. For each affirmation he offers a critique; in every criticism we are shown something to admire. The two gestures cannot be separated. We are left suspended and without direction in the space between judgments, hovering like wisps of down carried on a current of warm air.

The alternative future for dance that Bel proposes, then, cannot be said to leave history behind in search of a new or less contaminated movement idiom. His future dance features and foregrounds the impurity of cultural forms. As the swans vanish in the mist and the curtain falls, I want to make one final plea for the exploration rather than denial of complicity. The imperial history of ballet persists. We remain vulnerable to seduction by power. That same seduction is what compels me to chase feathers: they are beautiful and alluring; they promise transformation. And therein lies their political potential. They offer the foundational knowledge of the past in all its sadness, a certainty from which we can launch our own changing and reiterative futures.

Notes

1. Nonetheless feathers display a collective organization recognizable as variations on modes of linearity. Such linear variation subtends the genealogical fictions I unpack and so is mimicked in the structure of this essay.
2. *Veronique Doisneau* was filmed in performance at Paris Opera Ballet for French television; I originally encountered the dance through a YouTube upload of this film, available at <https://www.youtube.com/watch?v=OIuWY5PInFs> as of October 1 2016.
3. I discuss Matthew Bourne's all-male *Swan Lake* later, but focus on Nureyev's *Les Lac des Cygnes* because it provides the choreographic and narrative intertext for Bel's work. On Bourne, see Suzanne Juhasz, "Queer Swans: Those Fabulous Avians in the *Swan Lakes* of Les Ballets Trockadero and Matthew Bourne," *Dance Chronicle* 31, no. 1 (2008): 54–83.

4. Rebecca Schneider, *Performing Remains: Art and War in Times of Theatrical Reenactment* (London and New York: Routledge, 2011): 2; Elizabeth Freeman, "Packing History, Count(er)ing Generations," *New Literary History* 31, no. 4 (2000): 742.

5. Schneider 15.

6. Julian Carter, "Embracing Transition, Dancing in the Folds of Time," in *The Transgender Studies Reader*, Volume 2, ed. Susan Stryker and Aren Aizura (New York: Routledge, 2013), 130–44.

7. This neglect is changing: Mark Franko's *Handbook on Danced Reenactment* is anticipated from Oxford University Press in 2016. See also Andre Lepecki, "The Body as Archive: Will to Re-Enact and the Afterlives of Dances," *Dance Research Journal* 42, no. 2 (2010): 28–48.

8. Amelia Jones, "'The Artist is Present': Artistic Re-enactments and the Impossibility of Presence," *TDR: The Drama Review* 55, no. 1 (Spring 2011): 20–21.

9. Performance theorists have rejected this claim repeatedly for decades, which seems to have had little impact on its popularity. See Peggy Phelan, *Unmarked: The Politics of Performance* (New York: Routledge, 1993), 151–52; Amelia Jones, "Presence in Absentia: Experiencing Performance as Documentation," *Art Journal* 56, no. 4 (Winter 1997): 11–18.

10. André Lepecki offers a useful overview in "Concept and Presence: The Contemporary European Dance Scene," in *Rethinking Dance History*, ed. Alexandra Carter (London: Routledge, 2004), 170–81.

11. See, e.g., Christel Stalpaert's description of audience responses in "Reenacting Modernity: Fabian Barba's *A Mary Wigman Evening (2009)*," *Dance Research Journal* 43, no. 1 (Summer 2011): 90–95.

12. André Lepecki, "The Body as Archive: Will to Re-Enact and the Afterlives of Dances," *Dance Research Journal* 42, no. 2 (Winter 2010): 28–48, esp. p. 31.

13. See Jerome Bel's website at http://www.jeromebel.fr/eng/jeromebel.asp?m=3&s=8&sms=5.

14. *La Bayedere*'s tragedy ensues when a temple dancer resists the advances of the High Brahmin; *Giselle* is about a peasant girl who falls in love with a Duke; *Swan Lake*'s plot unfolds from a Prince's lack of interest in the marriage necessary for perpetuating his royal line. Merce Cunningham's abstract *Points in Space* would seem to be an exception, but Doisneau contextualizes her excerpt from that work with the explanation that dancing without music (as Cunningham required in this piece) is made possible by strict attention to all the other bodies onstage. Thus, in Bel's hands, the modern work is also "about" the importance of relative positioning within a larger order.

15. Actually this point applies beyond the re-enactment of *Giselle*; I would go so far as to say the whole dance is meant as a provocation to consider the traditional

hierarchies that structure POB as an institution. When POB commissioned Bel to make the company an original work, he responded with a dance that seems deliberately difficult to incorporate into the company's repertory after Doisneau's retirement. As an extended solo, the part would conventionally go to someone of a higher rank than Doisneau, but that dancer would then be required by the dance's text to disavow her success, claiming Doisneau's relatively modest career as her own. Alternatively, the role could be danced by another *sùjet*, but doing so would necessarily mean her being allowed to perform a major part without being promoted to the rank at which she becomes eligible to do so. If Paris Opera insists on its customs and rules of rank, it has wasted its commission; and if it relaxes them, it moves that much further away from its own institutional values and tradition.

The political discussion inherent in *Veronique Doisneau* is tightly linked to issues of re-enactment and medium. If Bel was thumbing his nose at POB by making them a dance they couldn't restage, they recouped their investment by freezing the moment of its staging and allowing its endless and unrestricted replay: *Veronique Doisneau* was filmed for public television and put into the digital public domain. Because Doisneau's farewell performance is easily available on YouTube, POB can be understood as continuing to restage the piece despite her retirement and without adjusting its values. Further, Bel's commentary on POB's internal hierarchy repeats itself without respect for changing times and circumstances, and in this respect the technology of its reproduction drags the dance into duplicating the stubborn persistence of social and aesthetic holdovers from absolutism that it critiques.

16. In 1993 POB acquired the right to stage Mats Ek's 1982 reinterpretation of *Giselle*, which has become a very popular part of its repertory. Thus, the Swedish choreography is part of the ballet's multiform past at POB, and well worth further consideration, but space limitations prevent examination of the way that Bel incorporates Ek's work into his own. On the Mats Ek *Giselle* at POB, see Patricia Boccadoro, untitled dance review (July 13, 2004). Available at http://www.culturekiosque.com/dance/reviews/mats_ek.html.

17. Mark Franko, *Dance as Text: Ideologies of the Baroque Body* (Cambridge: Cambridge University Press, 1993).

18. For *Swan Lake*'s basic libretto and history, see Selma Jeanne Cohen, *Next Week, Swan Lake: Reflections on Dance and Dancers* (Middletown, CT: Wesleyan University Press, 1982), esp. ch. 1. The Nureyev *Swan Lake* has been filmed by Paris Opera Ballet for public television and as of this writing is available on YouTube.

19. For more on the potential to read "latent homosexuality" into Nureyev's Siegfried, see the Nureyev Foundation website. Available at http://www.nureyev.org/rudolf-nureyev-choreographies/rudolf-nureyev-swan-lake.

20. Interestingly, Kent Drummond describes Matthew Bourne's pas for the Prince and the (male) Swan as a scene of instruction, as though that precludes eroticism. On the gayness of such moments, see David Halperin, "Deviant Teaching," in *A Companion to LGBTQ Studies*, ed. George Haggerty and Molly McGarry (Hoboken, NJ: Blackwell 2007) 146–167. "The Queering of Swan Lake," *Journal of Homosexuality* 45, nos. 2–4 (2003): 241.

21. Drummond has suggested that mass audiences, presumably largely straight, are able to respond positively to the portrayal of same-sex desire in Matthew Bourne's *Swan Lake* because the Prince is too childlike to be taken really seriously as a gay man; he is ultimately exonerated "of agency and even reality . . . [The ballet] can be read, in the end, as a sad, bad dream of sexual vagrancy: the misguided adventures of a child [who lacked] proper parenting" (251). In many ways I see Bourne's *Swan Lake* as a literalization of what remains implicit in Nureyev's staging.

22. Judith Jack Halberstam, *In a Queer Time and Place: Transgender Bodies, Subcultural Lives* (New York: NYU Press, 2005) 174.

23. Bel's foremothers in this area include, most notably, Yvonne Rainier, Trisha Brown, and Pina Bausch; Rainer's 1965 *No Manifesto* remains one of the most powerful verbal articulations of this choreographic vision.

6

Dancing Marines and Pumping Gasoline

CODED QUEERNESS IN DEPRESSION-ERA
AMERICAN BALLET

Jennifer L. Campbell

Among George Platt Lynes's many photographs of male nudes, one partic-ular image of a dancer in the role of Mac, the gas station attendant hero from the American ballet *Filling Station* (1938), offers a compelling visual paradox.[1] In the photo a young Jacques d'Amboise stands with his right leg propped up on a stool, clothed head to toe in coveralls, the type of long sleeved, one-piece safety garment often worn by mechanics and factory workers. Although the outfit covers the dancer's entire frame, the costume itself is fashioned from thin, translucent material, allowing Lynes to capture the nakedness of d'Amboise's body underneath. Because of its transparency, this loose-fitting, traditionally functional garment deftly serves an ironic purpose: although technically intended to conceal nudity, the clothing actually provides a peep-show of d'Amboise's chest and genitals, leaving little to the imagination.[2] When contextualized in ballet performance, the costume design achieves more than ironic statement: it connotes a hetero/homo duality, suggesting that Mac simultaneously inhabits two worlds—the typical, everyday life of the working man (coveralls) and a realm associated with something more provoc-ative, risqué, and "other" (see-through material).

Filling Station belongs to a group of several Depression-era ballets devel-oped by arts impresario Lincoln Kirstein for his troupe, The Ballet Caravan, and in this essay I offer a close reading of two of these works, *Filling Station* and *Time Table* (1941), teasing out the queering of masculine codes that occurs within these pieces.[3] Kirstein's philosophical approach to formulating new ballets—a perspective that viewed storyline, music, staging, and choreography as equally important parts—allowed him to shape works with a gay-friendly undertone.[4] He shifted the heroes from European princes to working-class American men who were, as dance historian Peter Stoneley states, the "emergent heroes of a queer American pantheon," and he forged ballets that could lead a double life, much like gay men themselves during this period.[5] Because of Kirstein's integrated method of ballet creation, I believe that parings of ballet components, specifically dance and visual art and dance and music, should be closely evaluated for their queer semiotic freight. Furthermore, I argue that in these works the interplay between working-class characters, cartoonish costumes, suggestive choreography, and campy burlesque music alludes to an underlying subtext that reflected aspects of homosexual behavior as practiced in New York during the first half of the twentieth century.

Evolving Codes of Masculinity on the Ballet Stage

Before delving into the Ballet Caravan examples, the evolution of masculine roles—defined specifically in this essay as male characters danced by men as opposed to male characters danced by women, like the travesty dancer—within the genre of ballet needs to be addressed. In the Franco-Russian classical tradition of *ballet blanc*, lead male roles existed largely in the context of heterosexual couplings. The typical plot of a ballet blanc, although it offered opportunities for various types of erotic expression, focused on heterosexual relationships, commonly revolving around the interactions of one man, the danseur, and one woman, the prima ballerina, or perhaps a love triangle in which the man had to choose between two women.[6] Marius Petipa, a French director/choreographer in Saint Petersburg, Russia, was tremendously influential in establishing the traits of Franco-Russian ballet, including its formal structure, dance movements, and mime gestures; Petipa and his choreographic assistants collaborated with composer Pyotr Ilyich Tchaikovsky, yielding some of the most famous ballets still in the repertoire today: *Swan Lake* (1877; 1895 Petipa/Ivanov choregraphy), *The Sleeping Beauty* (1890), and *The Nutcracker* (1892).[7]

In the neoclassical/modernist works of the Ballets Russes, a group that developed from and in reaction to classical Russian ballet, Sergei Diaghilev complicated the heterosexual emphasis of ballet blanc via the inclusion of effeminate male characters.[8] Ballets Russes dancer and choreographer Vaslav Nijinsky conspicuously fashioned sexually androgynous roles in *Schérézade* (1910), *Le Spectre de la rose* (1911), and *L'Après-midi d'un faune* (1912).[9] In the twilight of the troupe's existence, Diaghilev used sailors as main characters: three sailors in *Les Matelots* (1925) and one sailor in *Las Pas d'acier* (1927). To at least one critic, the sailor figure was no less emasculated as he merely "replaced the sex appeal of the [male] oriental slave; factories, dungarees and talc provided the glamour once sought for in fairy places and fatuous costumes; but the essential element of attraction remained the same," suggesting that these works had a homosexual underpinning.[10] The European public devoured these exotic boundary-pushing ballets, the eyebrow-raising androgyny going relatively unquestioned and failing to incite outrage, largely because Europeans considered the Russians and the oriental themes of the ballets as "other" and "foreign."[11] When the Ballets Russes toured the United States in 1916, however, several productions were sanitized of their sexual deviancy, and Nijinsky came under critical attack for his epicene characterizations.[12]

In the United States during the first half of the twentieth century, ballet offered an outlet to question political and social practices in Depression-era America, but allusions to controversial material tended to be covert, and effeminate male roles (especially the sexual implications of these roles) were largely driven into subtext.[13] Although it occupied the slippery position of being an exotic import and a gloriously entertaining leg show, ballet in the United States was primarily considered high art and connoted social prestige, perhaps necessitating that any references to potentially taboo topics such as homosexuality be minimally confrontational to the public-at-large.[14]

Especially in the mid-1930s and 1940s, references to homosexuality in the high arts were often coded and only obvious to those who were "in the know," even in one of the most culturally progressive urban areas: New York City. Although queer culture thrived in New York City in the 1920s, with pansy-act burlesque shows and cabaret revues in Times Square, lesbian performers in Harlem, and gay balls in Greenwich Village, these activities became viewed by authorities as perversions, leading to censorship by government officials and police.[15] In the case of the visual arts, specifically painting, discretion was advised:

> For a homosexual artist to make a painting about the experience of his subculture was to risk public exposure. Certain artists took that risk, but just as often the representation of homosexuality in American painting followed the model of society at large—that is, it was veiled.

Paintings about homosexuality made use of certain disguises that were *meant to be uncovered only by a particular audience* (emphasis mine).[16]

Ballet invited similar scrutiny in the United States during this period. Although not traditionally designated as "visual art," ballet combined the static visual of set designs and costumes (akin to the properties of a painting) with the ephemeral visual of choreography; any hint of non-heteronormativity in a ballet, therefore, was necessarily subtle.

Queering the Masculine in *Filling Station*

A discernable assertion of homoeroticism can be found in *Filling Station*, and an example from the visual arts helps illustrate the queerness in this ballet. With a plot by Kirstein, music by Virgil Thomson, and costumes and set design by Paul Cadmus, *Filling Station* valorizes the average working man: Mac, a gas-pumping proletarian hero, cartoonishly assists a family, truck drivers, a drunk, rich couple, and a state trooper, and helps arrest a gangster—all in the course of one day. Prior to *Filling Station*, Cadmus painted *The Fleet's In!* (1934), a work that depicts the antics of sailors and marines on shore leave (figure 6.1). He used Riverside Park in New York City as the setting for the painting, a location that has sexual implications. At the time, Riverside Park was a well-known site for illicit and queer sexual encounters; female prostitutes and male pansies frequented the area, offering docked seamen the promise

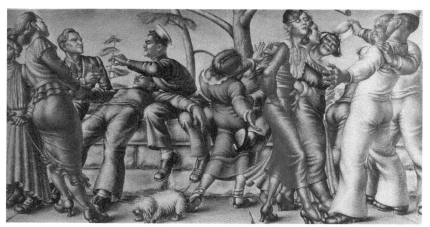

FIGURE 6.1 Paul Cadmus, *The Fleet's In!* (1934). Oil and tempera on canvas, 30 x 60 in. Navy Historical Center, Washington, DC.

of sexual activity.[17] Cadmus portrays all his figures in the painting, both men and women, with tight-fitting clothes that accentuate the posterior and groin areas, giving them a caricature-like appearance. Although some of the seamen are talking to women, Cadmus positions the sailors' buttocks facing outward, suggesting what art historian Richard Meyer has called "an anal-erotic logic of insertion and reception" and placing the potential for both homo- and heterosexual interaction on the male bodies.[18] Furthermore, Cadmus includes a direct reference to homosexual behavior: one particular male character, the dapper civilian on the left, whose presence seems incongruous with the staunch masculinity of the sailors and marines.[19] His red tie, which was a known code commonly used in certain New York circles to communicate interest in same-sex activity, coupled with his ringed fingers, his finely groomed eyebrows, and his blond, wavy hair all identify him as a fairy or pansy.[20] This suave gentleman offers a cigarette to a marine,[21] a variation of another code by which those interested in same-sex encounters could identify one another, and the lingering gaze between the two men suggests that further interaction will likely follow.[22]

Cadmus's visual presentation of characters in *Filling Station* largely echoes his imagery in *The Fleet's In!*, especially the caricature-like clothing designed for the performers. Dance historian Mark Franko interprets Mac's costume as suggestive of a homoerotic aesthetic, and refers to a publicity photo of Mac in which dancer Lew Christensen stands with legs apart, his hands in fists on his hips, his nipples and legs clearly seen.[23] Cadmus avoids the blatant inclusion of a red tie, instead using red piping to outline Mac's see-through suit. Mac's stance, which Christensen also integrated into his choreography, hints at the idea of an ironic superhero: by donning this outfit, a regular person adopts the "heroic" identity of a working man. The pose also exudes uber-masculinity, exemplifying an idealized male body type desired by both women and gay men.

Cadmus's portrayal of the truck drivers, with their tight pants and chest-baring shirts, also insinuates homoeroticism (figure 6.2). One design sketch in particular reveals a tall, muscular truck driver, smoking a cigarette and assuming the stance just described. The other truck driver, smaller in stature with wavy hair, gazes directly at his associate, his hand on his friend's shoulder, the other arm akimbo on his hip, and one leg crossed in front of the other— all coded suggestions of the second truck driver's sexual interest in his counterpart.[24] Cadmus's truck driver drawings anticipate the later beefcake genre, which were images published in magazines for gay men under the guise of physical fitness during America's censorship of gay erotica in the 1950s and 1960s.[25]

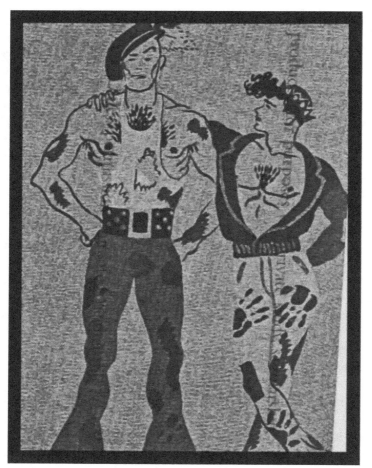

FIGURE 6.2 Paul Cadmus, *Filling Station*, Truck Drivers' Costumes. Art © Jon F. Anderson, Estate of Paul Cadmus/Licensed by VAGA, New York, NY.

When translated into choreography, the sexuality of the truck drivers and their relationship with Mac becomes ambiguous because of their physical interactions. The choreography during Scene 4, "Truck Drivers' Dance," combines graceful ballet movements with tumbling and exaggerated manly gestures, such as quasi-arm wrestling, producing a sexually undefined and campy result. As seen in the film version of the ballet, Mac and the truck drivers do more than occupy the stage and dance alongside one another; these men touch.[26] Some of the physical contact involves exaggerated displays of traditional masculinity. Other aspects of the choreography resemble naïve horseplay, such as the somersaults or when Mac is sandwiched between his two friends as they pretend to drive a truck, yet the bodily positions of these campy gestures invite an interpretation of queerness. Such bawdy humor would be expected on the vaudeville or burlesque stage, but these types of interactions make a more provocative statement in ballet: the somersaults situate the paired truckers with each person's head close to the groin of the other, while the forward-facing gesture with Mac between the two truck drivers mirrors the position of insertion-reception present in *The Fleet's In!* The use of lowbrow, comedic choreography in this ballet blatantly evokes the burlesque environment and the gay culture associated with it.[27]

The queerest aspect of this scene's choreography, however, is found in traditional ballet movement, when Mac and one of the truck drivers take turns acting as the cavalier for one another—taking on the traditional chivalrous role of the male dancer but for another man, not for a ballerina. Mac stands solid as the larger truck driver runs toward him; the truck driver leaps and Mac simultaneously lifts him high in the air, then throws him to the right-hand side. The smaller truck driver follows suit, first being lifted and tossed by Mac, and then by the other driver. This series of lifts, where one man supports the other, undermines the heteronormative masculinity of the two truck drivers by placing each of them in a lifted, fairy-like position—the smallest truck driver, the most effeminate, is lifted twice and never serves as the cavalier. This action, perhaps more than any of the other choreographic elements, calls the sexual identity of all three characters into question.

Enter Two Marines: Kirstein and his Balletic Men

As Ballet Caravan's artistic director, Kirstein was staunchly dictatorial, and his heavy-handedness made a clear imprint on the performance of masculinity in the works produced by his company: *Time Table* is certainly no exception.[28] Kirstein's decision to set *Time Table* to Aaron Copland's *Music for the Theatre* (1925) marked a fairly strong deviation from his typical musical choices. Since his inception of the American Ballet Company, and especially with the Ballet Caravan, whenever Kirstein constructed a ballet based on an American theme, he usually commissioned a new score from a current American composer.[29] Kirstein's use of *Music for the Theatre* stands apart as the only instance of him allowing an entire work composed nearly two decades earlier to serve as the basis of one of his American ballets, an anomaly that merits closer attention.

Taken collectively, the storyline, formal structure, and music of *Time Table*, as well as Kirstein's authorship and development of the ballet, work together in their queerness. Although Antony Tudor's choreography no longer survives, Kirstein's scenario for *Time Table* (initially called *Good-Night and*

Goodbye) helps supply details of the action in lieu of the missing physical movement.[30] The curtain rises to reveal a railway station in small-town rural America and a stationmaster walking the platform. During the "Prologue," a marine and his girlfriend enter followed by the arrival of other heterosexual couples at the station. The second part, "Dance" serves as a general dance for all the pairs of characters on the stage up to this point, while the third part, "Interlude," returns the focus to the marine and his girl.[31] "Burlesque," part four, introduces two new characters, both marines, one happy and one serious. The "Epilogue" finds everyone meeting the arriving train; the couples take their places at the platform; the men leave and the women say goodbye. Finally, the girlfriend is the only one of the lovers left. She dances a short solo, exits, and the station master returns to walking the railroad tracks with the lantern.[32]

Kirstein's scenario broadly adheres to the larger structure of Copland's music. The large-scale form of the work is arch-like, with Copland placing the "Prologue" and "Epilogue" at either end; the "Dance" and "Burlesque" in symmetrical opposition; and the "Interlude" in the center (figure 6.3).[33] Arch form typically refers to a ternary ABA form, or ABCBA when expanded, usually within the single movement of a piece of music. Letters indicate when the presentation of melodic and harmonic material is the same, and these letters also highlight the symmetry of the form. In an ABCBA form, the initial statement of AB is balanced by the return of that material as BA; the C section offers the most contrast. This formal construct provides clarity with regard to Copland's five-movement piece, although the A and B now represent pairings of movements sharing similar characteristics and styles as opposed to an exact return of musical material.

When Kirstein's scenario is overlaid onto the music, the action and entrance of characters shifts, queering the musical and dramatic emphasis (figure 6.4). Kirstein's plot involves an orderly introduction of characters in

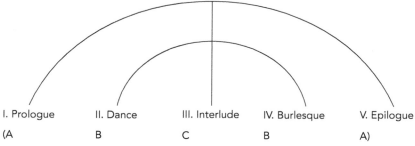

FIGURE 6.3 Musical form of Copland's *Music for the Theatre*.

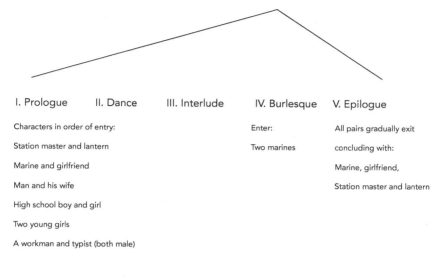

I. Prologue   II. Dance   III. Interlude   IV. Burlesque   V. Epilogue

Characters in order of entry:	Enter:	All pairs gradually exit
Station master and lantern	Two marines	concluding with:
Marine and girlfriend		Marine, girlfriend,
Man and his wife		Station master and lantern
High school boy and girl		
Two young girls		
A workman and typist (both male)		

All pairs dance in parts I, II, and III.

FIGURE 6.4 Dramatic form superimposed on *Music for the Theatre* by Kirstein.

the "Prologue"; no new characters appear until the "Burlesque," when the final two participants in the ballet, the two male marines, make their presence known. This twist knocks the balanced arch form of the music off-kilter by giving the "Burlesque" a heavier dramatic emphasis. Instead of the moody, bluesy, and romantic "Interlude" taking center stage, the "Burlesque," a dance for two men rather than a heterosexual couple, becomes the climax of the action.

The shift of focus to the "Burlesque" accentuates the music of this particular movement, which is one of the most oft-discussed sections of *Music for the Theatre* among music scholars. In this portion of the work, Copland combines elements of jazz and popular music to evoke the risqué environment that characterized burlesque shows in the 1920s. Copland's musical style has "gay-friendly connotations," and the "Burlesque" serves as one example of music as sexual allusion."[34] Beyond the obvious musical innuendo of the breast-baring girlie show, the locations of the New York City burlesque theaters, the types of entertainment performed in these venues, and the activities of the audience members who attended these productions also suggest non-heteronormative associations. As Howard Pollack observes:

At the time Copland wrote this piece, America's major burlesque houses were clustered in New York's Times Square area, that is in the heart of the city's gay ghetto. George Chauncey writes that burlesque itself attracted homosexuals during this period, not only because the theaters (especially the balconies) served as cruising and trysting places, but because their entertainment was so sexually transgressive (including frankly homosexual routines).[35]

Many routines included cross-dressing acts, women dressing as men and men dressing as women. The sexuality of Copland's music and all that it connoted would not have been lost on Kirstein.[36]

The inclusion of sailor images on publicity fliers for burlesque shows and Harlem theatrical productions strategically advertised the queerness of these performance spaces. One of the acts Kirstein frequented was that of Gladys Bentley, who mixed ribaldry, vulgarity, and cross-dressing of the burlesque with the blues of Harlem, and her shows embraced homoerotic content.[37] When she performed at the King's Terrace nightclub and the Lafayette Theatre in 1934, a promotional ad for the show displayed Bentley in her masculine getup standing behind six African American men dolled up in sailor suits. James Wilson describes the image and its relevancy to the gay community:

> The picture of the sailor chorus surely was a reference to the gay subculture, which transformed New York's waterfront into a legendary homosexual cruising spot. For gay men, the sailor on-leave was a symbol of masculine eroticism, pent-up sexuality, and rough trade.[38]

This type of homosexual coding within a publicity photo likely would have resonated with Kirstein, who saw both sailors and marines as potential partners for anonymous physical gratification.[39]

In *Time Table* Kirstein opted to introduce not just two men, but specifically two marines during the "Burlesque," shying away from the more obviously coded sailor character. Because of their exchanges with the female dancers, the two marines in this ballet are apparently not exclusively or overtly gay, but the marines do not have to be solely depicted with men in order for there to be a same-sex undertone.[40] The entrance of the two marines follows the "Interlude" in which pairs of heterosexual couples engage in romantic or domestic kinds of actions that indicate the status of their relationships. The two marines signify another "pair," interacting with one another as well as with the other characters. They try to distract their friend, the first marine, from his girlfriend in an effort to involve him in their antics. To be sure, these two characters add a humorous element to the ballet; Kirstein's scenario, however, gives dramatic weight to this section of the music, implying greater significance beyond that of comic relief. Very little information about the actual dancing exists, but one reviewer documented the following: "[*Time Table*'s] main fault is lack of choreographic development. The horseplay of the two young marines offered Tudor an excellent opportunity, but he gives them almost nothing to do."[41] Perhaps the horseplay of the marines resembled the homoerotic vaudevillian choreography of the truck drivers in *Filling Station*; if so, then the intended purpose of these marines extended beyond that of mere entertainment and offered a coded reference to inclusion aimed at the gay community

Queer Legibility or Titillating Subtext?

Performances of *Filling Station* and *Time Table* took place in the United States and South America, begging the question: Were any of these suggestions of queerness recognizable to audiences? Press reviews of *Filling Station*, when it was performed at various venues across the United States in 1938 and 1939, make no overt mention of this underlying agenda, but two reviews of the premiere in Hartford, Connecticut, use flowery vocabulary that imply possible cross-readings of the ballet as both queer and normative.[42] A critic for *Hartford Courant* declared the premiere a "scintillating performance" with "sheer flair" and "technical modishness that put a sting and tingle into the dance and turn it out with a flourish"; overall the ballet was "a gay, capering thing."[43] Writing for the *The Hartford Times*, Marian Murray used more suggestive terminology, calling *Filling Station* a "penetrating commentary of modern life, pointed up with that satirical but amusing tongue-in-cheek." She also connected the characters to a sexualized environment outside of the gasoline station, noting that the costumes were "cellophane oiled silk, printed cotton velvet tweeds and chiffons, creating slightly burlesqued accoutrements."[44]

Time Table was specifically created for Ballet Caravan's 1941 South American tour and the only staging of it prior to the troupe's departure was a dress rehearsal at Hunter College, New York.[45] Unfortunately, there are no extant reviews of the pre-tour exhibition. In South America the group performed *Time Table* only five times, and it received two brief mentions in the Brazilian (July 3, 1941, *Correio da Manhã*) and Argentinean papers (July 29, 1941, *Noticias Graficas*), but the explanations of the choreography failed to do anything more than rehearse the scenario.

Filling Station, on the other hand, was performed extensively on the South American tour, numbering twenty performances in all and the most of any of the modern American works in the company's repertoire.[46] It met with mixed reactions from South American audiences but not necessarily because of the issue in question. Newspaper reviews, correspondence, and embassy reports indicate it was largely the "modern" style of ballet dancing and the poor realization of the music that resulted in criticism.[47]

One person, however, reacted adversely to the modern American works. In a letter to Nelson Rockefeller, Coordinator of Inter-American Affairs for the US government, Kirstein documented the unexpected behavior demonstrated by the US ambassador to Brazil, Jefferson Caffrey. Caffrey had been "very nice until the first performance [in Rio de Janeiro]," but the following day he "turned on the project. He let it be known far and wide that he considered the whole affair non-representative and if he had only a little more interest he would have 'forbidden' us to present the American scores."[48]

The exact reasons for Caffrey's abrupt change in attitude toward the company remain unclear; however, his volte-face occurred after the Ballet Caravan's premiere of *Filling Station* in Rio de Janeiro. Perhaps Caffrey disliked Thomson's music or Kirstein's leftist-inspired plot. Or perhaps Caffrey belonged to what art historian Jonathan Weinberg called that "particular audience"—as someone who recognized coded references to homosexual behavior.[49] At the very least, Caffrey's sensitivity to queer representations in dance may have been elevated because of personal circumstances, his sexuality having been called into question while serving as the US ambassador to Cuba in 1934.[50] In 1940 the Roosevelt administration teetered on the precipice of public scandal when Caffrey's colleague and friend Sumner Welles, Under Secretary of State at the time, sexually propositioned a male African American train porter while on a work-related trip. Painfully aware of the situation, officials in Washington successfully kept this incident and rumors of other indiscretions in Welles's past from the press, but eventually forced Welles to resign in 1943. By the time the Ballet Caravan visited Brazil in 1941, Caffrey would have learned the circumstances surrounding Welles's tribulations. Whatever the reason, it was a North American, Caffrey, who took issue with *Filling Station* and not the Brazilian general public or press.[51]

In *Filling Station* and *Time Table*, Kirstein and his collaborators successfully queered masculinity on the ballet stage in a way that made a "both/ and" possible—a ballet could lead a double life, hospitable to those drawn to chivalrous heterosexuality and male homoeroticism at the same time. These works, however, offered more than merely gay social life adapted for the stage; the artmaking itself queered the performance space. The characters and costumes depicted gas station attendants, truck drivers, and marines, all of whom represented idealized masculinity but were also associated with rough trade, meaning "men who lived in the 'normal world' but had sex with other men."[52] The choreography in these selections included vaudevillian tumbling and movements found in burlesque shows, and, in the case of *Filling Station*, queer versions of traditionally heterosexual choreography. And in *Time Table* the music itself connoted the gay-friendly space of the burlesque environment. These components worked together in a way that shrewdly merged conventional masculinity and queerness shrouded in a cloak of discretion, causing audiences and critics in the United States and South America to interpret *Time Table* and *Filling Station* as modern, humorous, touching, and even profound works of entertainment—suggesting that the "other world" of the marines, Mac, and his truck driver friends remained carefully veiled to the public at large but subtly disclosed to those who could read or even sense the codes.

The transformation from coded queerness to more straightforward representations of homosexuality in ballet has been little discussed. As late as 1995, German dance critic Horst Koegler wrote, "[Ballet's] 'coming out' has taken an unusually long time. Actually we know next to nothing about the role homosexuality has played in the history of ballet." For Koegler, Jerome Robbins's 1962 ballet *Events*, which has an "explicitly gay pas de deux," signified ballet's official out-of-the-closet moment.[53] What Koegler and other dance historians have not extensively examined is the role covert queerness played in ballets prior to that. Koegler nods to Diaghilev's hints of homoeroticism in *Jeux* (1913) and *Les Biches* (1924), but no other works are mentioned, leaving the reader to conclude that gay ballet dramatically arrived on stage like a flamboyant diva queen. The close readings offered here help ameliorate the gaping historical record, but many more works should be revisited. Only by looking closely at queer codes embedded in the choreography, music, costumes, and set design will we clearly see the evolution leading up to ballet's eventual coming out.[54]

Primary Sources

American Ballet Caravan. Jerome Robbins Dance Division. New York Public Library for the Performing Arts. New York, NY.
Ballet Society Archives. New York, NY.
Rockefeller Family Archives. Rockefeller Archive Center. Sleepy Hollow, NY.

Videography

Ballet Caravan. Motion Picture, 1938–1940. Black and white film with excerpts of *Filling Station* and *Billy the Kid*. New York Public Library, Jerome Robbins Dance Division.

Filling Station. Motion Picture. NBC-TV "Your Show of Shows," 1954. Performed
   by members of the New York City Ballet. Jerome Robbins Dance Division.
   New York Public Library for the Performing Arts, New York, NY.
Filling Station. Motion Picture. *Jacques D'Amboise: Portrait of a Great American
   Dancer.* Max Liebman Presents: Sunday in Town October 10, 1954. DVD.
   Video Artists International. 2006.

Acknowledgments

Portions of this paper were presented at the Music, Gender, and Globalization
Conference at Cornell University (2011); at the Congress on Research in Dance
Special Topics Conference at the University of Michigan (2012); and at the meet-
ing of the International Musicological Society Congress in Rome, Italy (2012).

Notes

1. George Platt Lynes's photos are available in the Jerome Robbins Dance Division,
   New York Public Library, as well as at the Kinsey Institute for Research in Sex,
   Gender, and Reproduction at Indiana University. In the 1930s, Lincoln Kirstein
   and choreographer George Balanchine hired Lynes to create publicity materials for
   their ballet company. This particular photograph likely dates from 1953, when the
   New York City Ballet revived *Filling Station* and d'Amboise performed in the role
   of Mac.
2. When onstage, dancers Lew Christensen and Jacques d'Amboise wore a dance
   belt underneath Mac's costume.
3. *Filling Station* premiered in 1938 in Hartford, Connecticut, with music by Virgil
   Thomson, choreography by Lew Christensen, and costumes by Paul Cadmus.
   The work became a staple of the Ballet Caravan repertoire and was performed
   across the United States in 1938–9 and on the group's tour of South America in
   1941. It was also staged in 1953 by the New York City Ballet and later adopted into
   the San Francisco Ballet's repertoire. *Time Table,* set to *Music for the Theatre* (1925)
   by Aaron Copland with choreography by English dancer Anthony Tudor and costumes by James Stewart Morcom, was specifically created for the troupe's South
   American tour. It was performed at a pre-tour dress rehearsal at Hunter College,
   New York, and not performed again in the United States until a restaging of it
   in 1949.
4. *Filling Station* has endured considerable scrutiny, but queer interpretations typically hinge on two points: (1) the homosexuality of the collaborators, specifically
   Kirstein and painter Paul Cadmus and (2) the connections between Cadmus's
   painting *The Fleet's In!* and the costumes/set design of the ballet. Peter Stoneley

addresses both points in *A Queer History of the Ballet* (New York: Routledge, 2007), 93–124, while art historian Jonathan Weinberg focuses solely on the visual connections between the painting and ballet in *Speaking for Vice: Homosexuality in the Art of Charles Demuth, Marsden Hartley, and the First American Avant-Garde* (New Haven, CT: Yale University Press, 1993).

5. Stoneley 104. George Chauncey, *Gay New York: Gender, Urban Culture, and the Making of the Gay Male World* (New York: Harper Collins, 1994), 273. Chauncey writes, "They [Queer men] constantly moved between at least two worlds: a straight world in which they were assumed to be straight and a gay world in which they were known as gay."

6. Lynn Garafola, "The Travesty Dancer in Nineteenth-Century Ballet," *Dance Research Journal* 7, no. 2 (1985): 35–40.

7. For more about the history and development of ballet, see Jack Anderson, *Ballet & Modern Dance: A Concise History*, 2d ed. (Princeton, NJ: Princeton Book Company, 1992).

8. For information about the Ballets Russes, see Lynn Garafola, *Diaghilev's Ballets Russes* (New York: Oxford University Press, 1989). For details on Diaghilev, modernity, and queer identity, see Stoneley, *A Queer History of the Ballet*, 66–92.

9. Alexandra Kolb, "Nijinsky's Images of Homosexuality: Three Case Studies," *Journal of European Studies* 39, no. 2 (2009): 147–71.

10. Constant Lambert, *Music Ho! A Study of Music in Decline* (London: Faber and Faber, 1934), 53, 64, 105.

11. Stoneley, *A Queer History of the Ballet*, 66–92.

12. Ibid., 97–98.

13. Ibid., 96–97. In the late 1930s several dancers and dance troupes in the United States expressed overtly leftist political and social views through the radical aesthetic of modern dance, while ballet companies favored more conservative subject matter. For more on modern dance, see Ellen Graff, *Stepping Left: Dance and Politics in New York City, 1928–1942* (Durham, NC: Duke University Press, 1997) and Mark Franko, *The Work of Dance: Labor, Movement, and Identity in the 1930s* (Middletown, CT: Wesleyan University Press, 2002). On modern dance, race, and homosexuality, see Susan Manning, *Modern Dance, Negro Dance: Race in Motion* (Minneapolis: University of Minnesota Press, 2004).

14. Stoneley, *A Queer History of the Ballet*, 96.

15. For details about the prevalence of gay culture in 1920s New York City and the crackdown on pro-gay activities and establishments that followed in the 1930s, see Chauncey, *Gay New York*, 290–354.

16. Weinberg, *Speaking for Vice*, 19.

17. Stoneley, *A Queer History of the Ballet*, 182, 147. Also see Chauncey who points out that sexual distinctions made among men in the early twentieth century were not relegated to the binary categorization of homo/heterosexual. Throughout

his book, Chauncey explains several categories of sexuality, including as wolf, pansy, and fairy.

18. Richard Meyer, *Outlaw Representations: Censorship & Homosexuality in Twentieth-Century American Art* (Oxford: Oxford University Press, 2002), 40.

19. Weinberg, *Speaking for Vice*, 33–41.

20. Meyer, *Outlaw Representations*, 43. Meyer supplies a list of codes used by effeminate males interested in same-sex relations during this time period: "Indeed, Cadmus's treatment of the male civilian features a virtual catalog of period signs of the so-called pansy or fairy: pursed lips, rouged cheeks, ringed fingers, red tie, slicked-down blond hair, even the sinister cast of shaded eyes and brows."

21. The marine in Cadmus's painting also reinforces my later interpretation of homoeroticism in *Time Table*. Including a marine does not automatically indicate homosexual behavior, but Cadmus's depiction implies an openness to same-sex sexual behavior on behalf of the marine, an openness can be extended to the two marines in *Time Table* when combined with the musical and dramatic context in which they are presented.

22. Chauncey, *Gay New York*, 188. He notes, "A 'normal' man almost automatically averted his eyes if they happened to lock with those of a stranger, whereas a gay man interested in the man gazing at him returned his look." Furthermore, he states, "In order to confirm the interest indicated by eye contact, or as a way of initiating contact, men made use of a number of utterly conventional gestures. Perhaps the most common simply involved asking for a match or for the time of day."

23. Franko, *The Work of Dance*, 120.

24. Meyer, *Outlaw Representations*, 23.

25. *Physique Pictorial* was an example of a beefcake magazine.

26. I am basing my analysis of the choreography on a motion picture version of *Filling Station*. See *Jacques D'Amboise: Portrait of a Great American Dancer*, Max Liebman Presents: Sunday in Town October 10, 1954, DVD, Video Artists International (2006).

27. Howard Pollack, "The Dean of Gay American Composers," *American Music* 18, no. 1 (Spring 2000): 41–42.

28. See "Analysis of Ballet Theatre's Present Position," folder 3560, box 49, Jerome Robbins Dance Division, American Ballet Caravan/New York Public Library. When Lucia Chase, the former director of Ballet Theatre, requested an analysis of what might happen if the Ballet Caravan and Ballet Theatre merged, the assessment revealed that Kirstein's artistic philosophy was of considerable concern:

> Kirstein is firmly convinced ... that an artistic director must have complete artistic dictatorship in the production of a ballet. He alone chooses the composer, the scene and costume designers and the author. He has the

final word of approval on the choreography, lighting and casting. He does not believe choreographers have sufficient knowledge of music, painting, design, etc., to be given much latitude in the production of a ballet.

29. Kirstein asked Kay Swift to compose the music for *Alma Mater* (1935); Elliott Carter was commissioned for *Pocahontas* (1936); Paul Bowles wrote the score for *Yankee Clipper* (1937); and Robert McBride provided *Show Piece* (1937). These works were followed by *Filling Station* (Virgil Thomson, 1937), *Billy the Kid* (Aaron Copland, 1938), *Charade* (Trude Rittmann, 1939), and *City Portrait* (Henry Brant, 1939). Even though *Juke Box* was based on Alec Wilder's previously written *Octets* (1939–1941) and not entirely new, the score was at least crafted from recently written music.

30. Tudor initially traveled to the United States to work with Ballet Theatre, a rival company to Kirstein's that formed in 1939. While in the United States, Tudor accepted Kirstein's commission to choreograph *Time Table* for the Ballet Caravan. It is not fully clear whether Kirstein or Tudor suggested using *Music for the Theatre* or whether they mutually decided on that particular score. The descriptions of the plot are from Kirstein's detailed scenario *Time Table* (*Good-Night and Goodbye*) held in the Ballet Society Collection, RG6, file 3134, Ballet Society Archives (BSA hereinafter).

31. Copland opted for the term "part" instead of "movement" in the subtitle of the piece, *Music for the Theatre: Suite in Five Parts*.

32. The characters and plot outlined in *Good-Night and Goodbye* shifted slightly in the final version of *Time Table*; the general emphasis on heterosexual pairs and the entrance of the two marines during the "Burlesque" remained intact. See the list of characters for both scenarios in Ballet Society Collection, RG6, file 3134, BSA.

33. Howard Pollack, *Aaron Copland: The Life and Work of an Uncommon Man* (New York: Henry Holt, 1999), 128.

34. Pollack, "The Dean of Gay American Composers," 40. According to Pollack, Copland "never tackled overtly homosexual themes in his work nor did he openly discuss the relations of his music to his sexuality," but Pollack maintains that "certain prominent aspects of Copland's work suggest the positive and liberating ways in which his music may have spoken, if not to a gay-exclusive audience, to a gay audience nonetheless." Also see Gayle Murchison, *The American Stravinsky: The Style and Aesthetics of Copland's New American Music, the Early Works, 1921–1938* (Ann Arbor: University of Michigan Press, 2012), 116–19.

35. Pollack, "The Dean of Gay American Composers," 41–42.

36. Martin Duberman, *The Worlds of Lincoln Kirstein* (New York: Alfred A. Knopf, 2007), 83–84.

37. For more on Gladys Bentley, see James Wilson, *Bulldaggers, Pansies, and Chocolate Babies: Performance, Race, and Sexuality in the Harlem Renaissance*

(Ann Arbor: University of Michigan Press, 2010), 154–91. Also see Shane Vogel, *The Scene of Harlem Cabaret: Race, Sexuality, Performance* (Chicago: University of Chicago Press, 2009).

38. Wilson, *Bulldaggers, Pansies, and Chocolate Babies*, 177.

39. Kirstein realized that his encounters with rough trade would not yield any long-lasting relationship, which he had begun to look for when he made the statement, "Streets full of sailors and marines. I keep my eyes neatly averted, forcing on myself what I know and have known too long to be true, that it's no use" (Duberman, *The Worlds of Lincoln Kirstein*, 227). For Kirstein, gas station attendants also fell into this category (ibid., 276).

40. In *Gay New York*, Chauncey points out that having sex with another person of the same gender did not necessarily mean that person was labeled as or even considered himself to be homosexual. He explains that a category of "normal" was applied to men who tended to be very masculine and played the "husband" role in any sexual situation; "normal" had little to do with being strictly heterosexual (Chauncey, *Gay New York*, 66–68).

41. Robert Sabin reviewed the restaging of this ballet in *Musical America*, February 1949. Quoted in Nancy Reynolds, *Repertory in Review* (New York: The Dial Press, 1977), 63–64.

42. This methodology of historical spectatorship and cross-reading is drawn from Manning, *Modern Dance, Negro Dance*, particularly pp. xix and 75–83. Film reviewers during this time avoided direct mention of homosexual content, believing that "talking about homosexuality would adversely influence readers." This type of self-censorship may have taken root among those writing about music, dance, and art, which means that reviewers failed to address homosexual content directly but would have appropriated effeminate terminology to hint at a non-heteronormative subtext. For more on film, production codes, and reviews, see, Chon Noriega, "'Something's Missing Here!': Homosexuality and Film Reviews during the Production Code Era, 1934–1962," *Cinema Journal* 30, no. 1 (Autumn 1990): 20–41.

43. Review in *The Hartford Courant*, January 7, 1938.

44. Marian Murray, "*Filling Station* Wins Acclaim Here in Presentation by Ballet Caravan," *Hartford Times*, January 7, 1938.

45. For more on US cultural diplomacy and the Ballet Caravan tour, see Jennifer L. Campbell, "Solidarity: Music, Diplomacy, and Inter-American Relations, 1936–1946" (PhD diss., University of Connecticut, 2010).

46. Ballet Society Collection, RG6, files 3124, 3129, 3131, and 3134, BSA.

47. For details, see "The American Ballet Caravan," [Report], no date, page 4, 10, folder 966, box 101, RG 4L (NAR/Personal Projects), Rockefeller Family Archive/Rockefeller Archive Collection (hereinafter RFA/RAC) and Letter to

Nelson Rockefeller from Lincoln Kirstein, July 2, 1941, folder 966, box 101, RG 4L (NAR/Personal Projects), RFA/RAC.

48. Letter to Nelson Rockefeller from Lincoln Kirstein, July 2, 1941, folder 966, box 101, RG 4L (NAR/Personal Projects), RFA/RAC.

49. Weinberg, *Speaking for Vice*, 19.

50. Whether this was merely malicious gossip is unknown, but complaints about Caffrey from a Cuban citizen and a clipping from the Cuban press reached Washington officials. For details, see Eric Paul Roorda, "McCarthyite in Camelot: The 'Loss' of Cuba, Homophobia, and the Otto Otepka Scandal in the Kennedy State Department," *Diplomatic History* 31 (2007): 733–35.

51. The concern over homosexuals in government positions festered, and by the 1950s the State Department was accused of harboring "sexual deviants," leading to an internal antigay campaign that resulted in hundreds of workers being investigated and fired. See David K. Johnson, *The Lavender Scare* (Chicago: University of Chicago Press, 2004), 65–77.

52. Nadine Hubbs, *The Queer Composition of America's Sound* (Berkeley: University of California Press, 2004), 67.

53. Horst Koegler, "Dancing in the Closet: The Coming Out of Ballet," *Dance Chronicle* 18, no. 2 (1995): 232.

54. One such example is musicologist Carol Oja's discussion of Jerome Robbins's ballet *Fancy Free*. The work has long been accepted as heteronormative and absent of homosexual undercurrent. Oja, however, re-examines *Fancy Free*, looking closely at Robbins's scenario, choreography, and personal life, as well as the cultural context of the wartime sailor character, and she argues that *Fancy Free* connotes recognizable albeit coded same-sex references alongside the dominant male–female plot. She writes, "*Fancy Free* gave those gay GIs at the Metropolitan Opera House a staged vision of their own lives by dramatizing a bar where hetero-and homosexual partnering happened in overlapping spheres." See Carol Oja, *Bernstein Meets Broadway: Collaborative Art in a Time of War* (Oxford: Oxford University Press, 2014), 20–32.

7

Queer Spaces in Anna Sokolow's *Rooms*

Hannah Kosstrin

In the opening of a dimly lit scene set by a melodic exchange between piano and trumpet, a woman passionately runs among a handful of empty chairs and visits an imaginary lover in each one. Losing herself in her fantasy, she grabs hold of her skirt as if tearing off her dress and pulsates her hips while her fingers rain down her sides. Seeking a warm body to quench her desire, the woman approaches an empty chair from behind; with a turning flourish she satisfyingly flops into it as she broadly fans one leg open and lands her wide-flung heel with a heavy thud. Digging the ball of her foot into the floor with repetitive friction that resonates in a rocking motion deep within her pelvis, she emits palpable sexual tension in a moment of rapture. These images compose "Escape," a solo in American modern dance choreographer Anna Sokolow's postwar dance *Rooms* (1954), a work about urban alienation, isolation, and sexual despair.[1] In pre-Stonewall New York, social codes and law enforcement that policed gay people's bodies and actions further contributed to experiences of marginalization. Gay men and lesbians necessarily exchanged public desire in nuanced cues, building sexual tension that they could later commence in private spaces—or generating longing that they could not satisfy by themselves. In the solo's climax, the performer creates a bed by rearranging two chairs to face each other, where she shares a rocking embrace with the chair's invisible inhabitant. Supine, she traces wide arcs with an extended bare leg as her dress falls aside. She loses herself in fulfilling intimacy before she realizes that she is alone, and she thrusts the chairs aside. Dancers and scholars associated with this solo have long assumed this woman desired a man. A queer reading of this dance disrupts its presumed heterosexuality and shows that by staging queer desire in a closeted society, Sokolow wrote gay people into the dominant narrative of the Cold War by exposing the plight of all who drowned in wells of loneliness.

Sokolow (1910–2000) made dances for social change that exposed humanity in brutal circumstances. A nine-year principal dancer for the Martha Graham Dance Company and a leader of the workers' dance movement in the 1930s, she became known for mid-century dances of alienation that spoke to a US generation reeling from World War II. Sokolow conveyed searing content through abstracted form, gaining a reputation for making dances that appeared universal while attending to specific content. She fought for humanity in specific contexts by using contemporary subjects instead of showing a universal pathos of humanity through traditional archetypes as Graham did. Sokolow departed from Graham's thematic material and choreographic methods, while building her own work from Graham's codified vocabulary. In *Rooms*, abdominal contractions from the Graham lexicon originate spasms of sexual energy and become chasms of sensuous longing.

Sokolow presented portraits of raw, unromantic, painfully sensual, nonnormative sexuality through *Rooms'* vignettes that showcase urbanites' psychological isolation. Focused around eight dancers in eight chairs that represent apartments in a tenement building, *Rooms* presents nine vignettes of loneliness and unfulfilled desire. Sokolow shaped this piece with students at the Actors' Studio in New York, premiered it in Mexico City in 1954, and first presented it in New York at the 92nd Street YM/YWHA on February 24, 1955. Kenyon Hopkins's experimental jazz score for five-piece band, at times driving, at times dissonant, reinforces postwar unease and typifies the dance's modernity. Sokolow used what she saw as irony in the music's syncopations to present the grit, not the glitz, of New York.[2] For Sokolow, the dance "reflects," she said, "the tiny, awful loneliness of people shut up in their rooms in a place like New York."[3] This loneliness reflects postwar discontent under society's affluent surface and presents the vulnerability of people on society's margins. The vignettes represent the people's fantasies, which differ starkly from their realities outside their apartments.[4] The *Rooms* suite includes "Alone," "The Dream," "Escape," "Going," "Desire," "Panic," "Daydream," "The End?" and the reprise of "Alone." The dance's casting was explicitly tied to performers' expressed gender; only in contemporary reconstructions does a woman perform a man's role, for example, due to casting needs. The music's dissonance and the movement's psychologically induced turmoil embody alienation. Thematic movements include dancers sliding the soles of their feet along the floor and digging in their heels, vulnerable staggered leg shapes accompanied by arched backs, and vibrating fingers that convey nervous tension. The dance's scenes reinforce the unity among these characters without necessarily pointing to their gendered realities.

The possibility that homosexuality undergirds *Rooms* struck me as I read the dance from Labanotation score. Labanotation, a twentieth-century movement notation system conceptually similar to music notation, provides a map for the inside of the dance through a staff with symbols that show where the body goes in space and time, and how to perform specific movements. A notator attends rehearsals and is privy to instructions a choreographer gives to dancers. Ray Cook, whose membership in Sokolow's company during the 1960s gave him additional kinesthetic insight into the inner workings of her dances, notated many of her works. His Labanotation scores include written motivational instructions to the dancers for performing the movement. These kinds of notes in his *Rooms* score of "Escape" gave me pause: "Running to your lover. She is so lovely" followed by "Your lover is flying in at the window."[5] Cook later insisted "She is so lovely" was a mistake in the text,[6] yet the congruence of phrasing raises questions about this otherwise heteronormative solo within an otherwise heteronormative dance. Is the male lover, then, lovely? Or does "she" instead refer to the soloist? A lover flying in at the window suggests images of objectified feminine *sylphides* or Vaslav Nijinsky in *Le Spectre de la Rose* that are hardly normatively masculine.[7] In the 1970s, Sokolow said this soloist "thinks she is Greta Garbo waiting for a lover to come in."[8] This image of Garbo, the iconic actress and lesbian idol who is believed to have had relationships with women as well as men, suggests the soloist awaits a female lover.[9] As an empowered subject instead of a passive object, moreover, this woman's power queers the space through sexuality that challenges gender hierarchies and enables lesbian desire, as she delineates her space through her interaction with her absent lovers instead of allowing them to define her. The more I watched *Rooms*, the queerer it appeared.

Taken with *Rooms'* "Desire" section, wherein one man's chair turned toward another's quietly denotes homosexual desire, the sapphically cryptic pieces of information in "Escape" reveal implicit gay, lesbian, and non-heteronormative themes in *Rooms*. In this essay, I site these queer spaces among a broader consideration of *Rooms* within the context of the 1950s Lavender Scare in the United States to show that gay people defined the mainstream even as social stigmas marginalized them from it. *Rooms'* inhabitants' discontent stems from sexual dissatisfaction and an inability to connect with other people. These experiences were homosexual as well as heterosexual, and queer through the empowered positions of performers as subjects in charge of their own desire and in creating spaces of absent lovers who may or may not be of same or opposite gender. In the following discussion, I situate analyses of *Rooms'* solos "Going" and "The End?" that resonate with narratives of closeting, and the explicit portrayal of sexual longing in the sections "Escape," "Desire," and "Panic" within a historical context for *Rooms* and the Lavender Scare to demonstrate how these vignettes embody gender discourse and Cold War rhetoric. The 1950s climate of fear, which included anticommunist, anti-Semitic, homophobic rhetoric as part of the Second Red Scare and the Lavender Scare, specifically implicated gay people in addition to suspected Communists.[10] Sokolow's repositioning of bodies, desire, and alienated angst in *Rooms* defied Cold War surveillance.

Rooms' positioning of its spectator as voyeur—through audience members peering into the private, vulnerable spaces of the characters' apartments—invites a queer reading by not explicitly defining how a spectator should watch this dance. I invoke here theater scholar Stacy Wolf's "lesbian" spectatorship specifically and queer spectatorship more generally to queerly read *Rooms*. In her reading of Mary Martin as Peter Pan, Wolf's lesbian spectator "[reads] actively, against the grain, and through desire."[11] Unlike the elusive lack of sexual desire associated with Martin's "tomboy" Peter Pan and historically in lesbian narratives, the "Escape" soloist, donning an evening gown with her long hair flowing, is frankly forthright in her intimate cravings.[12] Although her sensuality easily reads as heteronormative, I read this solo against the grain as one that is sexually non-normative through the openly powerful sexual control the soloist portrays. In this and other *Rooms* vignettes, the dancers' perceived genders signify larger themes related to their onstage power, yet summoning dance scholar Jane Desmond's model for a queer framework that upends the centrality of concert dance's heteronormative assumptions complicates these significations beyond a one-to-one relationship of desire.[13] I further take gender theorist Teresa de Lauretis's tack of "queer" as a marker of critical distance to highlight non-heteronormative women's experience manifest in *Rooms'* vignettes, from women in charge of their own sexuality to making visible lesbian and gay male spaces, and dance scholar Suzanne Juhasz's use of "queer" as a verb that subverts gender conventions.[14] While queer discourses often privilege male experience, and *Rooms'* overt presentation of male homosexual desire reinforces lesbian invisibility, the centrality of women's experience to Sokolow's dance opens a space for all kinds of female desire wherein invisible queer(ed) women's spaces become visible.[15] A queer reading of *Rooms* points to moments ripe for queer spectatorship and also to instances of non-normative heterosexuality that reposition *Rooms'* function within early Cold War politics.

Sokolow embedded *Rooms'* queer codes within dominant recognizable tropes that aligned with cultural narratives of the time. These include Sloan Wilson's 1955 novel *The Man in the Gray Flannel Suit*, which presented a private postwar psychological vulnerability. The dance also connects back through time to Radclyffe Hall's 1928 novel *The Well of Loneliness*. This story was part of lesbian currency with feelings of societal exclusion for being queer, and its narrative aligned in time with the tenement houses of Sokolow's youth on which she based *Rooms*. Instead of rejecting it as deviant, critics embraced *Rooms* as dark but nonetheless universal, thus covertly accepting these queer spaces into mainstream representation and enabling their inhabitants to define the society that otherwise excluded them.

My interest in opening this discussion stems not solely from gay-coded moments in "Escape" and "Desire" but also in how Sokolow subverted contemporary expectations for gendered and sexualized bodies onstage. Sokolow was known for dating men and I have found no evidence to the contrary. Yet, *Rooms* encompasses a larger upset of normative gender expectations based on Sokolow's life choices and dances that do just that: she never married her romantic partners and she performed solos, such as *Case History No.—* (1937), *Lament for the Death of a Bullfighter* (1941), and *Kaddish* (1945), wherein she took on the power of men's roles and significations that challenged social conventions and subverted onstage gender hierarchies.[16] Moreover, as music theorist Nadine Hubbs notes in her study of gay modernist composers whose music defined American nationalism at mid-century, "for pre-Stonewall homosexual subjects to defy the dominant culture's paramount message to them—that they should not exist—was the most crucial form of queer social resistance."[17] *Rooms* is thus a site of social resistance because its characters exist and are not necessarily marked as queer: queerness is part of, not outside of, the generalized experience that Sokolow portrayed in this dance.

This kind of queer reading activates how the reputation of an established dance like *Rooms*, known for reflecting society, can reframe spectators' historically informed expectations. The social climate around *Rooms* has changed since its premiere, and its contemporary reception rubs against long-held associations with the dance wherein the abstracted movement dictates the meaning and negates markings of marginal themes. I conduct choreographic analysis to make meaning of the work at its premiere and how it has changed through time, and I cull information from varied sources to generate a full picture of the dance. I gather information about *Rooms* from the Labanotation score, film of the dance, dancers' reflections performing the piece, and critical response of the dance from the 1950s to 1960s. I also work from live performances of *Rooms*, and a studio session with Suellen Haag of the Sokolow

Dance Foundation, who coached my students in "Escape" and "The End?" which they staged from the Labanotation score. Cultural changes in US society around the dance initiate new readings of it. My reading of *Rooms* as a queer text does not displace the interpretations of the dance that circulated in the years before the Stonewall rebellion, second-wave feminism, and the gay liberation movement; rather, it amplifies these earlier interpretations by revealing the continued resonance of the work for dancers and spectators who came of age with different assumptions about gender and sexuality than informed Sokolow's generation and the generations of *Rooms'* first casts.[18]

Rooms and the Cold War

Rooms destabilizes normative representations of homo- and heterosexual desire within the 1950s cultural milieu of normalcy and the postwar choreographic tension that dance scholar Gay Morris defines as a "game for dancers," with movement that appeared to be only about itself instead of social critique so as to distract attention within an era of surveillance.[19] Postwar modern dance in the United States portrayed archetypal themes and emotions through abstracted movements that were perceived as universal. Choreographers drew many of these elements from the technical and compositional instruction of their mentors, who included Graham, Doris Humphrey, Katherine Dunham, Lester Horton, Hanya Holm, and Charles Weidman. *Rooms'* social statements stand out against other postwar choreography, such as that of Alwin Nikolais (who trained with Holm) and Merce Cunningham (who trained with Graham and with ballet choreographer George Balanchine), gay choreographers who arguably deflected spectators' interests in their personal lives with objective, abstracted choreography that denied fleshy coupling of any kind.[20] Similarly to the composition of Nikolais's and Cunningham's companies, Sokolow employed dancers who were highly trained, mostly in the Graham technique she taught coupled with elements of the Stanislavsky Method of Physical Action to draw movements from their own experiences. Dissimilarly to Nikolais's and Cunningham's choreography, Sokolow drew *Rooms'* movements from quotidian gestures and behaviors. This artistic choice cemented the dance in a gritty present that dance historian Rebekah Kowal points to as something that makes Sokolow's "ordinary" actions extraordinary through the specific, realistic struggles they convey.[21] As Sokolow challenged modern dance conventions in *Rooms*, a queer reading of *Rooms* requires pushing against the grain not only of the work's presumed heteronormativity but also against the hegemony of universality in postwar modern dance.[22]

The closet and modern dance's claims to be apolitical moved together in the Cold War. The postwar modern dance community and its dance critics, who counted significant numbers of gays, lesbians, Communists, and sympathizers in its ranks, protected its members while deflecting suspicions. This support included critic Gertrude Lippincott's 1946 call for apolitical abstract expressionism in dance the same year the US Congress reinstated the House Un-American Activities Committee (HUAC),[23] and critic Margaret Lloyd's assertion in her 1949 *Borzoi Book of Modern Dance* that though there were once left-wingers, "There are no reds in modern dance today."[24] Through their writing, critics shielded dancers amidst the panic that intertwined the Second Red Scare and the Lavender Scare. Nevertheless, the Lavender Scare's infiltrating fear caused dancers and choreographers to cover their identities. The dance world protected the "open secret" of homosexuality in its ranks, "while," as dance historian Susan Manning notes, "granting gay men and lesbians full citizenship and often leadership within the profession."[25]

Due to a shift in Sokolow's choreographic process, her dancers' actual experiences—homo- and heterosexual—contributed to the work's creation. After she stopped performing in the early 1950s from a chronic back injury, Sokolow relied on the Stanislavsky Method to build nonlinear narratives based on character studies for which the performers drew upon their own lives. Sokolow asked questions in rehearsal such as, "How does it feel to be near someone who is not there?" to generate movement material.[26] Although they were not credited as such at the time, the dancers' individual experiences became part of the larger work. While later in her life Sokolow claimed that each of the eight dancers represented facets of herself,[27] the onstage personalities presented a wider range of knowledge based on what the dancers brought to the piece.

Even though *Rooms* put forth a spectrum of sexual desire that was otherwise marginalized at the time, critics' laudations after the US premiere suggest that they supported its cry against an oppressive society of which repressed desire was an unmentionable part. Critics spoke in generalized terms about the dance's theme of sexual loneliness and its overall darkness. In *Dance Observer*, George Beiswanger described the work as a contemporary hell, while in the *New York Times* John Martin asserted that *Rooms*' "ultimate aim seems to be to induce you to jump as inconspicuously as possible into the nearest river," yet Doris Hering noted in *Dance Magazine* that "underlying its bleakest moments is the current of human generosity."[28] Although Sokolow portrayed a dismal experience, the piece retains an element of hope. Assessing the critics' reaction at the premiere, Morris connects this public embrace of *Rooms* with the dance's understood universality: "Audiences perceived in its alienation an essential element of modernity. As such, *Rooms* proved to be one of the rare instances in the 1950s when a dance of devastating critique was acknowledged as successful, even if its full implications were deflected."[29] One of these averted implications is that *Rooms* veiled individual identities within the larger climate of fear.

The Lavender Scare, which drove *Rooms'* inhabitants' anxiety, began in 1947 in what historian David K. Johnson defines as a systematic firing of suspected homosexuals from the State Department and subsequent witch hunt of gay men and lesbians inside Washington, DC in the name of national security. Gay people became scapegoats through the rhetoric of mapping Communism through their bodies. The discourse of the Lavender Scare was that gay people were morally and ideologically weak and posed a risk of leaking state secrets— and thus, as Johnson notes, they "needed to be systematically removed from the federal government."[30] Government hearings pitted gay men and lesbians against each other with pressure to name names in proceedings that mirrored hearings of suspected Communists. Gay people were no safer within the gay community than in mainstream society.[31] Historian John D'Emilio avers the conspiracy associated with gays and lesbians stems from the fear that since homosexuality is not necessarily marked on the body, gays and lesbians could invisibly infiltrate public institutions; within the discourse, no one was safe from gay people's stealthy, morally weak, highly sexualized bodies. Since the 1948 Kinsey report noted that a large percentage of American men were likely homosexual, and a large percentage of government workers fired in the 1950s on moral grounds were assumed homosexual, the penetrable homosexual body vulnerable to the Communist threat could permeate society.[32]

The voyeurism embedded in *Rooms* reproduces this government surveillance and anxiety within the space of the performance.[33] *Rooms'* solos "Going" (the fourth vignette) and "The End?" (the penultimate section) present ostracized individuals pressured to the end of their wits. Many gay people killed themselves during the Lavender Scare, when more homosexuals than Communists lost their government jobs.[34] The quiet suffering of gay men and lesbians closeted during the 1950s' suffocating climate of fear resonates in the feelings of isolated individuals Sokolow evoked with these solos. Within the postwar-influenced universality of this modern dance work, these characters' onstage fears reflect everyone's anxieties. Thinking about these Cold War gay suicides through dance instead of through empirical evidence or historical anecdote allows for a kinesthetic empathy that implicates its viewers in these characters' social and physical suicides. By distressing audiences, perhaps to rethink their own place in society, *Rooms* continues Sokolow's quest to enact social change through dance.

In "Going," a man fights—and loses to—a society in which he can never relax. He moves as if he does not have enough air to breathe. Jack Moore remembered that Sokolow coached him to perform the role as a prize fighter who could not win against the world.[35] In 1955 critic Walter Terry asserted the need for escapism when he wrote in the *New York Herald Tribune* that the dancer "soon becomes 'real gone' as he submits to hypnotic, self-mesmerizing rhythms of jazz."[36] Here, the music's syncopations represent restless unease. Indeed, Cook's motivational notes in the Labanotation score assert, "The more gone he is, the sadder it is."[37] The music, which until this section consists of a lonely trumpet against pounding drums of varying intensity, shifts to an orchestration reminiscent of big band swing with a quickly syncopating snare drum. The dancer retains a nervous resiliency in his joints, intermittently yet defiantly clapping his hands as if to snap us all out of his nightmare. He perches, twitters uneasily, quickly crosses and uncrosses his legs, twists his ankles and knees along jagged pathways performing the "shorty George," and boxes an invisible opponent. He is cornered; he never relaxes. He slides across the floor, seeking places to hide. He is alone in his room or hiding in an alley. Is he plotting something? Do his movements reveal feelings that belie his normative baseball jacket? Even at the end, when he sits on the floor and drops his arms more in exhaustion than relief, he remains tense.[38] The character's need to "become gone" and to lose himself in the privacy of his apartment—through music, drugs, or alcohol—displays his buckling under social pressures.

With similar feelings of desperation, in "The End?" a woman on the rooftop is driven to suicide with abrupt, aggressive, and self-destructive movement. Her vibratory fingers evoke the senseless chatter of a world closing in on her. She pulls and tears at her own face, chokes herself, thrusts her torso forward and back, and blindly throws herself forward over her chair. In the stark musical score a snare drum rasps sharply, but intermittently, and a trumpet screams, scolding yet foreshadowing. The soloist's pain manifests in deep dips of her head backward that expose the vulnerable angles of her neck. In a moment of silence, the dancer reaches skyward before falling in a heap on the ground with a sickening empty thud—twice. The last moment is eerily tranquil: the dancer, having gingerly climbed up onto the chair as if on a ledge, serenely moves her arms up and down, navigating an otherworldly ether. This upsetting but oddly peaceful image makes this woman's suffering visible while engaging the audience as witness to her death.

Queer Desires

The heart of *Rooms* beats in the fierce longing of rhythmic heel slides in the central section "Desire," paired with the unanswered, aching twists through the spine with arms grappling for someone to love them back (figure 7.1).

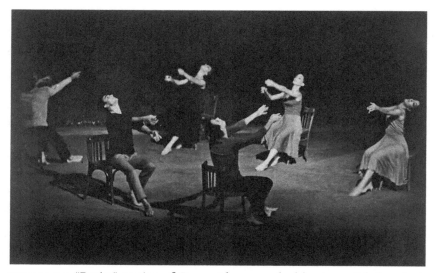

FIGURE 7.1 "Desire" section of *Rooms* (choreographed by Anna Sokolow, Lyric Theatre premiere 1963). Photographer unknown. Dancers include Moshe Romano, Avraham Tzuri, Yanun Neeman, Dahlia Harlap, Liora Hackmey, and Ze'eva Cohen. From the Collection of the Israeli Dance Archive at the Beit Ariela Library, Tel-Aviv.

In this vignette's explicit sexual desperation—"God damn it, why doesn't someone make love to me?" a motivational note in the Labanotation score cries—a mix of gendered couplings and overt sexual displays disrupts postwar dominant narratives of love and kinship.[39] In *Rooms*, women desire as much as men; while both are lonely, neither seem particularly available. "Desire" features three men and three women seated in facing rows of chairs sharply angled through the middle of the stage. They perform myriad presentations of overt, almost masturbatory, sexual cravings. Discourses of normative sexuality in the 1950s dictated gender roles for women to be driven by their emotions, dependent upon men, and sexually available to them but not sexually aggressive, and for men to be rational and emotionally aloof, which displayed social strength.[40] "Desire" portrays just the opposite. Through full-body pleadings and pulsing leg gestures that originate in the groin and desperately dig the heel into the floor, all with a gaze that is more self-deprecating than aggressively sexual, Sokolow staged raw, unromantic sexuality during an era that tempered women's public presentation of sensuality.

Sokolow reorganized modern dance conventions of gender presentation beyond her upending of the sexual longing people could express onstage. "Desire" counters popular theatrical heterosexual coupling in what Manning terms "mythic abstraction" in Martha Graham's and José Limón's archetypal narratives that covered over queer subjectivities.[41] By fitting dancers into clearly delineated heterosexual romantic roles, Graham's and Limón's dances portrayed a heteronormative status quo even if the dancers performing these roles were gay. With its raw desire and its portrayal of, according to Kowal, "typical people in recognizable situations," *Rooms* contrasts Graham's and Limón's chaste, abstracted epic choreographies.[42] Through offering an alternative to heteronormative mythic narrative, *Rooms* upsets mid-century modernism in many ways beyond its non-normative sexuality, with a non-sequential series of vignettes built on character studies instead of an archetypal chronology, movements built from everyday postures and gestures instead of an abstracted movement vocabulary, and a portrayal of the people next door instead of a satisfying and exotic mythic journey. *Rooms'* characters, as well as the audience, want an escape.

"Desire" highlights queer, more than normative, yearning. This begins, but does not end, with the facing of the man in the middle toward the downstage man instead of the woman opposite him to imply homosexual longing.[43] His craving sets the tone for the section: with a piercing gaze at the downstage man, he first slides his heels in silence and the others join when the music begins. While, according to Ze'eva Cohen, who performed *Rooms* during the 1960s, Sokolow never discussed this moment of homosexual desire with the cast, it seems to be an open secret among dancers who know this work.[44] A handful of gay men I have encountered who performed *Rooms* under Sokolow's direction report being cast in this role. Whether these men's experiences reflect a necessity for blurring the boundaries between art and life for a gay man to perform this role or whether it is coincidence remains unclear. Regardless of Sokolow's intent or the rehearsal room culture, this moment invites queer spectatorship by explicitly staging homosexual desire, as opposed to the implicit homosexuality in the dance's other vignettes.

The further-unfolding gay-coded movements in "Desire" disrupt heteronormative assumptions more deeply than the man with the turned chair. As the dancers lie supine in heterosexual pairs, two women end up next to each other. They all blindly reach for each other in space, sensuously undulate as they rise and return to the floor, and hug their knees in vulnerable, frustrated moments. Failing contact, the dancers rock back and forth, cupping their bodies in long contractions. The most upstage woman couples, pausing, with the woman of the middle pair who also swings with the man to her downstage side. While arguably this moment could be interpreted as lonely people experiencing universal longing, the significance of the gendered casting of this dances' roles, the silence of these two women connecting, and the fact that a viewer could easily miss this brief moment amidst the activity, renders this instance of lesbian desire barely visible. When the dancers reprise the heel slides, all but the original "gay" man pause, foregrounding his yearning against the rest.

Even though the spectator observes people in their apartments, these people in turn look inward on themselves and prevent a pleasurable return of the voyeuristic gaze. Critic Clive Barnes noted as much when he wrote in 1967, "The voyeur's eye view that Miss Sokolow offers us is not elevating but is salutary. No one could ever enjoy *Rooms*, but they might be all the better for being horrified by it."[45] These layers of looking produce a subjectivity for *Rooms'* inhabitants in which they expose, yet deflect the gaze of, their vulnerability. In the harrowing final image of "Desire," the dancers stand on their chairs with hollowed-out chests, hunched shoulders, limbs succumbing to gravity, and bodies rotating as if swaying in a gentle breeze. They appear to have hanged themselves to escape their pained and unquenchable needs. This shared fate envelops the dancers' differentiated desires into similar marginalization.

Lesbian Longing: Alone but not Lonely

If an absent lover does not have to be assumed to be of opposite gender to the desire-er, and if this absence can be productive, the "Desire" section of *Rooms* on which the full work pivots destabilizes the heteronormativity of postwar alienation instead of reinforcing it. In questioning a causal relationship between gender and sexuality in terms of identification and desire, gender theorist Judith Butler asserts, "The heterosexual logic that requires that identification and desire be mutually exclusive is one of the most reductive of heterosexism's psychological instruments: if one identifies *as* a given gender, one must desire a different gender."[46] The universality associated with *Rooms* manifests Butler's assertion: with the exception of the man in the turned chair, the dancers are assumed to desire members of the opposite gender because their lovers are absent. Spectators have traditionally considered this man gay because the man toward whom he reaches physically fills the space to confirm his yearning. Yet, an absent lover can also denote queer desire. Dance theorist Valerie Briginshaw argues that since dances with lesbian content exist outside heterosexual binary assumptions of self and other, a space created by an absent lover is a reciprocal partner in the desire and renders these women's desire productive instead of a lack.[47] She asserts: "space, desire and bodies need to be rethought as reciprocally productive, that is they continually produce and are produced by each other."[48] This productivity supports Terry's 1955 critical assertion that *Rooms* is about aloneness (a productive filling of the space) instead of loneliness (a desiring lack within the space): Terry aptly described *Rooms'* suite of dances as "examples of aloneness," so that not all who are alone are necessarily lonely.[49]

Two other solos, "Escape" and "Panic," reframe heteronormative expectations about desire through ambiguous or absent lovers. Both feature one chair set apart from four. The empty chairs of "Escape" offer space for queer reception through their co-production of desire, while the defined presence of the people in the chairs of "Panic" suggest relationships that take on many meanings. While in "Escape" the empty chairs only hold what is in the dancer's memory and imagination, in "Panic" four people fill the chairs, each staring placidly into space. In "Escape" the single chair is the space of reality and the four chairs are fantasy; in "Panic," the single chair offers solace and the four chairs present inescapable reality. In "Escape," the woman's illusion, or the reality that she cannot have it, disappoints her; in "Panic," a world full of real people with whom the man cannot communicate chokes his fantasies.

"Escape" retains its long-associated heteronormativity in the way dancers and coaches pass it down. When Ray Cook told me that the "Escape" in-score direction "Running to your lover. She is so lovely," is a mistake, and further that this dance has no lesbian undertones, I became skeptical about this dance's legacy.[50] Based on reported evidence, the "Escape" soloist generally desires men; the front matter of the notation score notes her interest in men, and Cohen remembered that in her performance of the fantasy she was glamorous and desired by many men.[51] In her coaching session with my students in October 2011, Suellen Haag took into account the fact that the all-women cast might themselves imagine a lover of various genders in the chair opposite them, yet it was clear from her coaching that the prescribed gender of the absent lover was male. The absence of a physical lover allows flexibility for the individual dancer to imagine any form of lover, and this freedom should apply to the spectator as well. As "Desire" portrays gay men's yearning, "Escape" enables lesbian desire.

What is perhaps more subversive about this solo, however, is the power and control that the soloist possesses over her own sensuality. As Cohen recalled, she is loved in the way that she wants to be loved, and desired in the way that she wants to be desired.[52] Moreover, Briginshaw notes, in lesbian-defined concert dance spaces, women as both subject and object control the voyeuristic gaze.[53] The raw moments of pleasure and pain in this solo, paired with a sexually empowered woman with her unidentified lover, create a queer space of sexual strength. The woman's disillusionment at the end of the vignette when she leaves the fantasy to face reality may be one of a lover scorned, and it may also engage her resentment of not being able to have such a relationship, with another woman, in the public space outside her private apartment.

Unlike the empowered spaces and absent lovers of "Escape," the people in "Panic" define the space with their presence. The movement and sound score for this section are stark and desperate. In his personal hell, the "Panic" soloist runs frantically among the people in the chairs, at once afraid that they will see him and frustrated that they do not. He takes solace in his set-apart chair, onto which he grasps as he kicks his legs like an ensnared rodent, before hiding his face behind his hands. Who are these people, and why does the soloist feel trapped? Are they lovers, friends, a wife or family who would not understand? After the soloist spins in painfully tiny circles, falling and repeatedly banging his head against the floor, the people in the chairs leave one by one. This deep-seated panic has dire consequences. Literally alone onstage at the end of the section, the soloist covers his face in anguish. Did his honesty drive everyone he loved away? Or did they refuse to see him for who he really is? With labored breathing, he bolts across the stage and grabs onto an empty chair, which previously held the man who was the last to leave. The lingering of this now-absent man suggests that he was the most significant person for the "Panic" soloist; he takes on the role of the desired man in "Desire." Was he a closeted lover? His new absence suggests that he slipped through the soloist's fingers. The soloist's desperate grabs for the empty chair vacated by a physical (instead of imaginary) man suggest that perhaps his panic is not just the pressure of postwar unease but also the fear of being outed, of losing the ones he loves, or the pain of being unable to honestly converse with the people around him.

Quite possibly, the people in *Rooms* and especially the soloist in "Panic" no longer felt welcome within their own community. The tangible fear in "Panic" reflected resulting behavior from the Lavender Scare's queer surveillance. Stigmatized public presence of homosexuals as "sexual perverts" featured prominently in newspaper articles during this time, and writers clearly coded the language in these discussions for all 1950s readers.[54] The 1950s also saw the beginnings of the homophile movement, which, as precursor to the gay liberation movement, worked to combat discrimination against gays and lesbians.[55] Groups like the Mattachine Society and the Daughters of Bilitis formed with the goals of creating a sense of gay pride within a national subculture. By bringing gay activism into the public sphere, these groups upset the divide between the underground (though subject to frequent police raids) spaces of gay subculture in bars, drag clubs, and private parties, and the homophobic mainstream. Mid-1950s tensions increased between the young activist movement and the long-standing gay bar culture, as the homophile groups further aligned themselves with mainstream US values by insisting their members dress and act like members of the heteronormative white middle class.[56] The shifting spaces of this gay community, with assimilationist actions necessary for political change that further marginalized non-conforming gender expression, paired with homophobic and racist rhetoric, intensified social pressures for those people, as in *Rooms*, who felt doubly alienated.

These anxieties came to a head in "Panic," where Sokolow reproduced the frenzied, irrational-feeling fear of being caught. For critic Beiswanger, "Panic" is unbearable. He exclaimed in 1957, "Dante perceived no hell, as *Rooms* does, in 'Panic,' the bottomless pit of total insecurity and its terror into which the 'untouchable' are callously thrust. Dante envisioned the love-lost but not the unloved."[57] *Rooms'* queer spaces surface in Beiswanger's review. Gay people were among the US's "untouchables" in the 1950s, and significantly, many men who performed this solo—including Alvin Ailey, Jeff Duncan, and Paul Sanasardo—were gay. The social undercurrent generated by the homophile movement's work to cultivate a national subculture, along with and via Sokolow's choreographic practice of drawing from the dancers' own experiences to create their characters, entered *Rooms*. "Panic" thus lives up to its name.

In challenging Cold War social hierarchies, *Rooms* revealed the insecurity of living under tight social and government surveillance wherein non-normative actions and associations had dire consequences. Juhasz has noted about British choreographer Matthew Bourne's 1995 queer re-envisioning of *Swan Lake*, wherein the swan *corps* of men becomes a metaphor for a yearning to feel safe within one's identity, that "the viewer is compelled to struggle over the real/not real issue clearly mimics the situation of queer spaces in everyday life."[58] In Bourne's *Swan Lake*, the swans provide an imaginary haven with real-world and dangerous implications; similarly, the socially constructed closet of queer life offers a kind of security by masking queer identity and actions from those outside the queer community. *Rooms* contains this struggle: it presents imagery combining reality and fantasy, or outwardly manifesting characters' inner feelings and fears. There is not one prescribed way to perform any of Sokolow's dances in terms of motivation. Although Ze'eva Cohen imagined men in the "Escape" chairs, another dancer could have imagined women. Similarly, not all dancers who performed "Panic" were gay. Sokolow's despairing vignettes strike chords of empathy and self-identification for spectators. Due to the perceived universalism in the movement, audience members who were not otherwise alienated by the work likely identified with it, whether they felt the clammy fear of "Panic," or awaited their "Escape" woman to come home.

The lack of defined lovers in "Escape," "Desire," or "Panic" provides a broader spectrum of possible interpretations of this yearning. These spaces in *Rooms*, queer through their signified desire and subverted gendered and sexualized norms, spite the Lavender Scare's threats by enveloping the Cold War's "untouchables" into a universalized experience. Since proponents of red and lavender fear-mongering linked homosexuality and Communism within its rhetoric, it is further remarkable that Sokolow chose to showcase images of so-called "deviant" sexuality when she herself was under close FBI scrutiny for her own Communist activities.[59] Back in the "Escape" apartment, the soloist cannot sustain her fantasy of freely loving and being loved in return. Lacking the satisfaction of fleshy comfort with a tangible lover, the woman leaves her fantasy and returns to grip the back of a single chair, where she stands staring into empty space, as if into a mirror or out a window onto the stifling street. *Rooms'* ambiguous lovers and universal frame enabled Sokolow to make direct, though coded, political statements in this environment. As *Rooms* embodied early Cold War sentiments with movement that was explicit but nevertheless about itself, so too did *Rooms'* queer outsiders define the mainstream.

Postscript

On June 18, 2016, I stood outside Sokolow's last apartment at One Christopher Street, just steps from the Stonewall Inn in the heart of New York City's old gay neighborhood. It was less than a week after a gunman killed forty-nine people and injured fifty-three others at a gay nightclub in Orlando, Florida. By turning around I could take in the street sign naming that end of the block Anna Sokolow Way, her building, and the banners announcing the upcoming Pride holiday. The neighborhood memorials for the Orlando victims resonated with the history of violence against the gay community and a resolve that rang from Stonewall through the area. Sokolow made *Rooms* more than ten years before the Stonewall rebellion, and twenty years before she moved to Christopher Street. In both acts she staked her allegiance to the gay community, first by enabling gays and lesbians to define quotidian Americanness, and second by residing in the gay neighborhood. Knowing red-baiting firsthand as a communist Jew, Sokolow was an ally in a time when allies were scarce. She drew from her proletarian roots to inhabit queer spaces in solidarity, enacting coalition on and off the stage. Sokolow's work distinguished its own place in queer history by enacting queerness within a homophobic environment.

Acknowledgments

Thank you to my colleagues in the 2012 Andrew W. Mellon Foundation Summer Seminar "Dance Studies in/and the Humanities," Reed College's 2012 summer faculty research group, and Susan Manning for feedback on earlier versions of this essay. Many thanks to Clare Croft for her generous feedback. Research was supported by The Ohio State University Melton Center for Jewish Studies and Department of Dance, the P.E.O. International Sisterhood, and Reed College.

Notes

1. For this description of *Rooms*, I consulted the following: Anna Sokolow, *Rooms*, WNET/New York, directed by Jac Venza and performed by Anna Sokolow Dance Company (1966), Sokolow Dance Foundation; Anna Sokolow, *Rooms*, VHS, performed by Contemporary Dance System (1975), Collection of Dance Notation Bureau Extension Office, The Ohio State University; Anna Sokolow, *Rooms*, VHS, performed by Juilliard Dance Ensemble (1976-1977), Collection of Dance Library of Israel; Anna Sokolow, *Rooms*, performed by José Limón Dance Company, *Anna Sokolow's Rooms: The Centennial Celebration*, presented by José Limón Dance Foundation, Inc., February 9, 2010, Baryshnikov Arts Center, New York City; *Reedies Read Rooms*, performed by Reed College Dance Department, October 28–29 and November 4–5, 2011, Reed College, Portland, OR; *Dancing History: Anna Sokolow's Rooms*, performed by Stanford University Dance Division, February 9, 2012, Stanford University, Stanford, CA; and Anna Sokolow, *Rooms*, notated by Ray Cook, 1967–1975 and 1983 (New York, Dance Notation Bureau, 1980; repr., 2003).

2. Anna Sokolow, quoted in Jean Battey, "The Dance—Choreographer Works Slippers Off Dancers," *The Washington Post*, January 18, 1967, n.p., Alan M. and Sali Ann Kriegsman Collection, Music Division, Library of Congress, Washington, DC (hereinafter MD, LOC). In my larger project, I show how *Rooms* is a site of Jewishness, Communism, and queerness, and how Sokolow's use of Africanist elements in the movement and the music reinforced her connection to Americanization.

3. Anna Sokolow, quoted in Doris Hering, "My Roots are Here," *Dance Magazine*, June 1955, 36.

4. Jack Moore, interview by Larry Warren, April 11, 1987, transcript, 3, Larry Warren Collection.

5. *Rooms*, notated by Cook, 50.

6. Ray Cook (dancer and notator) in conversation with the author, July 2, 2011.

7. In the title role of *Le Spectre de la Rose* (1911), Nijinsky donned a pink rose-petal bodysuit and visited a dreaming woman by ethereally entering and exiting through a window. Michel Fokine's choreography here referenced *La Sylphide* (1832), wherein a *sylph*, the enticing spirit of a half-dead girl, magically enters and exits through a fireplace to tempt the male protagonist as he sleeps. Nijinsky also became a queer icon in the twentieth century.

8. Anna Sokolow, quoted in Larry Warren, *Anna Sokolow: The Rebellious Spirit* (Princeton, NJ: Princeton Book Company, 1991), 150. José Luis Reynoso cites this passage when he argues for a socialist feminist reading of Sokolow's work, and specifically for homosexual themes in *Rooms* and *Poem*. Reynoso avers that due to the lack of a physical lover, the "Escape" soloist could desire a man or a woman. José Luis Reynoso, "Some Constitutive Processes in Shifting Feminist Subjectivities: Anna Sokolow in the First Half of the Twentieth Century," paper presented at "Dance Studies and Global Feminisms," annual meeting of Congress on Research in Dance, Hollins University, Roanoke, VA, November 14, 2008.

9. See Rodger Streitmatter, *Outlaw Marriages: The Hidden Histories of Fifteen Extraordinary Same-Sex Couples* (Boston: Beacon Press, 2012), 87–97.

10. See David K. Johnson, *The Lavender Scare: The Cold War Persecution of Gays and Lesbians in the Federal Government* (Chicago: University of Chicago Press, 2004); John D'Emilio, *Sexual Politics, Sexual Communities: The Making of a Homosexual Minority in the United States, 1940–1970,* 2d ed. (1983; repr., Chicago: University of Chicago Press, 1998); and Nan Alamilla Boyd, *Wide Open Town: A History of Queer San Francisco to 1965* (Berkeley: University of California Press, 2003). For the 1950s social climate, see Ellen Schrecker, *The Age of McCarthyism: A Brief History with Documents,* 2d ed. (Boston: Bedford/St. Martin's, 2002); David Halberstam, *The Fifties* (New York: Fawcett Columbine, 1993); and Haynes Johnson, *The Age of Anxiety: McCarthyism to Terrorism* (Orlando, FL: Harcourt, 2006).

11. Stacy Wolf, "'Never Gonna Be a Man/Catch Me if You Can/I Won't Grow Up': A Lesbian Account of Mary Martin's Peter Pan," *Theatre Journal* 49, no. 4 (1997): 495.

12. See Wolf, "'Never Gonna Be a Man,'" 499–500, 508.

13. Jane C. Desmond, "Introduction—Making the Invisible Visible: Staging Sexualities through Dance," in *Dancing Desires: Choreographing Sexualities On & Off the Stage,* ed. Jane C. Desmond (Madison: University of Wisconsin Press, 2001), 11.

14. Teresa de Lauretis, "Queer Theory: Lesbian and Gay Sexualities—An Introduction," *differences: A Journal of Feminist Cultural Studies* 3, no. 2 (1991): iv; and Suzanne Juhasz, "Queer Swans: Those Fabulous Avians in the *Swan Lakes* of Les Ballets Trockadero and Matthew Bourne," *Dance Chronicle* 31, no. 1 (2008): 58–59.

15. See Judith Butler, *Gender Trouble: Feminism and the Subversion of Identity* (1990; repr. New York and London: Routledge, 2006); Judith Butler, *Bodies that Matter: On the Discursive Limits of "Sex"* (New York: Routledge, 1993); Desmond, "Introduction—Making the Invisible Visible," 3–32; George Chauncey, *Gay New York: Gender, Urban Culture, and the Making of the Gay Male World 1890–1940* (New York: Basic Books, 1994); Lisa Duggan, *Sapphic Slashers: Sex, Violence, and American Modernity* (Durham, NC: Duke University Press, 2000); and de Lauretis, "Queer Theory," iii–xviii.

16. See Hannah Kosstrin, "Inevitable Designs: Anna Sokolow's Proletarian Dances," *Dance Research Journal* 45, no. 2 (2013): 5–23; and *"Kaddish* at the Wall: The Long Life of Anna Sokolow's 'Prayer for the Dead,'" in *Dance on Its Own Terms: Histories and Methodologies*, ed. Melanie Bales and Karen Eliot (New York: Oxford University Press, 2013), 255–81.

17. Nadine Hubbs, *The Queer Composition of America's Sound: Gay Modernists, American Music, and National Identity* (Berkeley: University of California Press, 2004), 94.

18. Thank you to Susan Manning for helping me articulate this idea.

19. Gay Morris, *A Game for Dancers: Performing Modernism in the Postwar Years, 1945–1960* (Middletown, CT: Wesleyan University Press, 2006).

20. See Susan Leigh Foster, "Closets Full of Dances: Modern Dance's Performance of Masculinity and Sexuality," in *Dancing Desires: Choreographing Sexualities On & Off the Stage*, ed. Jane C. Desmond (Madison: University of Wisconsin Press, 2001), 147–207; Susan Manning, *Modern Dance, Negro Dance: Race in Motion* (Minneapolis: University of Minnesota Press, 2004); and Rebekah Kowal, "Being Motion: Alwin Nikolais' Queer Objectivity," in *The Returns of Alwin Nikolais: Bodies, Boundaries, and the Dance Canon*, ed. Claudia Gitelman and Randy Martin (Middletown, CT: Wesleyan University Press, 2007), 82–106.

21. Rebekah Kowal, *How to Do Things with Dance: Performing Change in Postwar America* (Middletown, CT: Wesleyan University Press, 2010), 86–87.

22. Thank you to Clare Croft for helping me articulate this idea.

23. Morris, *Game for Dancers*, 5–8; and Ellen Graff, *Stepping Left: Dance and Politics in New York City, 1928–1942* (Durham, NC: Duke University Press, 1997), 167.

24. Margaret Lloyd, *The Borzoi Book of Modern Dance* (New York: Alfred A. Knopf, 1949; repr. New York: Dance Horizons, 1974), 173.

25. Manning, *Modern Dance, Negro Dance*, 181.

26. Anna Sokolow, quoted in Warren, *Rebellious Spirit*, 119.

27. Warren, *Rebellious Spirit*, 253.

28. George Beiswanger, "New London: Residues and Reflections," *Dance Observer*, February 1957, 21; John Martin, "Dance: Study in Despair," *New York Times*, May 17, 1955, 26; Anna Sokolow Clippings, Jerome Robbins Dance Division of the New York Public Library for the Performing Arts (hereinafter JRDD, NYPL);

and Doris Hering, "An Evening of Dance Works by Anna Sokolow: 92nd Street
'Y' February 24 and 28, 1955," *Dance Magazine*, April 1955, 75.

29. Morris, *Game for Dancers*, 105.

30. Johnson, *The Lavender Scare*, 9.

31. Ibid., 147–63.

32. D'Emilio, *Sexual Politics*, 40–53.

33. Thank you to Takiyah Nur Amin for this observation.

34. Johnson, *The Lavender Scare*, 158–60.

35. Moore, interview, 3.

36. Walter Terry, "American Dance," *New York Herald Tribune*, May 16, 1955, n.p.,
Lester Sweyd Collection, Anna Sokolow Clippings, JRDD, NYPL.

37. *Rooms*, notated by Cook, 66.

38. In February 2012, Nia-Amina Minor performed "Going" in a Stanford University
performance of *Rooms* set by Lorry May, artistic director of the Sokolow Dance
Foundation. The solo still appeared queer. Minor blended seamlessly into the
role, yet her use of strong weight, syncopated urgency, and her ability to take up
a lot of space—paired with the baseball jacket—appeared masculine in contrast
to her biologically presenting woman-ness. When I spoke to Minor backstage,
she was surprised to learn that a man traditionally performed the solo; that
detail did not surface when she learned it. She, it seemed, embodied "Going"
as an early twenty-first-century woman influenced both by second-wave feminism and post-feminism's "girl power." Or, she assimilated movement made for
someone else into her body in a short rehearsal period, disconnected from its
historical significance.

39. *Rooms*, notated by Cook, 84.

40. Kowal, "Being Motion," 98.

41. Manning, *Modern Dance, Negro Dance*, 183–84.

42. Kowal, *How to Do Things*, 116.

43. Ibid., 108; and Reynoso, "Constitutive Processes."

44. Ze'eva Cohen (dancer and choreographer) in telephone conversation with the
author, February 5, 2012.

45. Clive Barnes, "Dance: Sokolow 'Rooms'," *New York Times*, September 8, 1967,
n.p., Alan M. and Sali Ann Kriegsman Collection, MD, LOC.

46. Butler, *Bodies that Matter*, 239, italics in the original.

47. Valerie A. Briginshaw, *Dance, Space and Subjectivity* (New York: Palgrave,
2001), 77–78.

48. Briginshaw, *Dance, Space and Subjectivity*, 78.

49. Terry, "American Dance."

50. Cook, conversation, July 2, 2011.

51. Cohen, conversation.

52. Ibid.

53. Briginshaw, *Dance, Space and Subjectivity*, 92–94.

54. Johnson, *The Lavender Scare*, 5–7.

55. D'Emilio, *Sexual Politics*, 2–3.

56. Boyd, *Wide Open Town*, 179.

57. Beiswanger, "New London," 22.

58. Juhasz, "Queer Swans," 71.

59. The FBI followed Sokolow from the 1930s through the 1970s. For a 1955 interrogation, see Anna Sokolow, State of New York Affadavit, May 9, 1955, and transcript of FBI interview with Sokolow, November 1, 1955, US Department of State, FOIPA No. 1138496-000. Many left-aligned American Jews like Sokolow distanced themselves from their communist pasts during the anti-Semitism that accompanied McCarthyism. In *Honest Bodies: Revolutionary Modernism in the Dances of Anna Sokolow* (Oxford University Press, forthcoming), I explain the role of Jewishness in Sokolow's navigation of this postwar matrix of the Red and Lavender Scares.

PART II

Dancing toward a Queer Sociality

8

Queer Dance in Three Acts

thomas f. defrantz

⊙ *theoryography 4.5: we* [still] *queer here*
⊙ in conversation with thomas f. defrantz, Kevin Guy, Gina Kohler, and James Morrow

queer dance: being, doing, making.
sister, watch me work.

being

the **be-ing** is easiest for me: queer me dancing, enjoying a muscularity of longness in effect with my 6′4″ frame tearing through movements. plastic-man-like limbs and fingers in motion, hips swinging when i want, tossing my locks to accentuate the beat. dancing, i *am* queer mostimes, and this moving-being aligns with a consistent being-in-the-world realized through my queer identity, inevitably claimed in conversation or in obvious, recognizable action. i am that thing we call queer, and in the being of it, understand it as a sideward inevitability that puts me near some, but further from others. being queer—like being a dancer—puts me in readiness to perform queer contours; alert to possible queer disavowal; but attendant to queer's inevitable arrival and always-already-thereness.

doing

doing queer is harder. not in an "acting femme" sort of way (as if i were a macho butch of some sort, **not**), but in a "making more apparent what is already present" way. the doing is about *difference* from some other doing; doing it to be *marked as queer* in variance from some other (straight?) mode. doing the dance queerly—well, if I'm doing it, the gesture already has that capacity willy-nilly—but *this* doing suggests these not-always-present modes of being inside it, brought to the fore by effort. I'm not trying to *naturalize* my queer affect by calling out its already-thereness, my queerbeing is not necessarily part of some sort of *nature-nurture* paradigm. like breath, it comes and goes in time, and sometimes matters less to me than at other times. but i won't discount its importance to me either, this queerness; it tends to **be there**, so amping it up, to *do it more*, takes palpable effort. enlarging the recognizability of queer makes me work against my suppositions of straight, at least, to imagine how you might understand this to be queer. but i do notice that whether i experience my gestures as "doing queer dance" matters little; how you, my collaborators or audience, perceive them to be "done queer" marks their capacity. queer being reflects an orientation to another: a near and far, rather than an address; **queer doing** assumes an interaction of self and other. **doing queer**, then, becomes something always shared, always interpreted and recognized between/among, rather than the kind of essential status that might be embedded in queer as identity. i need you to see me do queer; without you i'm nothing, sandra bernhard/not necessarily queer in gesture.

making

making queer is something like doing queer on steroids (and, okay, i do love muscle). to move an action or a dance to the realm of queer, we assume that queer exists, and that an action of "making" can happen inside or outside of queer terms. in other words, we assume that there *can* be a "queer dance"— which surely does not go without saying. and we imagine a stability that might be possible around its queer contents and their affects. "aha, there! i see *a queer* dance!" we are challenged to ejaculate in the presence of a **queer-made**. there must be something sustainable inside the queer-made so that it might feel formed, structured, and relevant to the discussion of its capacity. queer-mades exist in time, through time, across shifts in temporal contexts. queer-mades prove queer remains, that queer *is-was-will be*. queer-mades tend not to be naturally-occurring; they arrive after extensive jostling and cajoling. and queer-mades come from academics as often as from artists or people in the street; they include the long-winded analytical essays that explain how something done queerly becomes a queer-made, in a sort of self-reflective, always-operating teaching-moment justification. queer-mades arrive from effort, by we who need its presence, whether we work as professors helping others understand queer resiliency, or as artists bringing queer creative evidence into the mainstream of creative commerce. as with the arrival of "negro" that frantz fanon endures at the provocation of a white child ("Look, a Negro!"), queer-mades come because we are determined to note their presence.

being, doing, and making typify the ways i experience *queer* brought to bear on dance performances and research. the ***being*** might be the most historiographic here, as in repeated requests to construct queer-positive biographies of dance personalities (Arthur Mitchell, Loïe Fuller, Katherine Dunham, Alvin Ailey, Merce Cunningham, Lucinda Childs); constructing useful histories to predict possibilities for queer identity in the world today. this is a sort of "queer as antidote" to straight, or a "proof of possibility" for queer within dance, mobilized to account for queer presence in the face of its disavowal. these histories confirm that queer exists within dance across generations, and queer dancers can achieve success not necessarily contained by their queerness. the presence of queers in history might mean experiential queer ontologies of being.

and we need queer ontologies within dance, because so often we are told to not ***do*** queer in dance. for we boys, we hear, "butch it up," which tends to mean "pare it down," a command that calls on our ability to resist non-normative movement behaviors. a queer *doing*, though, calls for extravagance of some sort, an excess so that the queerness will not be mistaken for some brand of errant straightness, or some sort of straight misunderstanding. by 2016, queer still feels rare enough to need an on-the-noseness in its ***doing***, as in the men kissing in the beginning of Kyle Abraham's "Brick" (2008), or the ambisexual children making out in Miguel Gutierrez's "Everyone" (2007), or Katy Pyle's fantastical *Ballez* inventions, or Yanis Marshall's devastating demonstrations of men jazz-video|pop-music dancing in high heels. their very obvious queer-doing stabilizes the being-in-the-world; and yes, we still need the doing to confirm the being.

making a queer theatrical dance for a general US dance-going public continues to be elusive and awkward. but let's leave the bourgeois concert-dance stage out of it: happily, the twenty-first century brings forward all variety of communities in motion who eagerly support mostevery kind of performance in non-general venues. queer dance and choreography festivals, queer hip hop dance television programming, queer line dancing, queer lesbigay bar cabaret shows all proliferate, and these events are populated by queer-mades. essays, blogposts, and books—like this one you read now—offer academic treatises that make queer acts of performance apparent. these gestures of queermaking may not be mainstream, and they may derive power from their particularity. but they really do happen, all the time now, and we are not at a loss to find representations of queer-made dance here, there, and everywhere.

so, how could these truisms that matter to me be useful to dance and its analysis? to start, i strive to never forget the being-ness of queer presence in dance, and the many ways its variegated contours hurt, surprise, annoy, replenish, and inspire. queer holds urgent currency in dance, and dance provides a measure of solace and refuge for queer being. our collective willingness to privilege queer presence, and to reflect on sexualities and gender in terms of dance, marks our capacity to imagine together progressively. the largest cohort of dancers in the context of the United States—including liturgical dancers, hip hop dancers, video, commercial and concert stage dancers, folk dancers—embrace queer people in their midsts, even when those same queer people might be rejected outside the context of their dancing. if i begin with queer, and assume our presence among, say, african diaspora dance companies as well as Black dance events, i can be comforted by an assumption of sexual diversity seldom experienced otherwise.

as example, kevin guy's study "this side faces room: a decolonization of the mind" (2013), performed as part of *theory-ography 4.5: we* [still] *queer here* (2013), draws on its creator's willingness to assume his queer body as an impetus and end to his dancing. the work begins with a brief dance film that scrutinizes his musculature, focusing on his broad shoulders and rippled torso, while he moves, a black man in black briefs and black leather shoes, contained by a white circular space. the film ends with the removal of the boots; guy appears live in the performance space in the same black briefs and no shoes, working in slow, thoughtful balance and physical extension to van morrison's song "ballerina." guy's clearly-marked be-ing queer, demonstrated by sideward glances amid the willful display of his gym-bunny body, juxtaposes a tall and buff black man's ruminative dancing to a white man blues singer's exhortations toward an offstage ballerina. guy does very little that is queer, or queerly-shaped, beyond the kern of dancing itself; rather he exemplifies queer by his already-thereness, moving in order to discover possibilities at once interior to his own physical process, but shared with the gathered audience as evidence, in and of itself, of queer black masculinity as a reflective, animated presence.

when i was a little boy and not allowed to get my way because of some adult or parental rule, my mother used to say, in the vernacular, *"it be-s that way sometimes."* guy dancing *be-s* queer, he also does queer at times, with the virtuosity of a finely-trained dancer's capacity. me, not so much. doing queer, i relax and allow myself to fail, mindful that targeted failure provides an important space for humor and irony. making big mistakes, some purposefully, i confirm a willingness to not try to control an outcome, or predetermine a line of communication. i might be cynical or wryly persistent in the pursuit in my queer gesture; extravagant to a literal fault that suggests the outside of achievement as its own end. a hyper-particularity of doing produces queer gesture for me; inevitably, that gesture fails to do what it seems to intend. that failure is usually humorous on some level, to underscore a distancing between attempt and achievement.

two examples help underscore executions of queer failure in dance. consider keith hennesey's bewildering reconstruction of the chosen maiden's solo from nijinsky's "rite of spring" (1913) in his queer version "bear/skin" (2015). toward the end of an hour-long invention, hennesey interpolates nijinsky's choreography: trying valiantly, but failing repeatedly, in his attempt to convey the austerity of personal sacrifice that marked the original ballet's rendering of group communion. moving with a brutal care, always unable to complete the predetermined gestures but trying valiantly again and again, hennesey's dancing inspires guffaws and concern from me in the audience. as he struggles to perform the choreography as part of a patently-fake "aboriginal ritual," his middle-aged, white, queer-maleness pushes against the ambition of the choreography, to accentuate his queer-doing of the dance. watching, i wonder: will he hurt himself? what drives him to keep going, even when the impossibility of the task is apparent? is it okay to laugh at his failure? he dances and fails, trying something queer in taking on the dance for a young "maiden," doing queer as the extended failure of a performance. this is queer failure as an impossibility of execution that all we in the audience are forced to encounter and consider. it is hard to watch, fascinating and disturbing for me; the gestures of a seemingly self-inflicted wounding of dance.

but gina kohler's "dream [factories]" (2009), also included in "theory-ography 4.5," thrives in the repeated failure of its performer to accomplish an entirely queer task. kohler appears naked, seated with her back to the audience on a small square of mirror. she pours blood (beet juice, actually) down her back slowly to the sounds of her bantering with her husband and son watching fireworks. as the soundtrack segues into madonna's "like a prayer," kohler, swathed in blood, and brightly lit and reflected by the mirror stage she now kneels upon, begins to slip and slide unpredictably. at times she seems able

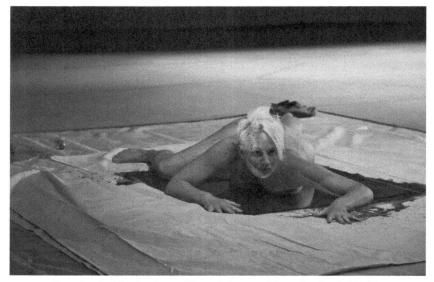

FIGURE 8.1 gina kohler in *dream [factories]*, 2013. Photo by Sarah Nesbitt.

to control her weight and its force amid the slippery fluids on the mirror, but as often as not, she skids into a turn or tumble, and finds her way back to face her audience. somehow, she thrives in her falls and recovery; we are invited to cheer when she controls her motions rhythmically. we smile as conspirators to her repeated failings in the impossible dance, queerly-done.

making queer calls up serious creative energy, as queer-mades have to be instantiated in the body as well as the imagination. to do this in dance, we create stabilized collections of gestures that are at once precarious and fussy, and then mobilize intellectual contexts that define those gestures as unequivocally queer. queer-made dances intend to stand as demonstrations of the variability of an outsider space, but at some point they also tend to look like well-made dances that just happen to be somehow queer. this is the challenge of recognizability; that **structure understood** is **structure normalized** and most likely *un*-queer. how to make something that continually demonstrates its non-normativity?

queer-mades push against normative gestural expression, even as they push against themselves. "11" (2011) created by james morrow, and included in "theory-ography 4.5," casts a queer contemporary dancer/b-boy into a series of elusive gestures reminiscent of catholic church practice, intercut with odd, loving manipulations of prop chairs. morrow dances away from the audience for much of this work, often exploring dramatic physical ideas without revealing his facial expression; sudden shifts in movement style signal a moody, always-fragmentary mode of queer production. at times, morrow's gestures fail and he repeats them, violently; but the dance as a whole fails to offer a coherent movement vocabulary or approach to its own contents. by the time morrow removes his shirt to retrieve a razor and shave his chest, revealing a prominent OBEY tattoo along his arm, his audience imagines an assemblage of experience that combine via their proximity within this performance. morrow's body engages these varied modes of moving; the work offers queer assemblage that ends with a full-color projection of a beating heart on the performer's exposed skin. b-boy movement, religious ritual gesture, neo-African dance, intimate personal grooming, and odd media projection collide in the performer's execution; queerly disagreeing with each as they each assert their presence in the dance. the queer-made of "11" emerges from the fizzy and mysterious montage of method that constitute its whole. morrow makes a queer world in his dance, where his ostensibly straight b-boy can collude with his selves as a contemporary dancer, former catholic altar boy, and sheperd fairey-admiring activist in a dance of unlikely affiliation.

sister, can you still hear me?

queer world-making has been popular among academic writers at least since lauren berlant and michael warner, *pace* José Esteban Muñoz, enticed us all with a weird utopic ability to imagine outlandish queer horizons, where complex intimacies and public sex could be simultaneously queer and private. but as a queer be-er of color, I've never been convinced that rampant worldmaking does the many things we might hope for. we might all imagine temporary queer worlds where we could be anti-racists and anti-misogynists—and still hot. but these ephemeral imaginary worlds aren't where i usually dance, drive—carefully, as a black man with dreadlocks—or even teach and present my creative work. queer world-making is fun to imagine, and useful when i try to take the time back from the un-queer structures of straight life. in general, i try to be pretty queer-going in an everyday sort of way. but the everyday worlds i go through are fairly constant in their need to reproduce non-queer normativity. SO, i disidentify in many of my daily encounters at work and in the world, resisting the pull of straight life as i can. but i also find this not to be very sustainable as a way of life; the hard work that queers of colors and others engage moment to moment as best we can.

to disidentify, i re-configure normative affiliations with my own, preferred, invented meanings and deploy these new mappings into the world. for example, like other choreographers, i make dances, but these works are usually open spaces that allow a group of collaborators to do what they want in response to the prompt of our shared labor. imagining a queer ground from which to move means that i work to reconfigure how a *choreographer* might be understood to function. as the project figurehead, a choreographer is often conceived as a political leader with ultimate veto power, and the ability to engage violence (cutting entire sequences of movement) to define the state (the final dance). choreographers make casting and editing decisions; they might define movement sequences or offer them up from their own bodies. i claim the role of choreographer in SLIPPAGE projects, but i disidentify from that oddly patrician array of responsibility to mobilize artists from whom i want to learn in creative practice. together, we make dances that are undisciplined; dances that resist pre-determination, but wonder at what might come of shared wit and unusual alignments of material and physical ideas.

as example, the multi-year "theory-ography" project emerged from this impulse toward collective queer creation. disidentifying itself as a stable work of performance, when it really isn't that at all, its varied manifestations share structural similarities among their iterations as embodied collecting pools for movement thinkers to explore textual and physical ideas together. "theory-ography" brings artists into collaboration around its theme to engage an improvised whole that always requires the participation of its audience. as a whole, the project is rampantly unruly and awkward. it insists on underestimating its potential, as it refuses to be rehearsed into a repeatable form. each iteration of the work contains "set pieces" contributed by participating artists, with the whole stitched together by a shifting set of tasks, texts, rules, expectations, and physical provocations provided by the performers, designers, technicians, and gathered audience members. previous versions of "theory-ography" have explored endings and beginnings (1.0: the end of the tale, 2008); the concept of the ready-to-hand (2.0: heidegger's hammer, 2010); theory as practice (3.0: we dance theory, 2011); queer presence (4.0: we queer here, 2012); and Black queer futures (5.0: *afro*FUTURE*queer*, 2015). imbued with queer intention, the work invariably emerges as a queer-made mobilization of being and doing in relation to a theme of shared interest.

for the 2013 *theory-ography 4.5: we* [still] *queer here* version, we created a short study that i performed, "the weight of ideas" as a live-processing experiment. clad in a business suit chosen to represent a queer public

academic/professional, a kinect camera followed my movements to produce data streams from my joints that were then affiliated with descriptive
words: performativity, mixed race, penis envy, anxiety, etc. a computer pro-
cessing patch, created in the visual programming language MAX by slippage affiliate kenneth david stewart, tied the words to different parts of my
body as i moved through the space in front of the camera; the words were
projected as dancing icons on a screen behind me. stewart discovered and
programmed the font types for the words and designed their sensitivity
to my gesture; i created a movement score that allowed for improvisation
around ideas of how labels attach to people as we see them, and return
to those people even as we might know more subtle distinctions of that
person's complexity. moving uncomfortably through the space, i felt the
weight of the words on my body; through a queer gesture of slapping my
knee, i could make one of the words vanish. i never knew which word/
label would disappear, and my physical improvisation grew in relationship to the revelations that the interface provided. we did establish one
unchangeable marker for the interface: when the last word was left on
the screen, i could control its visual scale directly through the movement
of my hands. the final word, *queerlove*, floats on the screen, and folds and
opens, like an accordian, as i move my hands toward and away from each
other. at the end of the dance, i open the word to its fullest width and with
open hands and arms, embrace the audience and move into its number.

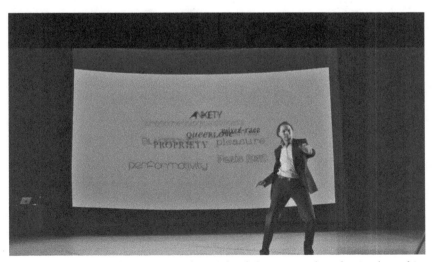

FIGURE 8.2 thomas f. defrantz in *the weight of ideas*, 2013. Photo by Sarah Nesbitt.

"the weight of ideas" ties words to gesture to underscore how viewers contribute to the actual making of queer, no matter the intention of the performer. in the revelation of this crucial relationship of object/viewed to viewer/interpreter, we confirm that queer is a collaborative assemblage; queer dance is a distortion, hopefully in a useful way, toward something unanticipated and awe-ful (awful) that exists *now, here,* and *for this gathered community.* dance enhances queer visibility. queer dance emerges from **being** and **doing**, perhaps, but its contents are brought into focus by the **making** of its various audiences who can narrate the queerness at hand.

being, doing, making. this works for me as a three-part exercise worth revisiting again and again. there is something called queer, and it can be done and made as dance. reading emerging theories, participating in dancemaking differently, and navigating queer desires, i shimmy through a shared creative craft with SLIPPAGE collaborators that continually enlivens. as this short essay demonstrates, our work is indebted to writings by lauren berlant, jack halberstam, bell hooks, Zora Neal Hurston, josé esteban muñoz, franz fanon, hortense spillers, and many others; we bring these sometimes-queer avatars into our conversations and creative practice as we move together.

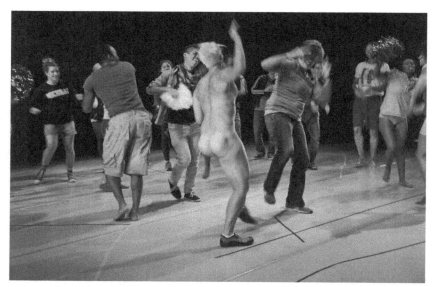

FIGURE 8.3 audience and performers dance together queerly in *theoryography 4.5: we* [still] *queer here,* 2013. Photo by Sarah Nesbitt.

we should all be so lucky. sadly, we aren't; and our perverse enchantments with queer dance are not easily available to the many people who might need them or enjoy their creation in the world. we don't all get to tell sexy stories in public, joke about queer life, publicly embrace our queer predilections, or collectively mourn our many losses and disappointments. our physical and emotional connections to the devastations of orlando, june 2016, vary. we don't all get to be, do, or make queer. if anything, the unmet challenge for queer theory and queer dance might be an opening of access for anyone who wants to think-move queer; an allowance for more people to understand strategies of queer [black/asian/trans/aboriginal] performance on our bodies, in our imaginations, and among our friends.

sister, i love you? this is for you. thankufalettinmebemiceelf—agin.

References

Berlant, Lauren, and Michael Warner. "Sex in Public." *Critical Inquiry* 24, no. 2 (1998): 547–66.

Fanon, Franz. *Black Skin, White Masks.* London: Pluto Press, 1986.

Halberstam, Jack. *The Queer Art of Failure.* Chapel Hill, NC: Duke University Press, 2011.

Hartman, Saidiya. "Venus in Two Acts." *Small Axe* 26.12, no. 2 (2008): 1–14.

hooks, bell. *Black Looks: Race and Representation.* Boston, MA: South End Press, 1992.

Hurston, Zora Neal. "Characteristics of Negro Expression." In *Negro, An Anthology*, ed. Nancy Cunard (London: F. Ungar Publishing 1934), 39–46.

Muñoz, José Esteban. *Cruising Utopia: The Then and There of Queer Futurity.* New York: NYU Press, 2009.

Muñoz, José Esteban. *Disidentifications: Queers of Color and the Performance of Politics.* Minneapolis: University of Minnesota Press, 1999.

Spillers, Hortense J. "Mama's Baby, Papa's Maybe: An American Grammar Book" Diacritics, Vol. 17, No. 2, Culture and Countermemory: The "American" Connection. (Summer, 1987), pp. 64–81.

9

In Praise of Latin Night at the Queer Club

Justin Torres

If you're lucky, they'll play some Latin cheese, that Aventura song from fifteen years ago. If you're lucky, there will be drag queens and, if so, almost certainly they will be quick, razor-sharp with their humor, giving you the kind of performances that cut and heal all at once. If you're lucky, there will be go-go boys, every shade of brown.

Maybe your Ma blessed you on the way out the door. Maybe she wrapped a plate for you in the fridge so you don't come home and mess up her kitchen with your hunger. Maybe your Tia dropped you off, gave you cab money home. Maybe you had to get a sitter. Maybe you've yet to come out to your family at all, or maybe your family kicked you out years ago. Forget it, you survived. Maybe your boo stayed home, wasn't feeling it, but is blowing up your phone with sweet texts, trying to make sure you don't stray. Maybe you're allowed to stray. Maybe you're flush, maybe you're broke as nothing, and angling your pretty face barside, hoping someone might buy you a drink. Maybe your half-Latin-ass doesn't even speak Spanish; maybe you barely speak English. Maybe you're undocumented.

Outside, there's a world that politicizes every aspect of your identity. There are preachers, of multiple faiths, mostly self-identified Christians, condemning you to hell. Outside, they call you an abomination. Outside, there is a news media that acts as if there are two sides to a debate over trans people using public bathrooms. Outside, there is a presidential candidate who has built a platform on erecting a wall between the United States and Mexico—and not only do people believe that crap is possible, they believe it is necessary.

Outside, Puerto Rico is still a colony, being allowed to drown in debt, to suffer, without the right to file for bankruptcy, to protect itself. Outside, there are more than 100 billstargeting you, your choices, your people, pending in various states.[1]

You have known violence. You have known violence. You are queer and you are brown and you have known violence. You have known a masculinity, a machismo, stupid with its own fragility. You learned basic queer safety; you have learned to scan, casually, quickly, before any public display of affection. Outside, the world can be murderous to you and your kind. Lord knows.

But inside, it is loud and sexy and on. If you're lucky, it's a mixed crowd, muscle Marys and bois and femme fags and butch dykes and genderqueers. If you're lucky, no one is wearing much clothing, and the dance floor is full. If you're lucky, they're playing reggaeton, salsa, and you can move.

People talk about liberation as if it's some kind of permanent state, as if you get liberated and that's it, you get some rights and that's it, you get some acknowledgment and that's it, happy now? But you're going back down into the muck of it every day; this world constricts. You know what the opposite of Latin Night at the Queer Club is? Another Day in Straight White America. So when you walk into the club, if you're lucky, it feels expansive. "Safe space" is a cliché, overused and exhausted in our discourse, but the fact remains that a sense of safety transforms the body, transforms the spirit. So many of us walk through the world without it. So when you walk through the door and it's a salsa beat, and brown bodies, queer bodies, all writhing in some fake smoke and strobing lights, no matter how cool, how detached, how over-it you think you are, Latin Night at the Queer Club breaks your cool. You can't help but smile, this is for you, for us.

Outside, tomorrow, hangovers, regrets, the grind. Outside, tomorrow, the struggle to effect change. But inside, tonight, none of that matters. Inside, tonight, the only imperative is to love. Lap the bar, out for a smoke, back inside, the ammonia and sweat and the floor slightly tacky, another drink, the imperative is to get loose, get down, find religion, lose it, find your hips locked into another's, break, dance on your own for a while—but you didn't come here to be a nun—find your lips pressed against another's, break, find your friends, dance. The only imperative is to be transformed, transfigured in the disco light. To lighten, loosen, see yourself reflected in the beauty of others. You didn't come here to be a martyr; you came to live, papi. To live, mamacita. To live, hijos. To live, mariposas.

The media will spin the conversation away from homegrown homophobic terrorism to a general United States vs. Islamist narrative. Mendacious, audacious politicians—Republicans who vote against queer rights, against gun control—will seize on this massacre, twist it for support of their agendas.

But for a moment, I want to talk about the sacredness of Latin Night at the Queer Club. Amid all the noise, I want to close my eyes and see you all there, dancing, inviolable, free.

Note

1. "Everything You Need to Know about the Wave of 100+ Anti-LGBT Bills Pending in States," *The Huffington Post*, April 16, 2016, http://www.huffingtonpost.com/entry/lgbt-state-bills-discrimination_us_570ff4f2e4b0060ccda2a7a9.

10

An Buachaillín Bán

REFLECTIONS ON ONE QUEER'S PERFORMANCE
WITHIN TRADITIONAL IRISH MUSIC AND DANCE

Nicholas Gareiss

▶ "Lafferty's"

▶ in conversation with Nicholas Gareiss

As the first strains of the reel emerge from the pin-drop silence of the hall, I step out from the wing, crossing upstage behind the fiddler to stand next to him. Continuing the momentum of that stride, I graze the worn and swiftly-wearing soles of my shoes against the stage floor, beginning my dance with a series of hushed half-time brushes and shuffles to mark the tempo. I can feel the surface of the wooden floor through the leather soles as I lightly push the balls of my feet forward, caressing the ground twice, then twice again, and finally once more before releasing the weight of my frame through a weight-bearing footfall on a downbeat. I can feel the sounds created by my contact with the floor slip inside my collaborator's already-established tempo. I can reside here.

I begin lightly punctuating and accenting the arcs and valleys of the melody. Following the first part of the reel, about twenty seconds after I make my entrance, I sculpt my steps to imitate the melody of the tune "Big Pat's." Assembling the small one- or two-sound rudiments of trebles, hops, and tip-steps in the moment, I imitate the phrasing of the fiddler's bow by anticipating, mirroring, and dueling the back-and-forth motion of his arm with back-and-forward gestures of my knee and lower leg. Our sixteenth notes coalesce. We are now sounding together, my collaborator and I.

I have long felt the presence of a nascent queerness within traditional Irish music and dance. This queerness is and is not spoken about; it exists in rumors and in whispers, tacitly undergirding the performance conventions of the genre. Nothing could be more phantasmal, more impossible, more queer.

My fifteen years of experience performing within traditional Irish music and dance have allowed me a rare glimpse into a part of Ireland to which many Americans are not usually privy. I feel fortunate that my technical expertise and acclaim have allowed me access to an upper echelon of professional performance in this realm, even as my national identity marks me as an outsider. As both a queer-identified person, and an American working in the genre of Irish traditional music and dance, I believe my not-quite insider/not-quite outsider status has revealed fascinating contradictions of this subculture that would not otherwise become apparent. From this parallax, it is possible to illuminate heteronormative paradigms within this idiom and its corresponding social scenes. It is my humble hope that through the positionality of a queer American working in traditional Irish music and dance, I can bring to light ways of subverting these heteronormative paradigms using performance, allowing nascent queer tendencies to susurrate.

Anthropologist Clifford Geertz writes, "You don't exactly penetrate another culture, as the masculinist image would have it. You put yourself in its way and it bodies forth and enmeshes you."[1] As both a dancer and an anthropologist, the notion of a non-penetrative ethnographer, or indeed one who is penetrated himself by the culture, resonates with me, envisioning powerful new implications for queer work in ethnology and performance. Geertz's cultural "enmeshing" proffers the potential for queerness that is culturally specific. His idea of a culture "bodying forth" and enmeshing the ethnographer, revealing its secrets in its own time, on its own terms, offers insight into the ways cultural forms perform their nascent queerness. I have experienced this in my very enmeshed relationship with Ireland and its music and dance traditions, as well as through the enmeshing of my ethnographic training with my career as a dancer.

Traditional music scholar Helen O'Shea asserts that "Irish" and "queer" are "mutually exclusive identifications" in the discourse of both Irish nationalism and the Irish music scene.[2] In this essay, I wish to dismantle O'Shea's assertion in two ways: by revealing the "already-queerness" within the forms of Irish traditional music and dance themselves, and subverting the "mutual exclusiveness" of Irishness and queerness through my own performances in Irish traditional music and dance, onstage and off. Here I depart from my previous research as an anthropologist interviewer to explore the experience of doing ethnography as a performer and queer subject.[3] This project turns the ethnographic gaze upon my own experience and artistic practice, the ways that I have worked corporeally in Irish traditional music and dance, in the hope of revealing both queer possibilities within these idioms and suggesting queer aesthetic interventions.

Implicated in the question of nascent queerness in Irish dance is the matter of the form's centrality to Irish culture. Michael Seaver, in "Counting Capital: The Real Value of Dance in Irish Society," writes, "It is clear that the dancing body in Ireland is firmly placed in the centre of our cultural land-scape and that dancers contribute to social and cultural discourse through the ability to theorise through the moving body."[4] Even before the 1994 debut of *Riverdance* and the subsequent deluge of similar Broadway-style Irish dance shows, the long history of dance in Ireland had already created a collective psy-chic precedent for this genre's movement vocabulary, locomotive quality, and canonical repertoire that continues today. Due in part to the fact that many children are taught Irish dancing at elementary school in Ireland, often Irish people who do not consider themselves connected to the arts are intimately acquainted with the modalities of this corporeal tradition. In my own experi-ence, Ireland is the only culture in which I can step into a taxi cab, inform the driver that I am a dancer, and have the driver's unseen assumptions about my work remotely resemble what I actually create. This includes the role of spe-cific body parts (the feet, legs, ankles) in the dance, as well as the form's sym-biotic relationship to the jigs, reels, and hornpipes of Irish traditional music.

Perhaps because of the cultural ubiquity of dance in Ireland, Irish music and dance have long been held as more than simply indigenous cultural forms, but somehow representational of Irish identity and seminal to its reification. For Irish citizens and visiting tourists, these practices are often cast as last ves-tiges of the "real Ireland," re-enacting a romanticized version of the country held a priori by Americans and, surprisingly, reified by many Irish people themselves. This romantic notion of Ireland was summarized by former Irish president Éamon De Valera, "a land whose countryside would be bright with cozy homesteads . . . with the romping of sturdy children, the contests of ath-letic youths, the laughter of comely maidens . . . the home of a people living the life that God desires men should live."[5] Despite recent developments in Irish marriage equality, these heteronormative cultural associations of home, family, and nation continue to manifest within current conventions of Irish dance performance.[6] I argue that these poise the form for disruptive queer performance activism because of the cultural capital the dance genre carries within Irish society.

Despite the strong psychic precedent for Irish step dancing in Ireland, within the genre of traditional Irish music and dance performance, dance is simultaneously a point of focus and marginal.[7] This simultaneity contributes to Irish dance's queer possibilities. In traditional music concert settings, professional Irish musicians often employ dancers for short segments of choreography—usually fast reels in 4/4 time—to punctuate the high points of the performance. A convention has developed: "roll on the dancers," the steel-shod, unwieldy team of bodies as spectacle (stroke sex symbol, stroke national icon) in the form of the red-haired *colleen* in the short black skirt or velvet trimmed, Book of Kells-spattered dress. "Just come on for the last 32 bars of the last number of the first half, the finale, and the encore," I've heard musicians say. This tokenistic use of bodies demonstrates dance in service of the entertainment aspect of the performance of Irish traditional music, and simultaneously, the performance of Irishness. During these short choreographic segments, the long line of erect dancers step in precision, arms at their sides, their upright comportment a perfect metaphor for the properness of postcolonial dignity.

Experiencing these shapes and choreographies within my own body, I realize that dancers can create tremendously effective and memorable moments as our watched bodies interact with music and with each other.[8] Further, due to both the corporeality of our art and the interplay of marginality/centrality of Irish dance in these contexts, step dancers can evoke strong statements of gender representation.[9] Within the contemporary performance conventions of Irish traditional music and dance, these statements are engineered to enforce theatrical depictions of compulsory heterosexuality and binary notions of gender, irrespective of the identities of the exponents.[10] Dancers are often tacitly directed to offset the possibility of queerness when employed by the Irish music industry's largely heterosexual roster of touring musicians. While working with an established traditional Irish band, one bandleader once asked me hopefully, "You don't do any dancing with a young girl, do you?" For him, a heterosexual *pas de deux* was the pinnacle of Irish entertainment, projecting the "correct" theatrical national sexual binary through the dance.

Compulsory heterosexuality and binary gender are also reinforced through Irish dance pedagogy. Former lead dancer in *Riverdance*, Breandán de Gallaí, related the story of an Irish dancing teacher telling their teenage male students to "butch it up a bit" when onstage. Another Irish dance teacher, choreographer, and producer I worked with will not even allow two boys to look at each other if performing together. In his shows, male dancers must look at the women onstage or at the audience. In his words, "boys have to be aggressive and hit the floor hard, they have to jump higher and wink at the ladies in the third row." Hearing such stories enforcing traditional gender roles makes me wonder if perhaps queerness could function as a site of aesthetic destabilization of these conventions, reframing the limits of gender expression in Irish traditional dance performance.

By considering the aesthetic and morphological trappings of these traditions, I set out to create performance work in opposition to these precedents of the genre, opening it queerly as a polysemic means of cultural and personal expression.[11] To do this, I drew inspiration from the nascent queerness I sensed in Irish traditional music. Similar to Irish dancing, Irish traditional music is sometimes characterized and valued by its masculine energy in which good equals masculine. A flute player once remarked to me on a younger female musician's style, "She plays great, for a girl." However, in stark aesthetic contrast to commercial Irish dance theater, there exist quieter subgenres within the musical tradition referred to as *goltraí* and *suantraí* (sad and hushabye tunes). In the performance of "slow airs," for example, musicians are permitted to exhibit moments of sensitivity, quietness, tenderness, or remorse. Within Irish-language *sean-nós* singing, there is a custom of singers—particularly men—engaging in a rare public display of same-sex intimacy through the act of hand-holding (called "winding").[12] These conventions critiquing traditional masculinity invite a queer reading of traditional Irish music, highlighting what fiddler Martin Hayes identifies as the genre's "subversiveness."[13]

The heightened sensitivity of slow airs and *sean-nós* singing seemed fertile territory from which to garner inspiration for a queer response to Irish traditional dance. Could I physically embody these rare exhibitions of emotions less typically construed as "masculine" in Irish dance movement? I wanted to take a nod from Irish music performance practice, in which men can sing vulnerably, tenderly, or bring each other to tears with a slow quiet melody played on the flute or accordion. In effect, to be queer enough to permit myself to portray what these men might be feeling but might not have been allowed to express culturally, and to do so through movement. My synesthetic aspiration of crossing Irish musical convention into the world of Irish dance was confirmed for me when one reviewer so flatteringly put it after one of my performances: I had become an "eye-opener for the ears."[14] The queer characteristics I sensed within the musical tradition, confirmed through Hayes's admission of the medium's subversive character, inspired a queer spirit of departure for re-imagining the conventions of Irish traditional dance.

With the strong cultural precedent of a hyper-masculinized, leather-clad, male dance archetype within Irish show dancing, any suggestion of male lightness, quietness, or possibility of simpatico response could prove strikingly queer. I became curious as to the possibilities of invoking queerness, not only in the sense that I am a queer-identified man but also by embodying a puckish suggestion utilizing the queer potentiality of the form itself. Far from a reactionary critique, I was interested in highlighting the attributes of the tradition that I had witnessed in other Irish cultural practices: the softness of traditional Irish song, the lightness of older dancers who were trained prior to the advent of commercial Irish dancing shows, and the almost amorous intimacy I had seen traditional instrumentalists embody when playing together.[15] These were aesthetic facets that I knew were present in the tradition, but my growing sense was that they were elided from contemporary Irish traditional dance performance due to heteronormative anxiety. This made me wonder what exactly a collaborative, quiet, responsive, intimate traditional Irish dance and music piece would look, sound, and feel like.

We begin trading variations on "Big Pat's," suggesting, referencing, sonically articulating notions of what might be possible within the phrases of the 32-bar tune. We repeat the form again, unfolding it further each time around. We move together downstage lock-eyed. The timbre of my sounds changes; both my skin and my ears pique with the audible and tactile sensation as I step close to the microphone downstage left. The sound causes the viewers to crane, sitting up in their seats, hoping to elucidate from where exactly the soft, sometimes gritty, scrapings are emerging. The melding sounds of the bowed strings and the leather shoes on wooden floor evoke within me a physical sensation that is both lush and invigorating. I can feel my torso release as my ankles, knees and hips busy themselves with the labor—and pleasure—of sounding out the ornaments and chassis of the melody I am playing with my onstage partner; his articulated through bow, mine with heels, toes, and the soles of my shoes. My focus remains fixed on my collaborator standing beside me, gaze alternating from his right arm drawing the bow, conjuring sinuous ghosts to underpin my scratchy trebles, drums, and toe fences, and, only a few inches higher, the musician's face, composed, and yet animated, in focused concentration.

To explore these queer aesthetic potentialities, I began experimenting with different aspects of my dance practice, beginning with footwear. Forgoing the use of fiberglass or steel taps, I began working in a pair of hard leather-soled shoes, resembling those I had seen worn by older dancers who were trained prior to the advent of standardized Irish dancing competitions and the later commercial Irish dancing shows.[16] The lack of taps on the toes and heels of the shoes expanded the palate of sonic textures I could achieve through my percussive dance movement, allowing darker tones that could blend and nearly disappear among the soundscape of fiddles, flutes, and accordions.

This facilitated a degree of audible dynamic potential that I had never experienced within Irish dance. Instead of being restricted to crisp, adroit, punctuating footwork, the leather soles granted access to a new world of queer timbres: sibilance, fricatives, shivers, scrapes, or silence. By sweeping the sole of the shoe, maintaining contact with the dance surface, I found I could imitate sustained instrumental resonance, allowing me to elongate the duration of my sounds.[17] Through a brush of the ball of the foot, very close to an onstage floor microphone, I could create barely perceptible, liminal murmurs. These new sonic components could be interwoven in footwork sequences of more conventional Irish dance choreography, or even more queerly, could make the dance fade in and out of audibility. Performance studies scholar José Esteban Muñoz identifies this queer propensity for near-imperceptibility, stating that queer dance is "hard to catch."[18] The change of footwear constituted a queer departure from Irish dance's current anxieties of needing to be clearly and unmistakably heard—anxieties of masculine virility and "hitting the floor hard"—allowing a once-prevalent, but now nascent, queer potentiality to literally susurrate.

In addition to reconsidering Irish dance footwear, I also began to evaluate the queer potential of working with a singular musician, rather than an ensemble. I found this changed the affective quality of my dance pieces dramatically, presenting the opportunity to highlight the onstage exchange between performers. With this simple shift came an adjustment in both positioning and proximity. Irish dancers, both soloists and ensembles often perform center stage, usually directly in front of the "accompanying" musician(s). With the reduction of the ensemble to one musician and one dancer, this spatial configuration no longer felt satisfying to me. Instead, I began to inhabit a movement space directly alongside my collaborator, often in very close proximity. This allowed both the musician and me to explore the communicative potential of gesture, mild changes in carriage, and eye contact.[19] Watching a musician's hands as he played, reading his body movement to anticipate musical ornamentation and dynamics lent a new simpatico to the experience of performing together. Rather than a hierarchical manifestation of soloist and accompanist emphasizing the virtuosity of the dance, the pieces became a responsive, same-gender *pas de deux*.

The spatial reconfiguration of dancing alongside my musician collaborator imbued the performances with a sense of legible rapport. One recurring comment from audiences was that the way we engaged visually was striking, even intimate. The notorious, "unspeakable" homosexual scandal made manifest and a rumor began circulating that my collaborator (a widely presumed heterosexual man) and I were sleeping together. I had no interest

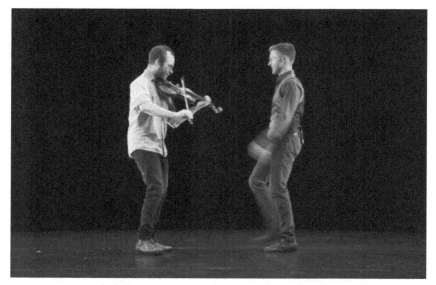

FIGURE 10.1 Nicholas Gareiss (step dance) and Cleek Schrey (fiddle). Photo credit: Sarah Nesbitt.

in verifying or denying this. The rumor itself demonstrated that the queer potential of enacting a collaborative intimate music-dance performance had been attained. Herein was the opportunity to present a sense of queer ambiguity and possibility within the recently homophobically strictured medium of traditional Irish music and dance. A simple performative choice to look at my male collaborator, rather than "wink at the ladies in the third row," had both aroused homosexual anxiety and simultaneously released that tension through an observable creative exchange between two performers.[20]

In my enmeshed relationship as both a performer and ethnographer, I noted the feedback these subtle performance shifts elicited from audiences and collaborators. This often incorporated remarks about my personal identity as an openly homosexual man.[21] After collaborating onstage, a flute-player friend stated, "You have the chops of an Irish dancer without the restrictions of being a heterosexual male." According to this comment, there was something aesthetically constraining about traditional masculinity in Irish dance movement. In the eyes of this interlocutor, my queer performance (onstage and off) alleviated this normative restraint, thereby opening new aesthetic possibilities. Further, his comment alluded that these possibilities were unavailable to the bodies of non-queer dancers. The contrasting aesthetic of my queer movement practice allowed for a perceived expressivity, constituting a slippage of the heteronormative masculine role typically performed by male

Irish dancers. A similar experience occurred during a pre-show sound check when a male member of a well-known Irish band I was performing with nodded to me and remarked, "*an buachaillín bán.*" The term translates in Gaelic as the "fair-haired" or "light-haired boy" and, in addition to being the title of several pieces of traditional Irish folk music, is also used colloquially in Irish-speaking communities to refer to homosexual men. Being "read" and identified as *an buachaillín bán* within this context confirmed hermeneutically the power of these performance choices in excavating nascent queerness within Irish cultural forms, a queerness that is and is not spoken, in whispers and linguistic obfuscation.[22]

The experience of having my performance of queerness observed and remarked upon brought Geertz's assertion into focus, collapsing my role as ethnographer-outsider and performing-insider. I found that presenting my moving body in performance allowed me to be penetrated by the gazes of audiences and fellow collaborators, becoming further interwoven culturally, as they projected their own background upon what they witnessed. Though for a long time I considered anthropological work and performance practice as separate modi, eventually I realized that my ethnography did not cease when I stepped onto the stage. Through performance, I was researching the meaning-making surrounding Irish traditional music and dance, even as I was interrogating norms of gender and sexuality. A queer-identified American outsider looking into the genre, I refused to become the penetrative ethnographer, eschewing the narratives of masculinist power and heterosexual stricture found both in the genre and in the binary anthropological history of ethnographer/subject, colonizer/colonized. Rather, by placing myself in the gaze of those familiar with the genres of Irish traditional music and dance, I found myself very culturally enmeshed indeed.

Through this Geertzian enmeshing I found space for queer aesthetic departure. Via a process that involved allowing Irish corporeal practice to inhabit my queer American body, I looked to other Irish cultural forms for what I perceived as a nascent queerness. Drawing inspiration from Irish traditional music, song, and pre-standardized, pre-commercialized Irish dance forms, I delved into these queer potentialities, exploring the ways they could influence my choreographic work. This de-interlaced Irish dance from its recent hyper-masculinized, heteronormative model, excavating a queer potentiality that was always there, but not articulated in the form. The process allowed me, as a performer within a roots genre, to maintain a connection to the cluster of practices associated with the history and geography of traditional Irish forms, while interrogating their tropes. It is my hope that this process can make space for other creative explorations by queer-identified exponents of Irish traditional forms, overwriting O'Shea's assertion of queer and Irish mutual exclusivity, and making the danced whispers of one *buachaillín bán* generative to this end.

The fiddler turns the tune, slipping from "Big Pat's" into "Dan Breen's Reel," arousing new rhythmical motifs within my body. There is sensuality, a physically rewarding coitus of melody, sound, and improvisational proposal. Though I am the only dancer onstage and he is the only fiddler, somehow I do not feel like a soloist, but rather his dance partner . . . and though we are playing phrases in the cadence of duple meter, we are holding each other like waltzers: lifting, bearing each other's weight, initiating sound and gesture through a reflexive, mutually-dependent process of affectual suggestion.

Notes

1. Clifford Geertz, *After the Fact: Two Countries, Four Decades, One Anthropologist* (Cambridge, MA: Harvard University Press, 1996), 44.
2. Helen O'Shea, "'Good man, Mary!' Women Musicians and the Fraternity of Irish Traditional Music," *Journal of Gender Studies* 17, no. 1 (2008): 66.
3. See Nicholas Gareiss, "Queering the *Feis*: An Examination of the Expression of Alternative Sexual Identity in Competitive Irish Step Dance in Ireland" (Master's thesis, University of Limerick, 2012).
4. Michael Seaver, "Counting Capital: The Real Value of Dance in Irish Society," *Dance Ireland*, 2012, February 10, 2013, http://www.danceireland.ie/content/pubs/Counting-Capital-The-Real-Value-of-Dance-in-Irish-Society.pdf
5. Éamon De Valera, *The Ireland That We Dreamed Of*, speech, March 17, 1943, January 12, 2012, http://www.rte.ie/archives/exhibitions/eamon-de-valera/719124-address-by-mr-de-valera/. The fact that Irish dance is marketed to tourists (the dance form is often called to duty to represent Catholic, rural, home and hearth Ireland) perpetuates the recycling and restaging of these heteronormative conventions. This is reified through dance scholar Jane Desmond's idea of "staging the natural": "tourists attending folkloric shows see a performance of 'traditional' (i.e., 'naturally occurring') behaviors which celebrate the difference and particularity of the performing group." Jane Desmond, *Staging Tourism: Bodies on Display from Waikiki to Sea World* (Chicago: University of Chicago Press, 1999), xvi.
6. For many, the Irish marriage referendum of 2015 signaled a cultural shift by granting marriage rights to same-sex couples in Ireland. While my fifteen years of fieldwork that informs this essay occurred prior to the much-publicized vote, it remains to be seen how the 2015 legislation will impact conventions of Irish traditional music and dance performance. Can state-sanctioned equality penetrate the heteronormative and binary gender-enforcing performance conventions

within traditional Irish dance? How will this shift in policy, enacted by popular vote, embolden queer Irish dance practitioners to explicate the nascent queerness underlying the form? Can Irish dance, so central within Irish culture, now queer the ideas of home, nation, and family it has traditionally been associated with? What other formerly unspeakable queer subjectivities will be elided from (or domesticated by) Ireland's recent same-sex equal rights agenda? I am eager to observe how the nascent queerness I sense within Irish cultural practices will be negotiated and performed in a post-referendum Ireland.

7. Folk knowledge suggests that most of the music in the Irish traditional music canon was once used for both soloistic step dancing and group social dancing. It is held as tacit among many musicians that step dance, though often currently disconnected from the traditional Irish music scene because of competitive dance contexts, still embodies an integral symbiosis with Irish traditional music.

8. I have found this to be especially true in my performances as a solo dancer. In a solo, it is possible to create tremendously expressive moments while subjecting one's body to the gazes of viewers and interacting with the audience and on-stage musicians. Within such performances, the Irish dance soloist references cultural mores and themes. Ethnochoreologist Catherine Foley argues, "when these practices are performed by step dancers in contexts appropriate to their performance, they generate meaning." For me, Foley's assertion that Irish dance performance has the ability to reify or disturb cultural norms, serves as a provocation for the performance of non-normative gender and sexuality. Catherine Foley, *Step Dancing in Ireland: Culture and History* (Farnham, Surrey: Ashgate Press, 2013), 19.

9. See Judith Butler, "Performative Acts and Gender Constitution: An Essay in Phenomenology and Feminist Theory," *Theatre Journal* 40, no. 4 (1988): 519-31; and the introduction to Jane Desmond's volume, *Dancing Desires: Choreographing Sexualities On and Off the Stage* (Madison: University of Wisconsin Press, 2001).

10. In my Master's thesis, "Queering the *Feis*," I make the case that these depictions of binary gender and heteronormative sexuality are often choreographed on the bodies of queer dancers, stricturing the physical articulation of non-normative sexuality. I demonstrate the falsity of O'Shea's assertion of queer and Irish mutual exclusivity through the textual act of publishing ethnographic interviews of over forty LGBT Irish step dancers collected while I was living in Ireland. I aver that the Irish step dance's appropriation by nationalist institutions has imposed a heteronormative framework on the form that is subverted by the prevalence and expertise of queer practitioners within traditional Irish dance today.

11. In considering the performance conventions of these genres, I realized that the stage would be the most salient environment in which performers might legibly queer traditional forms. To quote Desmond, "the feminization of spectacle, of putting oneself on display (without the cover of sport's masculinity-authorizing

violence), feminizes male dancers." This seemed especially applicable given the role of competition in the history and pedagogy of Irish dance. Desmond, *Dancing Desires*, 19.

12. Gráinne Campion, "Performance Style and Practice in the Sean-nós Singing Tradition" (Undergraduate thesis, St. Patrick's College Dublin, 2012).

13. Jacob Blickenstaff, "The Gloaming's Unlikely Convergence: Martin Hayes and Thomas Bartlett on their Multigenerational Irish-Music Powerhouse," *Mother Jones*, August 14, 2014, http://www.motherjones.com/media/2014/07/contact-thomas-bartlett-and-martin-hayes-gloaming-interview.

14. Paul O'Connor, "Back and Forth between Tradition and Abstraction at the Cobalt Café," *Last Night's Fun* (blog), February 8, 2011, https://lastnightsfun.wordpress.com/2011/02/08/899/.

15. Catherine Foley describes such pre-standardized Irish dance practices as embodying a softer carriage and a personal expressive response to music in *Irish Traditional Step Dancing in North Kerry: A Contextual and Structural Analysis* (Listowel, Co. Kerry: Red Hen Publishing, 2012).

16. The soles of these shoes were softer than traditional fiberglass-tipped "hard" or "heavy" shoes, but still harder than "light dance" shoes. "Light shoes" are used for a non-percussive style of Irish traditional dance incorporating aerial, nearly balletic movement. While there exists repertoire within the light shoe genre danced by both men and women, in traditional dance competitions, or *feiseanna*, women alone are allowed to compete in slip-jigs, a dance tune type in 9/8 time considered graceful, light, and too effeminate for boys. The shoes themselves also illustrate a fixed gender binary: "light" soft shoes worn by girls resemble lace up slippers or *ghillies*. In contrast, light shoes worn by boys have a fiberglass heel attached, which is utilized in a series of virtuosic stamps and clicks in the male versions of contemporary light shoe steps. Another genre of Irish dance which historically utilized leather-soled shoes is *sean-nós* ("old-style" in Gaelic) dancing, a regional style found in Irish-speaking *gaeltacht* area of Connemara, West Galway. The style is known for its percussive articulation, improvisation, and corporeal release into the floor. *Sean-nós* exists in stark contrast to the lifted and often airborne Munster-originating forms of Irish dancing taught by *An Coimisiún Le Rincí Gaelacha* and other competitive Irish dancing organizations. While historically many *sean-nós* dancers wore leather-soled shoes, during my time in Ireland all of the dancers who identified themselves as such, including my teacher, wore steel taps, rather than the fiberglass "tips" worn by the *Coimisiún*-style dancers.

17. This aspect of sustained, foot-to-floor fricative sound-making facilitated exciting new mimetic connections with instrumentalists. I could now "hold" my "notes" the way a fiddler or piper would, lending a new queer intimacy to my working

with musical collaborators through the often in-the-moment decisions of how long to sustain pitches.

18. José Esteban Muñoz, *Cruising Utopia: The Then and There of Queer Futurity* (New York: New York University Press, 2009), 81.

19. Pragmatically, this provided a tremendous increase in the ability to make decisions with a musician in an extemporaneous way in performance.

20. Thanks to Jill Dolan, who, after attending a presentation of an early draft of this paper and observing a video of my performance, wrote that my turning toward my collaborator onstage resisted the stricturing enforced by the prohibition of male Irish dancers never being allowed to look at each other. Simply by looking at my same-gender musician co-performer cultivated a visual regard of public intimacy, "rewriting the more frontal and heterosexual conventions of the dance." Jill Dolan, "Queer Dance at U of Michigan, " *The Feminist Spectator* (blog), February 22, 2012, http://feministspectator.princeton.edu/2012/02/22/queer-dance-at-u-of-michigan/.

21. While Ireland is distinctly noted for its "soft-pass," in contrast to American cultural hypermasculinity, there was nothing in my identity presentation that was attempting to "pass" as heterosexual.

22. In what Nancy Scheper-Hughes calls her "failed ethnography" of the rural west of Ireland, *Saints, Scholars, and Schizophrenics*, she identifies the Irish cultural predilection for "skill with words, metaphor, veiled insult," as "doublespeak," stating that she encountered conversations "laden with double-talk, obfuscations, interruptions, and non sequiturs, which make it difficult for the uninitiated outsider to follow and participate." Being "read" in this double-spoken way was a striking confirmation of the queer tendencies of Irish traditional music and dance. Nancy Scheper-Hughes, *Saints, Scholars, and Schizophrenics: Mental Illness in Rural Ireland* (Oakland: University of California Press, 1979), 158.

11

Aunty Fever

A QUEER IMPRESSION

Kareem Khubchandani

ironic that dance / my ticket to assimilation / my way of amusing / then winning / acceptance by whites / [how many of us have followed this path] / that the same steps were now
my passage / back home.

—MARLON RIGGS, *Tongues Untied (1989)*

▶ "Sari"

Origin stories matter.

They matter to us as queer people. Coming out scenes. First crushes.
Celebrities we masturbated to. Infatuation with mom's lipstick. Dad's tool
belt. Remembering these primal scenes provides us beginnings in a narra-
tive-driven world that doesn't have story arcs to reflect our lives.[1] Our non-
queer friends remember similar scenes, but they are not imbued with the
same gravitas that we give them. The shame they may have felt around such
improper attachments dissipates, or perhaps rests, upon securing and enjoying heteronormativity.[2] On the other hand, queer shame potentially inflames
when we put on a leather harness, bind our breasts, or take a PrEP pill,
reminding ourselves of the margins we continue to play on. Changing policies and access to rights have not made queers equals, and our bodies, desires,
and daily lives continue to be violently coerced into various gender and sexual
norms. Sometimes by our own shame—that's how hegemony works. Creating
stories about where we come from and how we're made gives us footing on
a delicate marley of gender and sexual normativity, fiercely policed and sanitized by religion, family, and government alike.

Origin stories matter to us as dancers. The first time we witnessed a virtuoso. Watched our sisters in the cipher and wanted to break like them. Home

videos and family legends of baby-you keeping time with complicated beats. The uncanny freedom we felt in the discipline of form. Such memories serve as punctuations that anchor our passion for art and practice. Such stories provide roots for our desire to make, especially when these desires lie beyond the logics of capitalist productivity or anthropological function. They help us and others make sense of and even love our strangeness. Our queer compulsions.

As queers, as dancers, as queer dancers, we are success stories, errant futures predicted in origin stories that could not be curtailed by propriety and respectability. Origin stories allow us to claim resilience, to facilitate and further our queer dancing futures without rejecting diasporic, immigrant, working-class, Third World pasts. More than just convenient nodes that naturalize our bodily desires (dance, gender, sexuality) in childhood formation, origin stories are pools of sentiment from which we continually draw aesthetic and erotic inspiration.

I want to tell you about my origin stories, about who populated them, about the women who made me want to dance. I want to recognize their labor and instruction that has given me the creative tools to survive as a brown boy navigating a racist and femmephobic America.[3] I want you to hear this story because when you see me perform as LaWhore Vagistan, the radical-feminist-bicurious-Bollywood drag queen, I'm worried that you see someone who has nicely arrived in a good gay identity as a temporary settler in the United States. Who performs a respectable multicultural identity, diversifying the gay bar with that *Slumdog*-realness. But I want you to know that (some of) my queerness—the strange ways I like to move on a dancefloor, to exhibit my body on stage and in public—comes from a time before my queerness had clotted into identity. Even before I called myself "gay" I was cultivating a queer sensibility. I knew to be embarrassed by my love of *The Sound of Music*, paisley prints, *Marie Claire* editorials on how to achieve orgasm, and the Vengaboys. But I reveled anyways. I still do.

So much of what is queer about me comes from my aunties.[4] When you see me dance, I hope you see more than just a liberated Third World homosexual who has arrived to fuse East and West by mixing Bollywood and US drag to please a multicultural audience. I hope you see that my earliest trainings were in the style of my Indian aunties, making beautiful dances in Ghana. Their style inhabits my muscles and shapes my taste. I dance in tribute to them.

I am a mama's boy. The youngest of three boys, the "mistake," the "love-child," the one who was supposed to be a girl. I stayed close to my mother, accompanying her to dance practices with her friends. Many of these Indian women had, in their twenties or even late teens, traveled to Accra, Ghana, from across the Sindhi diaspora, to marry their Indian husbands. While there are exceptions to the rule, men stay put and women leave their childhood homes. They arrived with origin stories of an elsewhere self. Memories that would help and hinder building a new life.

Once or twice a year, the Indian Merchants Association in Accra held large community events at the local temple, at the British High Commission, at rented ballrooms. At these events, the women always danced. Husbands were welcome to, but they hardly volunteered. They could be convinced, though I never learned how. Maybe using sex? I like to give my aunties such lysistratic agency. As a mama's boy, and as one of the only Sindhi boys in my age group, I was privy to my aunties' dance rehearsals. I pretended to do homework as I watched my aunties create and repeat movements. Twisting wrists against each other into flourishing arcs that traveled from hip to hip over the head. Regularly shifting weight on to the left foot every downbeat. Bumping heels of hands against each other to rattle imaginary bangles.

These simple steps are the foundations of my drag. When LaWhore prepares, she has gestural choreography to match the saucy lyrics of "Munni

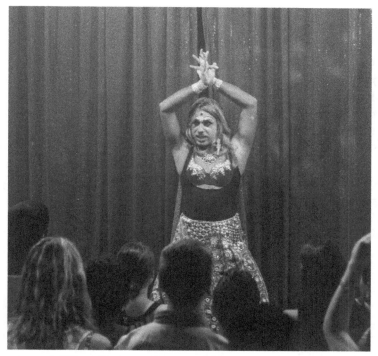

FIGURE II.I LaWhore Vagistan. Photograph by Tanay Dubey, courtesy of Kareem Khubchandani.

Badnaam" and "Fevicol Se." Running her hands over her mouth at the mention of "wet lips," pulsing her breasts outward when a "heartbeat" is mentioned. But Hindi film songs leave long instrumental sections between verses. My aunties' simple steps have become the instinctual fillers to those interludes in my Bollywood choreographies. Most drag queens would use such moments to collect tips. But so many audiences don't think that an Indian drag queen should be tipped. "She's just performing her culture." For some, culture is not art. In those empty moments, I have these fond repetitive steps to fill the difference between drag and culture.[5]

I was too young to attend the balls and galas, held after my bedtime, where Johnny Walker flowed freely. And so I relied on videotapes to see the finished products of these dances. At dance practices, I watched my aunties scoop hand-held lamps around their bodies, rehearsing the path of least burn. I never got to see the full effect of the fire-lit *diyas* in rehearsal. On video I could watch the choreography finally make sense under dimmed lights. On video, their regalia—gold-bordered saris, diamond jewelry, highlighted hair—sparkled in the flickering fires. I watched these videos incessantly. My aunties were my idols, transforming on stage from the makers of chutney sandwiches and chai, to satin-clad sex bombs and chiffoned nymphs. Transforming into men. So often my aunties played the parts of men in dances because husbands wouldn't perform. During their rehearsals, I observed the gestural language—balled fists, wide stances, and cocked heads—that made masculinity.[6] But on video I could watch my aunties in full drag, long hair tucked into hats or behind a shirt collar. Flirting with other aunties to much applause. From my aunties, I learned a Bollywood masculinity: flashy, smirky, effusive, and unabashedly sexy.[7]

When I dance, my face does the labor of entertaining the audience. I don't have great full-bodied coordination. But my face can tell the story of the song, even if the rest of my body belies my ineptitude. To some, this looks like good drag training rooted in lip-synch, camp, and melodrama, which tends toward over-exaggeration and satire. To others it signals training in classical Indian *abhinaya*, expressing the desires between mythic lovers. In reality, it is a skill learned from my dancing aunties, a technique that allowed them to exceed everyday limits placed on their gender. Their age (and sometimes weight) gave them an excuse not to indulge in highly aerobic choreographies. Instead they acted out scenes and stories based on song lyrics, using purposeful gestures and exaggerated facial features. A bit lower-lip was seductive. An index finger on the dimple was innocent. A cupped hand over a furrowed brow was searching. These externalized emotions, culled from the heroines of Hindi cinema, were not in excess of the choreographies my aunties did, they *were* the choreography.

My aunties also taught me how to dance. When there was a community event early enough in the evening to include kids, my aunties choreographed for my friends and me. I was schooled in the Twist and Mash Potato, and in Rock 'n' Roll turns, because those were the dances they loved as kids. Origins, sentiments, and repertoires transferred across generations. My mother's signature Twist shifts weight from right to left, and pauses on either side for a double leg lift with pointed toe. I've kept that. My aunties also insisted that I dance *as* a boy. But again, they were the ones who taught me how a masculine body moves, through their own instruction. By demonstrating on *their* bodies.

Since I've been old enough to attend those nighttime galas, my aunties are also the ones who give me permission to occupy the dancefloor. I feign reluctance knowing that boys are not supposed to dance. When I was a teenager, my mother and I were watching a cousin's wedding video brought over to Ghana from Hong Kong. She pointed out one guy on the dancefloor. "Everyone thinks he's gay. He's a very good dancer." But all my aunties know I love to dance. They've witnessed my penchant since those rehearsals in their living rooms in Ghana. They will always pull me up from my seat, and make me dance with them. I am easier than their husbands. I am willing (after a little persuasion) to become a spectacle and they love this about me. I don't take this to mean that they love and accept my gayness per se, nor are they making a spectacle of my flamboyance. Rather, they create a space on the dancefloor to transgress certain norms, to seriously enjoy dancing, to be queer through dance.

I have queer politics because of my aunties.[8] I understand the perils of heteronormativity and gender inequality because I have spent so many Saturday afternoons listening to them. They talked about meager allowances from their husbands. About manipulative in-laws. Affairs. Possible entrepreneurial ventures that wouldn't occlude their husband's status as breadwinner. Sometimes they just cried in each other's company. I witnessed that too.

Origin stories matter.

Now I am invited to dance festivals, teach in dance programs, and am published in dance anthologies. Now I am on boards of LGBTQ organizations, a scholar of gay nightlife, and a visible drag artist. It may seem like I have, just now, arrived. Origin stories remind me that well before my queer dance was validated by a variety of institutions, media, and audiences, I was dancing queerly. That I continue to dance queerly is not just a matter of individual resilience. It speaks to the care and pedagogy of those around me—lovers, mentors, friends, family, and yes, aunties—who have fought for space for me on the dancefloor, and who have their own origin stories that justify such queer acts.

Notes

1. Judith Roof, *Come, as You Are: Sexuality and Narrative* (New York: Columbia University Press, 1996).
2. Taylor Mac's *Young Ladies Of* (2008) describes the rituals through which young white men are inducted into proper heteronormativity by ridiculing and abandoning such improper attachments. R. Justin Hunt, "Queer Debts and Bad Documents: Taylor Mac's *Young Ladies Of*," in *Queer Dramaturgies: International Perspectives on Where Performance Leads Queer*, ed. Alyson Campbell and Stephen Farrier (New York: Palgrave Macmillan, 2016), 210–22.
3. Dwight A. McBride, *Why I Hate Abercrombie & Fitch: Essays on Race and Sexuality* (New York: New York University, 2005).
4. The title of this essay is a play on Jacques Derrida, *Archive Fever: A Freudian Impression* (Chicago: University of Chicago Press, 1996).
5. See the section titled "When Drag Is Not Drag" beginning on page 1053 in Jabir Puar's essay. Jasbir K. Puar, "Global Circuits: Transnational Sexualities and Trinidad," *Signs: Journal of Women in Culture and Society* 26, no. 1 (2001): 1039–65.
6. I was learning that gender could be disarticulated from sexed bodies well before I read Judith Butler's *Gender Trouble: Feminism and the Subversion of Identity* (New York: Routledge, 1990).
7. As J. Halberstam has argued, women also make and perform masculinity. J. Halberstam, *Female Masculinity* (Durham, NC: Duke University Press, 1998). Additionally, José Muñoz explains that despite his ambivalence around masculinity given the ways it was vigilantly policed in his childhood, it is around butch lesbians that he is most comfortable. José Esteban Muñoz, "Gesture, Ephemera, and Queer Feeling: Approaching Kevin Aviance," in *Dancing Desires: Choreographing Sexualities On and Off the Stage*, ed. Jane Desmond (Madison: University of Wisconsin Press, 2001), 428.
8. E. Patrick Johnson, "'Quare' Studies, or (Almost) Everything I Know about Queer Studies I Learned from My Grandmother," in *Black Queer Studies: A Critical Anthology*, ed. E. Patrick Johnson and Mae Henderson (Durham, NC: Duke University Press, 2005).

12

Last Cowboy Standing

TESTING A CRITICAL CHOREOGRAPHIC INQUIRY

Peter Carpenter

▶ "Last Cowboy Standing"
▶ In conversation with Peter Carpenter

A thin, white man walks across the stage toward the audience. He wears jeans, a white, sleeveless western-snap-front shirt, and one worn cowboy boot on his right foot. His left foot remains bare. The asymmetry of his footwear produces an uneven gait, recalling the rhythm of a limp. He looks toward a series of individual audience members throughout the space, and gives them a small nod, acknowledging their presence in this dance.

Queerness drives my choreographic work, explicitly prompting content and embodied/compositional experiments to counter the straight mind's oppression.[1] At times queerness provides a framework for research or a lens through which to see a (dancing?) body's agency. Other times queerness reminds me that my own white, gay male, privileged body cannot assume queerness—I attend to queerness through uncomfortable processes that say "yes" to perspectives beyond my own. Queerness serves to keep me working outside of my own navel-gazing and to remember to engage sex and gender within contexts of class, race, and globe. Put another way, when I dance queerly I remember the political limits of dancing alone.

Queering the expectations for concert stage performances historically predisposed to invalidate same sex desire occupied the center of my attention from early in my career. I began making dances in 1992, as friends and mentors of mine were dying of AIDS. Early works valued confrontation, grief,

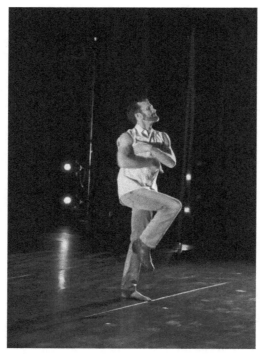

FIGURE 12.1 Peter Carpenter in *Last Cowboy Standing*. Photo by Sarah Nesbitt.

and stigmatized isolation. Today, queer methodologies—which have grown alongside my exposure to discursive strains in queer studies and dance scholarship—continue to shape my choreography. In particular, I appreciate the ways that queer theory has exposed and interrogated the privilege afforded to white, male, First World artists in the context of neoliberal inequities. With this essay, I intend to provoke a bit of methodological trouble, contextualizing the dance "Last Cowboy Standing," a solo I choreographed and performed for the first time in 2006, as part of a critical choreographic methodology that includes ethnographic fieldwork, detailed analysis of precursory choreographies, and sustained engagement with scholarship from dance studies, queer studies, and related fields. In this, I hope to reveal the historicizing practices that steep critical choreographic inquiry and vivify the possibilities for multidirectional exchange of knowledge production between scholar, choreographer, and subject.

The thin stature of the dancer and his wobbly walk betray his association with the cowboy's authoritarian masculinity. He arrives downstage and faces the audience with his arms at his sides. He stands ready to draw an imaginary gun, or maybe he stands frozen with fear. Ronald Reagan's voice comes over the sound system and the audience hears, "those who say that we're in a time where there are no heroes, they just don't know where to look." Reagan's voice echoes through the space. The dancer slowly (reluctantly?) steps around himself in a circle. His bare foot forms an unstable compass needle, anchoring the booted foot as he strides. His uneven cadence disavows Reagan's reference to heroes, even as his solo presence on the concert stage affirms the dancer's power.

I choreographed the dance "Last Cowboy Standing" as part of a larger research project on queer, danced iterations of the cowboy icon during the Reagan–Bush era (ca. 1980–2008). This work began as an ethnographic research project that I conducted at Oil Can Harry's, a gay country-western bar in Los Angeles' San Fernando Valley from 2001 to 2004 while I attended graduate school in Los Angeles. I have also looked at concert dances by artists such as Ishmael Houston-Jones, Fred Holland, Joe Goode, Marianne Kim, and Lee Anne Schmitt; each has taken on the cowboy with queer agendas. In choreographies on the concert stage and on the social dance floor, I have admired the complex relationship between critique and homage that marks numerous strains of ambivalence with cowboy masculinity. Finally, I have looked to popular culture—including mainstream film, gay independent cinema, and reality television—for ways in which the cowboy has emerged as a landmark of idealized gay masculinity and desire. The products of these interests have taken numerous forms, ranging from performative lectures to choreographic works to essays. "Last Cowboy Standing" is one installation of this ongoing methodological experiment.

"Those who say that we're in a time where there are no heroes, they just don't know where to look." This text repeats over the sound system in various, digitally edited incarnations. The dancer steps lightly, as if being blown up and back into space, curving and spiraling in the torso, before resting in a bound, weighted stance. His arms cross in front of his chest tightly. He might be containing the volume of his breath, or wearing an imagined straight jacket. Simultaneously, his bare foot darts at the floor and then at the boot he wears. His toes scrape up his shin, revealing the ankle of the tan boots as he pulls up the pant. Is the foot getting the boot's attention? Is the boot weathering the foot's abuses? What kind of conversation might occur between boot and foot?

I read the cowboy boot in the context of a metonymic chain of associations wherein cowboy-ness accrues symbolic resonance in consort with US national identity; the boot is not just the boot of the cowboy who performed hard labor in the nineteenth-century United States but also the cowboy that symbolizes Manifest Destiny, and the Hollywood appropriations of the cowboy swagger. This boot also gestures toward the anti-gay political associations cowboy-ness accrued in the Reagan–Bush era. And perhaps more to the point, the iconic cowboy imagery that I deploy does not reference any of the above in isolation; rather the cowboy imagery I work with is iconic in the sense that it draws power from all the referents above. The boot symbolizes a hegemonic, non-queer nexus of power relations and oppression that the choreographies in this project work to disrupt with physical and compositional acumen.

Offsetting the symbolism of the cowboy boot, the bare foot of the male dancer brings vulnerable effeminacy and kinetic possibilities. The bare foot provides an unguarded counterpoint to the masculine normativity the boot procures. And it gestures additively as well, toward the effeminacy and non-normative masculinity historically associated with the male dancer. In the context of the Reagan voiceover, this symbolism extends to AIDS.[2] Symbolically, the power embodied in the cowboy image meets, uncomfortably, the effeminacy and non-normative masculinity of the male dancer marked by the possibility of AIDS.[3]

The choice to prominently feature Reagan's voice in the sound score is based on my assessment that Reagan stands as one of the most important—if reviled—figures of queer life in the late-twentieth century. I draw this assessment from the importance of AIDS on the lives of LGBT people and the central role that Reagan's presidential neglect played in the development of the AIDS crisis. Here I join numerous queer scholars, activists, and Reagan's own biographer in attributing Reagan's lack of attention to the disease as a result of his othering of the gay men and intravenous drug users that were the first localized casualties of a plague that quickly became pandemic in scale. Biographer Edmund Morris describes Reagan as reflecting on AIDS as divine retribution for society's moral failings, on one hand, and cracking homophobic AIDS jokes, on the other.[4] More pointedly, public health worker Jan Zita Grover reads Reagan's lack of action in the early days of the AIDS crisis as driven by his assessment that AIDS was not a threat to the American public that he saw as his citizenry.[5] In limiting his view of the American public to straight, white, upwardly mobile Christians in whom the future of the nuclear family could be safely assured, Reagan staunchly maintained a blind spot to the health care needs of Americans deviating from the norm. Activist groups such as the AIDS Coalition To Unleash Power (ACT UP) marked his negligence through copious visual references to Reagan's image in protests that disrupted business as usual.[6] By placing my own thin, effeminate body in a cowboy boot and dancing with and against Reagan's voice, I intend to remember and re-mark Reagan's role in the epidemic while revising Reagan's conceptions of the American public to include queers.

The dancer develops a kinetic vocabulary from the stuttering steps and shifts he executed at the beginning of the dance. Slides, leans, and falls intersect within the body to propel him through space. He reaches his arms through space, scoots his feet underneath to catch up, and then stops. He walks (limping) toward the audience again. The dancer opens his mouth to lip-synch with Reagan as the audience hears, "I believe there is a plan, somehow a divine plan for all of us. I know now that whatever days are left of me, belong to him." The man moves his mouth in time with Reagan's voice; he is Reagan's puppet for a moment. He closes his mouth tightly and clenches his jaw on the "m" of "him," then rapidly opens and closes his mouth. At the same time he points his finger up to the sky, referencing the "him" of god to whom Reagan refers. This god finger turns to a pretend gun and the man plays at shooting three members of the audience. This dissolves into a sequence of gestures wherein the dancer touches himself from his head to his toes. His postures replicate someone shading his eyes from the sun, to a patient checking for swollen glands around his throat, to a citizen pledging allegiance, to a street hustler grabbing his crotch, to a ranch hand cleaning dirt out of the heel of his boot. Throughout this, his feet march in a steady rhythm. This series of gestures and stomps repeat again and again, accelerating to a mechanized fury.

I learned to sift through the politics and poetics of cowboy embodiment from a bunch of gays and lesbians at a bar in the San Fernando Valley. They taught me that cowboy-ness is a learned vocabulary and not a natural essence. As such, the majority of them encouraged me not to take this cowboy thing too seriously. We really just come here to dance, they would remind me, as I asked them questions about their disidentifications with the cowboy icon.

Yet I attend seriously, in spite of informants who told me the dancing was just for fun, to the ways that oppressive structures manifest themselves within queer cowboy choreographic histories. Gay country-western dancing became an identifiable social dance practice at the same historical moment that Reagan was elected to presidential office on an anti-gay, cowboy political agenda. In the late 1970s and early 1980s, cowboy-ness emerged as an entertainment destination not confined to western or rural America, nor concerned with heroism. Rather, country-western music, films, television shows, and dancing became a mainstream commodity, and film and television provided audiences with a contemporary, urban West, replete with sex and moral failure. Perhaps paradoxically, the gay rodeo movement, which developed alongside the popularity of gay country-western dancing, contemporaneously emerged from philanthropic impulses in the interest of improving the image of gays to mainstream America.[7] These destabilized moralities aptly reflected and arguably fed America's ambivalent relationship to cowboy-ness in the wake of Vietnam, the lingering shadow of the sexual revolution, and the advent of the Reagan presidency, which became known for a fervent advocacy for and enforcement of socially conservative, or "family," values. Throughout this project, I look at the ways in which queer cowboy choreographies point toward Reagan's moral imperatives that denied the humanity of citizens deemed untouchable in the early days of the AIDS pandemic. In "Last Cowboy Standing," the cowboy becomes a lens through which to interrogate Reagan's propagation of anti-queer cowboy politics.

After a sequence of careening, uneven steps, the dancer assumes a bound, stoic pose. Arms now down by his waist, he tries to flex his arm muscles for a moment, to lock this masculinity in place. A second later he jumps into the air and lands sprawled on the floor facing down. He immediately flails his arms and legs in a violent scrabble. His arms brush the floor as if trying to sift through an arid terrain, as if wailing on a gravesite, as if trying to push the ground away. His wiry frame bumps and scrapes audibly against the floor, the boot punctuating the irregular meter. Over this, the sound score scrambles Reagan's voice into a cacophony of empty, fragmented declarations. This collision of violent movement and disconnected sound recalls the confused logic of AIDS dementia and a restaging of Reagan's mind during Alzheimer's simultaneously. He then takes his weight into his feet and transitions from striking at the floor to a nonchalant brushing off of his boot and foot. He continues this gesture up his shins and thighs, crotch and torso. His facial expression betrays smugness, while his body recalls a Teflon surface, unaccountable to constituent or legacy.

While my choreographic research into the cowboy began at a gay country-western bar, I explored the compositional possibilities of bringing queerness and cowboy-ness together in the rehearsal studio. At times I worked from the codified pedestrianism of line dancing as a base for vocabulary, while at other times I worked with images and scenes from classic western films as source material. These sources developed unexpected political resonance. When studying the iconic cowboy masculinity of John Wayne in *Red River* (1948), for example, I became interested not only in Wayne's distinctive performance of masculine ruggedness but also in the way that this performance shaped masculine performances in generations of American men, including Reagan.

I find it ironic that both Reagan and I looked to Wayne as a model, but from different ideological and historical perspectives—whereas Reagan emulated Wayne's mannerisms, I sought to interrogate them. Over time I began to delight in how close the cowboy swagger could come to an effeminate swish. In choreographically combining these unlikely bedfellows, I intend to disidentify with the political conservatism associated with cowboy masculinity and reconfigure the cowboy's power to work for queers. Following José Esteban Muñoz's theory of disidentification, I try to use the code of heteronormative cowboyness "as raw material for representing a disempowered politics or positionality that has been rendered unthinkable by the dominant culture."[8] Indeed, who else but a queer choreographer would find such a swish in Wayne's swagger?

In the choreography described above, I intend the masculine authoritarianism of the cowboy to extend in multiple directions: toward the Reagan presidency, toward AIDS, toward queerness, and toward a potential for American democracy that I still want to believe in. And, in turn, I intend these sites to refer back toward cowboy-ness, coloring the possibilities for what the cowboy, and a cowboy dancing, might mean. "Last Cowboy Standing" creates these shades of meaning and layered resonances in synchronicities and disconnections between body and text, between presence (my body) and absence (Reagan's voice signals his absence from the space), between the official word of state ideology (isolated pieces of rhetoric in the sound score) and queer dissent (the choreographic resistance to the text). Queering the cowboy image has been the goal of many of the choreographies I have studied, and this experimental methodology which blends ethnographic fieldwork, choreography, concert dance analysis and extensive reading from pertinent scholars has attempted to reinforce the work of my precursors and develop the project through a surgical placement of queer cowboy choreographies next to the voice of Reagan as an indictment of Reagan's inaction during the early days of the AIDS pandemic. The autodescription of "Last Cowboy Standing" provided here serves as a further development in this inquiry.

This critical choreographic methodology did not occur in isolation or even by design. Rather, like many queers and dancers who end up producing public discourse, I simply tried to understand my own experience through connecting with other queers and other dancers. Sometimes the connections were cordial, sometimes heated, sometimes intellectual, sometimes sexual, sometimes gestural, and usually kinesthetic. Thankfully, queer studies and dance studies share an admirable history of connecting discourses to bodies, and scholars and choreographers alike have been relatively welcoming of my queer moves. Perhaps due to the youth of the fields, or due to the inter-disciplinary moment that we live in, or due to a valuing of corporeal knowl-edge, I have received great support and acceptance of my desire to work out of bounds. Even as some viewers and readers rightly question the queerness of my work due to my white male body taking center-stage, no queer or dance scholars have ever told me to get back in line. Rather they have reminded me to attend to my own privilege in the interest of pushing forward a radically queer, embodied politics. Their critique and conversation sponsors a multi-directional exchange of knowledge production, queering stage, page, and subject.

Notes

1. I take "the straight mind" from feminist scholar Monique Wittig's seething assessment of the negating effects of patriarchy for women, and I connect her critique of binary sex/gender systems to queers dwelling in the possibilities that exceed heteronormative templates for living. See Monique Wittig, *The Straight Mind and Other Essays* (Boston, MA: Beacon Press), 21.

2. AIDS Activist and dance scholar David Gere writes persuasively about the poten-tial for male dancers on the concert stage to have been assumed as carrying AIDS in the early years of the disease. Through a conflation of gay male with male dancer and gay male with AIDS-infected, men who danced were frequently assumed to be positive, see *How to Make Dances in an Epidemic: Tracking Choreography in the Age of AIDS* (Madison: University of Wisconsin Press, 2004), 47.

3. In addition to this symbolism, the boot and foot also deliver a kinetic discourse on the possibilities of the hybrid. In movement terms, the boot offers a slippery surface as well as the leverage of a lightly elevated heel. The foot counters these assets with traction and a more nuanced intersection with gravity.

4. See Edmund Morris, *Dutch: A Memoir of Ronald Reagan* (New York: Modern Library, 1999), 457–58.

5. See Jan Zita Grover, "AIDS: Keywords," in *AIDS: Cultural Analysis/Cultural Activism*, ed. Douglas Crimp (Cambridge, MA: MIT Press, 1988): 23–24. Grover theorizes the self/other distinction embedded within concern for the general pop-ulation in reference to Reagan's entire malaise with leadership around the di-sease. She writes, ""Gary Bauer, President Reagan's assistant, told *Face the Nation* that the reason Reagan had not even uttered the word AIDS publicly before a press conference late in 1985 was that the Administration did not until then per-ceive AIDS as a problem: 'It hadn't spread into the general population yet.'"

6. Gere analyzes the presence of burning effigies of Ronald Reagan as part of the1988 ACT UP occupation of the Food and Drug Administration in Rockville,

Maryland. Gere discusses the protest as a choreographic response to the FDA's conservative approach to experimental drug therapies in the early years of the disease. He writes that the burning of Reagan images—central to the visual and symbolic potency of the protest—were fueled not only by Reagan's ineffective leadership but also by the perception that Reagan was openly hostile to queers and people living with AIDS. See Gere, *How to Make Dances in an Epidemic*, 63–76.

7. For a nuanced triangulation of queerness, cowboy-ness, and Reagan, see Christopher Le Coney and Zoe Trodd, "Reagan's Rainbow Rodeos: Queer Challenges to the Cowboy Dreams of the Eighties America," *Canadian Review of American Studies* 39, no. 2 (2009): 163–83. Also see the website for the International Gay Rodeo Association: http://gayrodeohistory.org/. I first found this information in a printed program distributed at an IGRA event in Reno, Nevada, that I attended in April 2004. Another site detailing this history can be found via Dennis McBride, *Out History.Org*, "Reno Gay Rodeo": http://outhistory.org/exhibits/show/las-vegas/articles/rgr

8. José Esteban Muñoz, *Disidentifications: Queers of Color and the Performance of Politics* (Minneapolis: University of Minnesota Press, 1999), 31.

13
_____

RMW (A) & RMW from the Inside Out

Jennifer Monson

▶ *RMW(a) & RMW*: Performance #1
▶ *RMW (a) & RMW*: Performance #2
▶ in conversation with DD Dorvillier and Jennifer Monson

Interior prologue—the warm up

Dark room, blue light, fishing around for ground.

Last minute wig adjustment and make-up. Holly Hughes is ready for lesbian deer hunting
big guns, big eyes.

The backs of the audience, pressed against chairs. I'm waiting for the empty.

As we walk onstage, the audience adjusts to our wigs, our legs, our frumpy sex affect leaning in toward them.

RMW (A)

a space

I start to dance following the quick adjustments of being seen. Leaning into DD's watching, making something for her, abrasive, hitting back what the audience sees.

You are my cipher, my love, my cook, my combatant, my advisor, my bed, my protagonist. I am your heat, your smell, your eyes, your interpreter.

The timer goes off. You join me, take my stance, my move, myself and move it on. I watch you titillate, swivel, arch an eyebrow and a lip, become more beautiful, become me, become unholy. I'm seduced.

The timer goes off. I tread across the space to you. Fill you, imagine you, and head off.

another space
Exterior (the audience)

I look at as many of you as I can. Look you in the eye. You are hot, I want you, I will have you, I want to be on you, in you, fuck you hard, and then I'm turning. Face, face up, face down, face in DD's ass. Hair slapping her ass cheeks. I'm on my knees. She has always allowed me to beg. She is the empire state building, a vast dark lake, my ripple, a quiet sound from underneath, hunting me on.

We intermingle. We shine each other up. And slap our bare backs on the dark. DD is always better than me. Her music is everywhere.

Darkness, Transition. Changing Into Levi's and T-Shirt

RMW

I'm on the floor, like something hit me, waiting. You pick me up by the edge of my coat, I grab your hands and together we throw me away. Down stage left. It happens again, pulled, longing, thrown, bounced, shirt sleeves, slippery.

I hunch into the weight of my own body and compress it into yours. To help you toss me, slide me, putty in your pink hands.

I'm careful with you. Remembering instructions. Following technique to send you where you need to go. I crash onto you and roll to the side, pull at your jacket and devour you. Holding, squeezing, sliding up your belly, rolling you. You attend to me like a starfish, multi-legged, extending in and out.

Till you stop atop me. Unzip and decoat me. Roll me like taffy up to your lips. We kiss for a long time with so much movement it's a circus.

Our lipsticked lips locked together, feet pad up and off the floor as pants sail off the legs. I'm your beast of burden. Will hold onto you, hold you up, hold you out. Till you tower above – the stage on my back.

Down we fish flop around, bellies lifted, music of skin and floor, paying attention to sound only, throats closed.

I lift you up over my body, you sink and rise. Your weight settling my nerves, my bones.

In 1993 DD Dorvillier and I were commissioned to create a collaborative work for the Movement Research Sexual I.D. series curated by Jaime Ortega. At that time New York was a powerful seat of queer activism—Queer Nation,[1] ACT UP,[2] WHAM,[3] Lesbian Avengers.[4] George Bush Sr. was president and people were taking to the streets and demanding changes in drug laws, fair treatment of people with AIDS, access to abortion, and freedom of sexual expression. *RMW* was made in that spirit of immediacy, activism, and sexual openness. It played with a sensual confrontation between tenderness and brute force, and an ambiguously gendered sexuality.

In 2004, we were commissioned to re-create *RMW* for the HOWL! Festival at Performance Space 122 in NYC. The necessity for us to absorb and articulate the artistic, personal, and political shifts in the previous decade gave way to a second part, *RMW (A)*. Since then we have continued to perform the work as a diptych almost annually. The piece is a tool for calibrating the shifting landscape of desire, sexuality, and gender in both our individual lives and those of our larger cultural and political contexts. In a press release for a performance festival in 2011, we wrote, "Now in the age of Obama, internet organizing, and digital communication, the piece evolves into an exercise of listening and witnessing. The exterior space of the streets has been replaced by the interior space of the internet."

Both sections of the work continue to evolve over time and in relation to each other but in distinctly different ways. In *RMW (A)* we continue to use the body as a means to effect social and political readings through an immediate and reflective improvisational score. *RMW* keeps a steadier form through set, choreographed material. As time passes I experience *RMW* more like an object, a choreography, that DD and I enact with detailed precision but that changes with necessity as our bodies and our audiences change. *RMW (A)* is a structure of timed improvised actions and responses that gives space for new material to emerge. As the nature of queer evolves over time, I see the queer "object" and the queer "action" of the two sections responding to an evolving and mutable understanding of queer—one that, in this case, continues to destabilize the terms of gender and sexuality as our two differently female bodies move in and out of overt and covert movements of desire. Both parts of this diptych illuminate a particular kinetic sensibility evolving out of the time they were conceived.

February 2012, Ann Arbor, MI

At the performance of *RMW (A) & RMW* at the CORD conference, Meanings and Makings of Queer Dance at University of Michigan, there was an entirely queer audience arriving at the end of a dense and sophisticated co-mingling of academic, performative, social, scholarly, philosophical, political conversation and exchange. In the performance this allowed for a certain space to open up that gave me a completely new experience as a "queer" performer. DD and I start the performance with *RMW (A)*, the section of the piece that was created in 2004. Our costumes in *RMW (A)* are built around large wigs, drag make up, and clothes that expose our legs. At the conference—where the assemblage of drag would be well worn, well known, and well critiqued—I came into my own. Barefoot, big white legs, long blonde wig, bright red lips, long, languid eyelashes. I stabbed my gaze out into the audience and for the first time ever didn't wait for the audience to stare back or accept me or my invitation to come on in. Instead I went directly out—straight out on some limb that took me up close to every person. I had an overpowering feeling that I could "have" each one of these people—that I could want them, seduce

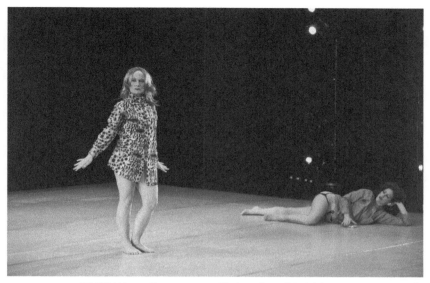

FIGURE 13.1 *RMW(A)* performance at University of Michigan, 2014. Jennifer Monson (*left*), DD Dorvillier (*right*). Photo by Sarah Nesbitt.

them, hold them in my desire in a way they couldn't turn back. I wasn't afraid of the stakes of being taken up on it.

The strategies that I use to access vulnerability are particularly DYKEY I think. They are about a specific kind of power and physical prowess, about endurance and obstinance that demand a physical risk-taking that is not precarious, but it is unstable. I find at the edge of the vulnerability an energetic frequency that pushes beyond representation into a different kind of desire that for me often exceeds the human, and at times also drops me into the bucket of erotic humor. The beyond-human is explicit in different ways— surging up through the dancing. The erotic humor feels like an uncanny return that I didn't even know I could return to. Improvised eroticism is comedy. It is titillating, unsettling, the seducer/seduced is in flux, a constant negotiation and surprise.

These strategies push past the subjectivity of the ego and the personal. Once that level of vulnerability has been passed the stakes are raised. It's no longer about me, or even my relationship to the audience. The borders have been crossed in order to map out the possibility of mutually constitutive experience. It is a bit like building trust, but it is also like clearing the brush with a machete and we are taking turns with the swing.

RMW (A)

RMW (A) is a structure of time. DD and I take turns dancing while the other holds a timer and witnesses the dancing. The time score is set in advance and fluctuates from five to one minutes. We exchange roles three to four times. (In the performances so far, I always begin. DD always ends.) At the end of each designated time segment the performer with the timer enters the dance by replacing—taking the place of—in the fullest way possible—the other performer. The new performer continues the dance from the moment the timer goes off while the other performer becomes witness. Roles are switched each time the timer goes off.

The structure of the piece is built around the triangulation of the roles of witness, doer, and audience. We watch each other, we let the audience watch us watch each other, we watch the audience watch us watch each other, and we watch the audience watch us. The transmission of information comes from the witnessing between DD, myself, and the audience. This exchange of witnessing and being witnessed both projects and absorbs the fleeting handles of personae, identity, and/or thingness alive in the dancing. It keeps multiple emerging desires on the move.

Practice and Preparation

There is a particular kind of preparation for the piece that is about looking in the mirror. DD helping me with the eyelashes and the eyeliner. We touch each other's faces. Put on nail polish and often remove it. Sew, comb out wigs, and iron shirts. I spend more time in the dressing room than for other performances. It is a production. The wigs come on last, slid over hair tucked under a wig cap.

This prepares us for the open-ended nature of the "practice" of the piece. It is a way for us to practice knowing each other and loving each other in the way of aesthetic intimacy that exceeds any notions of sentimental or romantic attachment. We are in conversation about ways in which we are making sense of the world through dance and that conversation can only be had in the dancing itself and in the witnessing of the audience. DD and I often talk about the piece as being like a folkdance—a kind of folklore that persists, bringing along histories, ways of knowing places and people that change over time as we continue to perform the piece. It is distinctly different than a piece in repertory. It restores me to a past and a historical way of moving and simultaneously lets me be in the present. And lets me imagine a future somehow.

There are multiple kinds of spaces or stances created between DD and me and the audience. There is an intimacy in the space between DD and me that we are discovering through the structure of the work as well as through our decades-old history of dancing together. We are, in part, revisiting our relationship and inviting the audience in to witness, but we are also reliant on the audience to help us address each other. The intimacy is not sentimental. It is based on years of hard-earned trust—of testing and accepting each other's aesthetic questions and demands as well as a shared commitment to use those questions to respond to the political contexts we find ourselves in. The work is about desire—the recognition and mobility of desire is constantly shifting in the spaces between the performers and the audience. We stand, sit, move, pose as a way of taking a stance toward each other and the audience. This allows all of us to be becoming lovers, strangers, critics, drag queens/kings, beasts, friends, toys, desires, and pure image and movement.

Different from *RMW*, in which we are dressed in similar clothes of jeans and t-shirts, in *RMW (A)* we wear distinctly different costumes but each are posing and perhaps practicing different strategies of drag. The costume provides a foil for me to literally dance myself into and out of any convention of gender or sexuality. DD spurs me on. In attempting to become her in that moment of transition when the timer goes off, the possibility of becoming anyone or anything opens up. Our costumes hold the signifiers of female, dyke, drag queen, poser. Temporality, authenticity, and/or representation are not legible or stable in these outfits. We find ourselves inside the external destabilization of the costume—it both physically dislodges us from a normal stance through the extra weight of fake eyelashes on the lid of the eye, the wigs on the skull that shape the use of the head and balance, the nakedness of the flesh on the legs, the smell and taste of lipstick, hairspray, and newly ironed clothes and through the play of becoming each other through taking on each other's movement.

I feel unlocatable in the wig, make-up, and dress until I start dancing. The dancing is where I make love, where I access the threads of desire shot across the stage from the many eyes and feeling bodies in the room. My body picks up on the waves and vibrations of this uncertain desire and rapidly makes it into an unfolding dance. For DD I am on display. For the audience, I haven't figured that out yet.

1993—DD and Jennifer at the Matzoh Factory

DD and I had been living together in the Matzoh Factory at 319 Bedford in Williamsburg, Brooklyn, for about two years when we made *RMW*. We were both somewhat active in the burgeoning queer activism of the time—participating in ACT UP and WHAM actions, and I was a fairly devoted member of the Lesbian Avengers. The Matzoh Factory was the place we lived, made work, had parties, had sex, and held workshops and performances for our friends and community. Other influences of the time included Circus Amok, Jennifer Miller's queer outdoor summer circus; Open Movement and Music Dance at Performance Space 122;[5] and the work of Yvonne Meier, Ishmael Houston-Jones and John Bernd, Mark Ashwill and the Spitters, as well as some of the work that I was developing (primarily *Tackle Rock* and *Finn's Shed*) that was based on physical limits of impact between bodies that was simultaneously fearless and vulnerable.

DD and I had been dancing together for five years or so. Although we had been dancing in a variety of contexts, *RMW* was the first time we solely collaborated on making something with each other. The intimacies of our relationship were forged through dancing and living together. When Jaime asked us to create a work for the Sexual I.D. series, it was both an invitation and opportunity to articulate and structure the collective influences that were shaping our artistic interests at the time.

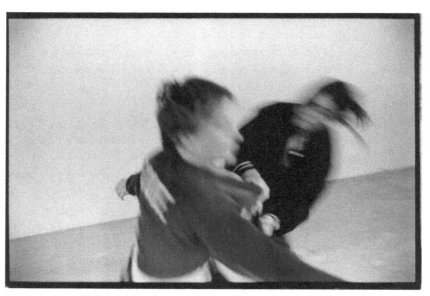

FIGURE 13.2 *RMW* rehearsal at the Matzoh Factory, Brooklyn, 1993. © 1993 Carolina Kroon.

Due to the AIDS epidemic, the early 1990s were a time that demanded an eruption of sexual liberation. Gay sex was defined as a death sentence, lesbian sex was barely visible, any kind of sex was dangerous and immoral, abortion rights were at stake as well as access to sex education. DD and I were exploring our sexualities with different partners and configurations and the energy of the erotics of that time fueled the choreography of *RMW*.

That year I had presented Tackle Rock, Hinge of Skin, *and* The Lesbian Avengers Pounding Dance *at Danspace Project at St. Marks Church. One of the performances was a benefit for Treatment Alternatives Program (TAP), an organization that Jon Greenberg had helped found. We didn't know each other well but Jon had reached out to a wide range of folks to think of ways to fundraise and bring awareness to the projects TAP was working on. We were doing what we could to expand our resources and networks to support the cause of fighting HIV however possible. It is hard to imagine that Jon died so soon after that event. He was such a powerful force to me in our political community and was fearless and generous as an activist.*

On the hot day of July 16th, I remember standing next to my friend, the choreographer Neil Greenberg, Jon's brother, in Tompkins Square Park after we had marched there with Jon's coffin from 1st Ave and 1st Street.[6] We were amidst the throngs of enraged, devastated mourners. The energy of collectively creating a space for public mourning through defying the police and moving in the streets together gave us a charged sense of joy. In that moment we were calling on each other to create a ritual that could contain the multiple layers of feeling and respect for Jon's and the many other lives unnecessarily lost.

The moment with Neil was like a pool of water. It was quiet and reflective. We stood in the space as dancers, sensing the movement around us, highly aware of emotional currents sweeping around us yet protected in the private, personal sense of Neil's loss. I couldn't imagine what it was like to experience one's dead brother's body in this public space that was activating, moving, and rallying so many people. It was one of the few times I have seen a dead body in public. It was wrenching—that moment, and I felt so honored to be there with Neil feeling his privacy and his responsibility to his family and to his community. There wasn't anger. There was an almost palpable joy at being able to celebrate together and witness and honor death together at the same time igniting our will to stop the dying and find a cure.

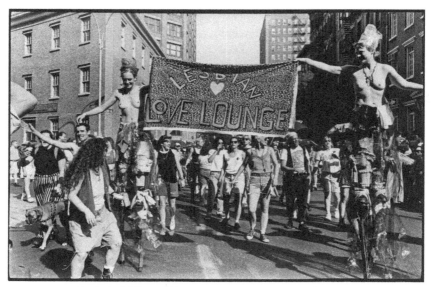

FIGURE 13.3 Lori E. Seid's Lesbian Love Lounge, Gay Pride 1993. © Dona Ann McAdams.

I don't want to be righteous or romantic or superimpose my own per-
sonal feelings about that time on this piece or on this writing. I was thirty-
two years old—five years younger than Jon Greenberg. My first good friend
with HIV had died in 1988 when he was thirty-five. (John Bernd—an
amazing artist and choreographer). This was our life then—to watch our
friends and the artists in and around our community gradually sicken
and die or take their own lives. We demonstrated in response. We took
over streets, we yelled, we chained ourselves up. Many other people have
narrated this story and were more involved than I was. I feel like I was on
the periphery of ACT UP, showing up at demonstrations, going primarily
to Lesbian Avenger meetings because I wanted to be around more women
and that was also a very hot and sexy time. DD and I had been living in
the Matzoh Factory for two years and were both more or less single and
having a lot of sex.

RMW (A) is RMW—Action is Object

RMW (A) reconceives the original *RMW*, adapting to what couldn't be conceived of in 1993 and to the unaccountable histories our bodies hold in relation to each other. The structure of the piece organizes meaning and memory

from the frequencies that are resonating in the space between us and the space between the two of us and the audience. This is a practice of transmission and reception delivered out of the obstinate structure or object of *RMW*.

Unlike in *RMW (A)*, in *RMW* we are always moving together in proximity and almost always touching or in a unison energy. We wear similar clothes; we do the same or related movements. We are the object that is a duet. The dance feels like a thing. It has a beginning and an end. *RMW* is the object from which the action/transmission of *RMW (A)* was born.

The sensibility of risky physicality is embedded in *RMW*. We were bent on making a thing—this thing I now call a queer object because to me it feels like you can pick it up and look at it and identify certain signifiers of a particular queer history. We wear the ACT UP uniform of Levi 501s and white t-shirts. We are obvious in our desire, like the queer kisses that were on display on the sides of buses in the safe sex education campaign of Gran Fury's "Kissing doesn't kill: Greed and Indifference Do,"[7] as well as their "Read My Lips" campaign. These images were gorgeous and sexy, the bodies kissing were sensual, exceptional, and the scale of them on the buses hailed us with our own erotic potential.

For me *RMW* has that same kind of graphic presence. It skirts a kind of representation of the erotic at the same time as the materiality of our bodies, sweating, bracing, sliding, throwing, and sucking constructs a kinesthetic object that the audience both sees and feels.

An object has a structure that reproduces a shape of erotics. It is a physical relationship that depends on being in the right place at the right time. The technical articulation that DD and I create is precise and we shape each other's bodies through touch. Whereas, in the action of *RMW (A)*, we shape each other's bodies through a transmission of presence. This queer action of transmission has a structure that reimagines a space and a shape of intimacy every time. It is a becoming; it is about a transmission of shape-shifting, a moving in and out of the transition of one being to the other or others. There is an echo of possible presences made available as the audience watches us transform the movement of one dancing body to another. We take hold of the existing desire in the other's dancing and move it somewhere unexpected.

RMW

In *RMW*, we start with an almost violent sequence of throwing each other helter-skelter across the floor: picking each other up by jeans and jackets, slamming and spinning in and out of the floor. Eventually I tear off DD's jacket and devour her until she stops sitting on top of me. She takes off my coat. She spins my head until we end in a kiss that we playfully extend into a contortionist duet. We get almost naked; we show our sweat. We create anticipation and erotic charge through falling and releasing, devouring and baring, opening and closing in a legible language of dyke desire. This scaffolding of choreography—this morphable queer object—holds the history and potential of our changing bodies each time we revisit the piece. It is a moldable object, fitting back into our bodies as they have moved through time—a bit more delicate, a bit more stiff, a bit more sophisticated, a bit more worn and husky, a bit more sexy. The lights never dim. When the piece is finished, I release DD's back onto my belly. We pause. We roll to the side and get to our feet.

Notes

1. Queer Nation is "a direct action group dedicated to ending discrimination, violence and repression against the LGBT community." It was founded in 1990 by activists working with ACT UP in New York City. Queer Nation, http://queernationny.org. The manifesto is available at http://historyisaweapon.com.

2. ACT UP NY, founded in 1987, is "a diverse, non-partisan group of individuals united in anger and committed to direct action to end the AIDS crisis." ACT UP, http://actupny.org.

3. Women's Health Action and Mobilization, or WHAM!, was "founded in 1989 in response to the U.S. Supreme Court's decision in Webster vs. Reproductive Health Services of Missouri, which granted states more power to restrict women's access to abortion." "Women's Health Action and Mobilization," https://en.wikipedia.org/wiki/Women%27s_Health_Action_and_Mobilization.

4. The Lesbian Avengers began in New York City in 1992 as a direct action group focused on issues vital to lesbian survival and visibility, http://www.lesbianavengers.com.

5. "Open Movement" was started by the artists who founded Performance Space 122 and was a weekly space for open improvisation. "Music Dance" was similar but included improvising musicians and dancers. The process was more rigorously structured. Specific improvisational scores were created, tried out, and discussed. At Open Movement, discussions were informal and there was no music and no decided-upon score. It was purely open space to move in.

6. "ACT UP Capsule History 1993," ACT UP NY, http://www.actupny.org/documents/cron-93.html.

7. Image that was posted on buses June–December 1989 as a project of Creative Time, NY, http://creativetime.org/programs/archive/1989/Kissing/Kissing.htm.

PART III

Intimacy

14

Futari Tomo

A QUEER DUET FOR TAIKO

Angela K. Ahlgren

I seldom consider myself an artist, even though I have been playing taiko for over fifteen years and writing about it for over ten. But today I write from my perspective as a queer white woman engaged in the creative act of crafting new taiko performance and in doing so, of making and remaking new possibilities. As a player, I enjoy the visceral pleasures of taiko—the obvious ones like moving my limbs and coaxing sound out of the drum, but also things like sweating together in rehearsal, packing up equipment in an unscripted choreography, and enjoying beer and sushi as we rehash the mistakes and triumphs after a performance. But some of my deepest satisfactions as a taiko artist are those momentary connections that spark between performers and spectators, the ones that suffuse a theatre with possibility, the ones that spill into the realm of the intimate, the sensual, and even the erotic. Perhaps all forms of performance-making enable these kinds of communion, but in this essay I want to foreground the space taiko has made for queer intimacies.

Watching a grainy DVD recording of my ex-partner and me performing together compels me to consider the queer acts that weave through my taiko experience, both on stage and off, part of the vast range of intimacies forged through performance. I draw the term "queer act" from performance ethnographer Ramón Rivera-Servera, who writes, "Being queer is never a completed journey but a continuous process of becoming queer that requires queer acts." As strategies for navigating a heteronormative world, these acts range from everyday practices to staged performances to modes of reading and spectating.[1] As for Rivera-Servera, my thinking about queerness is grounded in

materiality—lived experience—rather than abstraction, as well as in intersectionality.[2] This essay considers how racial difference and gender performance are entwined in my process of making and performing a taiko duet
for two women. In the following pages, then, I consider a series of queer acts,
centering on "Futari Tomo" ("Two Together"), my 2007 queer—or perhaps,
lesbian—duet for taiko. The inspiration for a queer taiko duet was drummed
and danced into being far before I ever decided to make the piece, or perhaps
I should say that taiko is a practice through which queer possibilities took
shape for me, both on and off stage.

Taiko is not an inherently queer or feminist practice. In fact, often its embodiment of masculine power has been put to heteronormative and nation-
alistic use.[3] But its sonic, visual, and kinesthetic boldness also make taiko
an appealing feature in gay pride parades and festivals, as well as in protests
calling attention to social injustices and anti-racist activism.[4] Taiko is a form of
ensemble drumming that originated in Japan in the early 1950s. It was taken
up by Japanese Americans in the late 1960s in California and has become
increasingly popular in recent decades in the United States, Canada, Europe,
Latin America, and now in other parts of Asia.[5] It was, in part, its impossible-
to-ignore sonic and visual qualities that made taiko so appealing to Asian
Americans in the late 1960s and 1970s and later, bolstered efforts to challenge
prevailing stereotypes of Asians as quiet and passive.[6] Recent data collection
efforts by the Taiko Community Alliance show that women comprise roughly
64% of taiko players who responded to the survey, and its feminist appeal is
well documented in taiko scholarship.[7] Yet this is not an essay about taiko as
explicitly activist performance, but an exploration of the potentialities of taiko
as a site for queer desires and intimacies, and therefore the political potential
in the erotic and the everyday. I have elsewhere explored ways of reading taiko
performance through a queer lens,[8] but here I elaborate on my history with
taiko and how it is intertwined with my understanding of myself as a queer,
white woman. The queer acts I narrate in this essay unfold not in isolation,
but in relation to other bodies, ideas, and practices: me and taiko, her and me,
then and now.

I. Two Together

In 2006, I moved from Minneapolis, Minnesota, to Austin, Texas, for graduate school. I moved away from Jen, my partner of six years, and from Mu
Daiko, the taiko group I had grown to regard as a family. One of the first
things I did was to create my first taiko composition, a duet for Jen and me to
perform. We developed it long-distance, working it out together during visits

in both cities, and rehearsing on our own in the spaces between. I wanted the song to ruminate on the tension between distance and proximity, and to somehow capture the connection and longing between us, two women. Often in taiko songs, the drums remain more or less stationary and the drummers move around them, but we placed these drums on casters and made them mobile, so that our proximity could be underscored as we expanded and contracted the space between us during the performance. In the piece, we begin on opposite corners of the stage, our individual rhythms intentionally not quite synced. By the end, after various positional and rhythmic shifts, we drum together, whirling past each other in a fast-footed dance between the faces of our two drums.

As I watch us perform on DVD, the wide shot makes us look small and far away, and the drumbeats sound bare without the chest-jolting there-ness of live performance. I feel exposed and vulnerable, more so now as I watch alone than when I performed it live in front of hundreds of people. Yet along with this vulnerability lives a shadow of the excitement I felt when I performed the piece, a bit of the elation that comes with performing live, the crackle and anticipation that builds between performers, between partners, and between the beats. In the piece, two separate pools of light appear, one on Jen downstage left, one on me upstage right. At first, the drums obscure

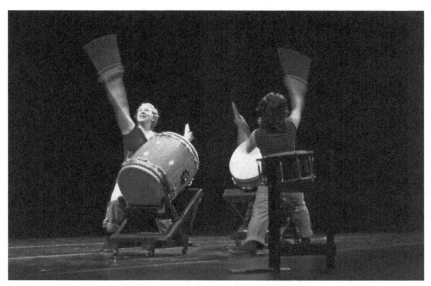

FIGURE 14.1 Angela Ahlgren (*left*) and Jennifer Weir (*right*) in the final section of "Futari Tomo" (2007). Courtesy of the University of Texas at Austin, photo: Ben Aqua.

us from view as we kneel behind them. I rise to the syncopated pattern Jen plays on her two drums. On the recording, my arms look almost liquid as they flow in X-patterns across the drum face: they sweep diagonally from left to right and back, then both arms unfurl into alignment for a moment before finding the next beat. It looks effortless, but I remember kneeling behind the drum, knees aching, awaiting the moment I could lift my *bachi* (drum sticks) skyward, the precise count on which I could begin to unfold my legs and rise into the pool of light, my face tilted toward its warmth. Each beat seemed so far apart. I wanted to jump ahead to the satisfying unison and up-tempo ending, to bridge the rhythmic dissonance and the gulf of stage floor between us.

Our costumes are intentionally more athletic than traditional, an attempt to look more sport-dyke than Japanese folk-dance. We wear baggy grey cargo pants and black athletic tanks from REI, along with black *tabi*, the split-toed, rubber-bottomed footwear popular among taiko players. My long blond hair lies in braids down my back, and Jen's short dark hair is loose. No makeup. Just the black expanse of the floor, our drums, and our pools of light. We are two women alone together on stage.

The two of us have different physical and emotional dimensions to our taiko playing, which emerge at different moments in the piece. We are playful with each other, smiling and smirking, and we call out to each other during solos. I focus somewhat shyly on the drum, particularly in the slow, opening moments. Even in faster solos, my tendency as a performer is to either channel my energy toward the drum or gaze out beyond the audience's heads. Jen looks right at the audience and flirts, her animated face and shining smile inviting them to respond. I root my feet to the ground and allow my arms to do the work, while Jen leaps around with energy bursting from all four limbs. I am careful; she is wild. I am precise, and she is a dynamo.

Despite these differences in style, our low stances and expansive arm movements cohere in unison moments. The strong, swift gestures create moments of physical and emotional largesse, a kind of fullness and richness I had glimpsed vicariously when I first saw taiko performed. Our emotional connection is clear. Here we are, the two of us together on stage, not separated as performer and spectator. We accompany each other musically: I keep a steady beat while she solos, and she drums for me while I move. And we accompany each other physically: our arms arc and swoosh in time, and we stay on stage together the whole time no matter how far apart or near to each other we get. We, the two of us together, collaborate in this queer dance, a performance of public intimacy between two women.

II. Music-as-Dance

When I first began taking taiko classes, before we even pulled out our practice drums, we learned to move our bodies. Before we hit the drum, we needed to know the *kata*, the basic physical form, of taiko. First, we did a warm-up. Jumping jacks, three sets of ten, counted out loud in Japanese (*ichi, ni, san, shi* ...). We swung our arms in wide circles to loosen our shoulders, we stretched our calves, and we rolled our wrists. The tape-wrapped tires mounted on folding chairs that served as practice drums remained on the periphery of the room. We stood in rows and learned how to align our feet, our hips, torsos, and arms, orienting ourselves toward an imaginary instrument. We learned how to swing our arms toward the drum, one body part at a time: first the hips, the belly, then the elbow, then the wrist, and finally the *bachi* (the drumsticks) propelling toward the drum head. Right, then left, right, then left. One, two, one, two. *Ichi, ni, ichi, ni.* This was "air taiko." Still the drums remained on the sidelines. We needed to absorb the choreography before we could make music.

With the emphasis on gesture and large-scale choreographed movement that is part of this musical practice, taiko lends itself to—indeed, requires—thinking about music and dance together. Taiko thus makes manifest the troubling of boundaries and the slipping out from under definitions that is central to this volume and that raises the unanswerable question of what constitutes queer dance. Some taiko players see themselves as musicians, others as movers, and still others as simply and only taiko players. Taiko is music and dance, music-as-dance, or as longtime taiko player Jeanne Mercer puts it, "music in motion."[9] Many kinds of music-making might be read as dance because, in the words of ethnomusicologist Matthew Rahaim, "when people make music, they move: a finger slides along the neck of a violin, a palm whacks a drumhead, a laryngeal cartilage tilts back and forth as air is pushed through the vocal folds."[10] In other words, there can be no music-making without movement somewhere in the body. In taiko, as in other musical genres, the body moves and sounds simultaneously; without movement, sound would be impossible. But taiko is both things together, music-as-dance, in a way that not all music practices are. Drums are configured in different visual patterns for each piece, and the drum placement facilitates a variety of movements and choreographies. While some movements are simply a matter of producing sound (the arm must move up or back in order to create enough force to produce the resounding *don* on the drum-head), others are designed to create stunning visual effects, or to emphasize the musculature of the player's body. Each piece, in other words, is choreographed both in terms of creating stage pictures through the arrangement of performers on stage and through the performers moving their own bodies while they play. Rahaim calls the music-making body in motion a "musicking body." Taiko bodies are both musicking and dancing, sounding and moving bodies, as well as sensual and sensing bodies.

It is this combination of music and motion that produces such undeniable kinesthetic effects on taiko audiences and performers alike. It was this combination that drew me to taiko in a queer act of spectatorship, the first queer dance between Jen and me. Queerness as a category is capacious, one I can move around in, push against, and try on as a series of stances. Women and people of color are often marginalized within this category, yet its capaciousness allows me to understand my own shifts between lesbian and bisexual as temporary and also bound together as a series of acts. North American taiko, too, in its relative newness and lack of agreed-upon gendered conventions and social meanings, leaves space for competing identifications and identity performances.[11] How might taiko in its multiple valences—as music and dance, as community practice and public intimacy—make room for queer acts between women?

III. Me and Taiko, Me and Her

The first time I witnessed a taiko concert was in December 1998. I was twenty-two. In those days, I stage managed often for Theater Mu, an Asian American theater company in Minneapolis whose Artistic Director, Rick Shiomi, had recently started a taiko group that would eventually become a major part of the organization. I was asked to fill in for the regular stage manager on this show, just for one night of the group's second annual taiko concert at the Southern Theatre, a beloved Minneapolis venue with dilapidated, crumbling-brick charm. By 1998, taiko had already developed a large following in the United States, especially on the West Coast, but to this white girl in Minnesota, it was still brand-new. The appealing unison movement, the rolling thunder of drumbeats, and the anticipation-filled space between beats (what I would come to know as *ma*), held my attention like no other performance.

One of the pieces that captivated me was "Pounding Hooves," a six-minute song written by Rick Shiomi that builds speed through unison movement while allowing individual performers to distinguish themselves through solos. It starts out with a slow and sultry swing beat, one drummer, then two, then three, unfolding from bent knees with a flourish of outstretched arms, softly beating their rhythms on the large barrel-shaped taiko while a fourth drummer keeps the *ji*, or base beat, on the upstage *shime-daiko* (high-pitched rope tension drum). Low martial-arts stances match the angle of the drums, forty-five degrees. The left knee bends toward the audience and the right leg stretches long. After each drummer has played her section introducing the song's major rhythms, the three finally cohere in unison sound and movement: three arms, three *bachi* (drumsticks), and three flashes of blue happi coat sleeve zing toward and away from us on alternating beats. *Don! Don! Don! Don!* Arms reach for the heavens, and shouts animate the space between beats. At the crest of a crescendo, the bachi crack out a sharp "ka, ka!" on the rims of the drums, as the drummers sweep their arms down and around, propelling a turn to the other side of the drums. The seven beats of silence while the drummers' arms whoosh and feet box-step around the drums fills the theater with anticipation. I watch carefully from my perch in the light booth, trying to discern the beginning of the next section in anticipation of the light cue. On the last silent beat of the *ma*, the drummers leap into the air as they unfurl their arms, expand their chests, and shout *HA!* Their bachi land on the drumheads as the drummers' feet reach the floor, and the moment is pure satisfaction.

As stage managing gigs go, this was easy. The performers needed minimal help moving drums at intermission, and they responded cheerfully to my announcements of "thirty minutes," "ten minutes," and "places." And it was there in that tech booth that I first felt the rumble of drums in my chest and acknowledged a prickle of possibility as I took in the performance. Hanging out on the periphery of the theater—backstage, in the tech booth, and in those strange, empty hallways in between—always felt like privileged territory, spaces from which I could view things not everybody else could see. These spaces offered their own queer perspectives, ones that were slightly askew but nonetheless a little more than what the average spectator could access. The booth itself, where I perched on an old stool in front of the lighting board, was a palimpsest of the building's history: flat black paint peeling where duct taped signs had been ripped off the wall; yellowing cue sheets and reminders not to leave food in the booth hanging on past their useful life; dried-up Sharpies and rolls of tie line heaped in darkened corners. No glass separated me from the audience settled into the 200 or so threadbare, red, once-velvety seats or the exposed brick wall that served as backdrop to the performance I was to run for the night.

Watching the six or so Asian American women and men move with such grace and power, I had no idea if this was something white people even did. Yet I was moved to find out. About three minutes into the song, the solos begin, and my eyes are drawn to Jen on the stage-left drum as she bursts into her solo with fierce joy. No longer constrained by the song's choreography, she throws herself into every strike of the drum and every fling of her arm with intense abandon. A Korean American woman of 5'2", Jen transforms before me, larger than life. She leaps to face the drum head-on and lifts her face to the audience, opening her mouth in a silent *roar* as she beats an X pattern on the drumhead before spinning around and laying out the rhythm that signals the end of her solo. I understand now that she had been playing taiko for only a few years, but that night her performance transformed me.

Most taiko players I know have a version of this love-at-first-sight story, how they saw taiko and wanted to play. This is mine, and it is erotically charged with both the pleasure of watching a woman perform and the desire to perform alongside her. Virtuosity, as performance ethnographer Judith Hamera writes, organizes the performer and spectator into a social relationship propelled by "the power of the vicarious."[12] Describing the performer Oguri's dances, Hamera writes, "The effects are more than visually arresting; they invite visceral, corporeal empathy."[13] Watching Mu Daiko from the tech booth, I responded kinesthetically to the performance. I wanted to be able to do what the drummers were doing. Their power and fluidity seemed unattainable, and I had no sense that I could achieve such feats of artistry and athleticism. And still, I wanted to. It looked effortless, yet also impossibly difficult—athletic, musical, powerful, beautiful, larger-than-life. Something about the joyful ferocity with which Jen propelled her whole body into the drums was appealing on a gut level.

Watching her, I was not only longing to drum and to perform. I was also longing for her. Hamera writes, "This longing across a gulf of physical difference is glorious and terrifying," a relationship in which the spectator can be "swept away by an upswelling of affect . . . by one's own insurmountable distance from, and connection to, the performer who inspired it."[14] And I was swept away by Jen's virtuosic performance, even though she had only been playing for one or two years. In retrospect, they were all mere beginners, but to me Mu Daiko's performance represented something completely beyond the scope of my own abilities—and beyond the bounds of whiteness. The longing and the "gulf of physical difference" between us (me and taiko, me and Jen) was complex because it was not only about technique and skill, and not only about queer longing, but also about racial difference.

I was swept away in a queer act of spectatorship, and swept into a longing for connection, longing to move alongside Jen and the other drummers. Ethnomusicologist Deborah Wong describes her first encounters with taiko from her perspective of an Asian American woman. She writes, "I had been moved many times by Asian American music-making, but watching taiko was one long extended moment of wanting to *do* that, wanting to *be* that—a deep urgent desire that I can now only describe as a truly performative effect. Watching taiko made me want to do it and all that that means."[15] What Wong hints at but does not quite say is that her experience of watching taiko was erotic, a kind of kinesthetic spectatorial experience that urged her to move and to act on the desires the drumming instilled. Her double entendre, "made me want to do it and all that that means" indicates an urge both to play taiko and to satisfy erotic desires. As for Wong, my first experience with taiko was a deeply visceral and sensual experience that was wrapped up in wanting to do what the performers were doing, to be with them, and to be what they simply *were*: strong, graceful, and unfettered.

But this "longing across a gulf of physical difference" between me and taiko, and between me and Jen, was about more than just skill and sensuality. It was also about race. Taiko did not answer a call to know my racial identity in the same way it has for Wong and other Asian American taiko players.[16] In that first encounter, thinking about the small group of Asian American performers before me, I wondered if it would be audacious for a white person to think about joining the group. Did white people play taiko? At this time, my question was not one of cultural appropriation or white privilege, but about observing the boundaries of a company with a specific mission to create work by and for Asian Americans. Mu Daiko was part of an Asian American theater company dedicated to creating roles for Asian American actors and producing plays by Asian American playwrights.[17] It would have seemed perfectly reasonable to me that the group would also prioritize the development of Asian American taiko players.

Yet the longing remained.

I was attracted to taiko for many reasons. It was powerful and graceful, and I could understand it as a bridge between my years as an athlete and my love for theater. The clean-lined, unadorned costumes that neither exposed nor entirely concealed the performers' bodies resonated with my ever-evolving sense of myself as a budding bisexual-lesbian and a feminist who eschewed things that seemed either hypersexualized or too obviously feminine. I also enjoyed the sense of ritual and discipline that is often part of taiko practice, if not always part of our specific group's practices. And certainly some of my attraction to taiko was part of an unconscious Orientalism, seeing the discipline and rituals of taiko practice as distinctly Japanese, different from the kinds of bodily and behavioral discipline required by basketball or tennis or play rehearsal, the practices of my Midwestern girlhood. As a girlfriend pointed out to me many years later, seeing women drum was also remarkable because drummers in pop music and even our own junior high and high school bands were overwhelmingly male.

Over time, my understanding of my own racial identity was profoundly shaped by taiko, but these insights came later. Within a month of that concert, I took my first taiko class. The charisma Jen wielded as a performer that night would later captivate me and evolve into a mutual off-stage attraction. A year after my first taiko class, I was performing on the stage of the Southern Theater with Mu Daiko rather than watching from the tech booth. And a year after that, I was dating Jen, not merely admiring her. After five years together, a wedding, and a house, I moved to Texas for graduate school, making our relationship a long-distance one.

It was my taiko practice and being half of an interracial lesbian couple that led me to study Asian American performance during graduate school. During our partnership, Jen and I indulged one another's interests and absorbed each other's histories and preoccupations. As she articulated to me recently, "you just kind of get on board" with your partner and what's important to them. As in the trajectory of "Futari Tomo," relationships ask their participants to negotiate distances, to move in and out of synch with one another, and to play in unison as much as possible. I began to understand how, although we both grew up in the rural Midwest, my experience being raised by my own, white Minnesotan birth parents was vastly different from her experience as an adopted Korean raised in a white North Dakotan family. We moved through the world differently—off stage and on. The intimacy of our relationship, along with the more casual intimacies between me and other Mu Daiko performers, propelled me to "get on board" and to adopt an Asian Americanist stance in my scholarship and in everyday practice whenever possible. Of course, despite these intimacies, differences never disappear—not in a marriage and not in a performing group—and the "getting on board" is a lifelong negotiation, a never-complete process that (like queerness) continually requires new acts.

IV. Here and There, Now and Then

"Futari Tomo" means "two together," yet it was really always about being apart. In taiko, as in many Japanese genres, the space between beats is not mere silence; it builds tension and lends shape to the whole composition. Dance scholar SanSan Kwan describes this meaning-laden emptiness, called *ma*, as "an in-betweenness of space and time [that] . . . is not empty and not negative but full of meaning and experience."[18] In "Futari Tomo," the physical space between the two performers contracts and expands throughout the piece, finally culminating in a section in which the two drummers whirl between two drums quite close together. Yet they never touch, and the space between them—between us—remains full of the tension built throughout the song.

We performed "Futari Tomo" for the first time in the spring of 2007, but by the time we performed it for the last time in 2008, we had broken up. Those later performances contained our new distance from each other as well as the palpable connection we shared. It is hard to read our chemistry in the wide shot of the recording I have, but I know it is there. Even after we broke up and continued to perform the piece, I cherished those moments on stage with her. In the nine-minute span of the song, we had little choice but to draw on the familiarity of our years together, not to mention our common training, to bring the piece to life. Performing required us to put quotation marks around our relationship and rely on our lived experience to realize the aims of the work.

Watching this queer duet now, several years after the performance was recorded on DVD, it takes some discipline not to want to jump into the screen and fix the tempo, adjust the technical aspects, not to mention refine our off-stage relationship. I am both distant from and deeply connected to the performance—my ex, myself, my taiko practice. Performance does slip away, as Peggy Phelan insists.[19] But I want to ask, along with Judith Hamera, "Why must we abandon the desire to envelop performance and hold it to us, or the desire for it to envelop us?"[20] Those moments on stage with Jen, even after our breakup—*especially* after the breakup—fulfilled the promise taiko offered when I first encountered it. When theater scholar Jill Dolan writes about utopia in performance, she writes about the effects of performance on spectators.[21] Yet those moments of vicarious longing, the queer desire, the glimpses of utopia I experienced when I first encountered taiko as a spectator, propelled me onto the stage. That performance practice compelled me to adopt a revised worldview. And in those nine minutes of performing this song, Jen and I could be just the two of us together, lifted out of the mundane details of breaking up, of distancing ourselves, and into the no-place of a bare stage where we could imagine a better future—no longer a future together, but perhaps not permanently estranged either. These moments on stage were delicious in their complexity. All the pain and disorientation of a breakup, the newfound concern over what was mine and what was hers, the uncomfortable practice of being apart: this was all channeled back into a mutual generosity that would have been impossible off stage. Performing with Jen allowed me to love her in those moments as the friend she was before we were together and the friend she would be again later. To hold on to this fraught performance is also to recognize that, as queer people and as women, we are always bound together, in cultural critic Maggie Nelson's words, by the "shared, crushing understanding of what it means to live in a patriarchy,"[22] and by the necessity of creating new queer acts.

At its core, "Futari Tomo" stages a deep longing, which permeates the gaps between two people, a longing that fills the distance between two people and compels them toward each other. Yet revisiting this duet now is not a longing for that moment in time or for that relationship, but rather an acknowledgment of the material—and transformative—effects of performance. When I wrote the song, I wanted nothing more than for Jen to finally move to Texas with me, to start something new together. In the last section, we whirl between the drums, always swishing close to one another, but never touching. I can't think of a taiko piece in which you'd touch another person. If this were modern dance, we'd probably eventually touch—embrace, roll around, share weight. If it were musical theater, our voices would harmonize. But in taiko, the most we could do was play in unison, look at each other, smile, and hope that the tension in the *ma*, this longing of one woman for another, made our performances crackle on someone's queer frequency.

Notes

1. Ramón H. Rivera-Servera, *Performing Queer Latinidad: Dance, Sexuality, Politics* (Ann Arbor: University of Michigan Press, 2012), 27.
2. Ibid., 27–28. Here, Rivera-Servera joins E. Patrick Johnson, José Muñoz, and others in his critique of queer theory's focus on white gays and lesbians.
3. Paul J. Yoon, "Asian Masculinities and Parodic Possibilities in Odaiko Solos and Filmic Representations," *Asian Music* (Winter/Spring 2009): 100–130. Yoon establishes the ways taiko, especially the style of playing the large *o-daiko*, is coded as masculine in both Japanese and American contexts. He contextualizes his discussion of Japanese o-daiko playing within a post–World War II context in Japan.
4. See, e.g., the image of a taiko player at an event commemorating Vincent Chin's death in William Wei, *The Asian American Movement* (Philadelphia: Temple University Press, 1993), 167 and cover.
5. Taiko is a Japanese word for drum. I use the term "taiko" here to describe the contemporary ensemble form of drumming that some might call "kumi-daiko" or group drumming, or the term used more commonly in Japan, "wadaiko," which distinguishes this particular style from other types of drumming. I use this generic term because it is the most common way for North American practitioners to describe their art form.
6. See Angela K. Ahlgren, "A New Taiko Folk Dance: San Jose Taiko and Asian American Movements," in *Contemporary Directions in Asian American Dance*, ed. Yutian Wong (Madison: University of Wisconsin Press, 2015), 29–61; Masumi Izumi, "Reconsidering Ethnic Culture and Community: A Case Study on Japanese Canadian Taiko Drumming," *Journal of Asian American Studies* 4 (2001): 35–56; Paul Jong-Chul Yoon, "'She's Really Become Japanese Now!': Taiko Drumming and Asian American Identifications," *American Music* (Winter 2001): 422–24.

7. "State of the Art Census Results Webinar," 2016 TCA Taiko Census, Taiko Community Alliance, September 24, 2016, http://taikocommunityalliance.org/events/census/. [Released under the Creative Commons Attribution ShareAlike International 4.0 License.] For discussions of the feminist potential of taiko, see Deborah Wong, "Taiko and the Asian/American Body: Drums, *Rising Sun*, and the Question of Gender," *World of Music* 42, no. 3 (2000): 67-78; Izumi, "Reconsidering Ethnic Culture and Community," 44–46.

8. See Angela K. Ahlgren, "Butch Bodies, Big Drums: Queering North American Taiko," *Women and Music: A Journal of Gender and Culture* 20 (2016): 1-26.

9. Jeanne Mercer, Life History Interview, January 24, 2005, Life History Interviews (transcripts), *Big Drum: Taiko in the United States* exhibition, Hirasaki National Resource Center, Japanese American National Museum, 369 East First Street, Los Angeles, CA 90012 (hereinafter HNRC/JANM archive).

10. Matthew Rahaim, *Musicking Bodies: Gesture and Voice in Hindustani Music* (Middletown, CT: Wesleyan University Press, 2012), 1.

11. I place taiko's relative openness in contrast to forms like ballet (one example of many), the gendered codes of which have been thoroughly critiqued by feminist dance scholars. See, e.g., Susan Leigh Foster, "The Ballerina's Phallic Pointe," in *Corporealities: Dancing Knowledge, Culture, and Power* (London: Routledge, 1996), 1–24. I distinguish North American from Japanese taiko here to acknowledge that in Japan gendered codes for taiko have developed along a different trajectory. During a presentation at the 2015 North American Taiko Conference, for example, former KODO member, dancer, and taiko artist Chieko Kojima related (via translator Yuta Kato) that in her early years performing with KODO, she danced, but was not allowed to drum because the drum was gendered female; thus, for a woman to play the drum would be wrong (i.e., lesbian).

12. Judith Hamera, *Dancing Communities: Performance, Difference and Connection in the Global City* (New York: Palgrave Macmillan, 2007), 40–41.

13. Ibid., 54.

14. Ibid., 57.

15. Deborah Wong, "Moving: From Performance to Performative Ethnography and Back Again," in *Shadows in the Field: New Perspectives for Fieldwork in Ethnomusicology*, 2d ed., ed. Gregory Barz and Timothy J. Cooley (New York: Oxford University Press, 2008), 79, italics in original.

16. See, e.g., Wong, "Taiko and the Asian/American Body," 74–75; and Jong-Chul Yoon, "'She's Really Become Japanese Now!'," 417–38.

17. In the fall of 2016, Mu Daiko announced that they will split from Mu Performing Arts at the end of the 2016–2017 season. Mu Performing Arts will focus its energies on theater, and the taiko group will continue under the auspices of a new organization, Taiko Arts Midwest.

18. SanSan Kwan, *Kinesthetic City: Dance & Movement in Chinese Urban Spaces* (Oxford: Oxford University Press, 2013), 85.

19. See Peggy Phelan, "Introduction: The Ends of Performance," in *The Ends of Performance*, ed. Peggy Phelan and Jill Lane (New York: NYU Press, 1998).

20. Hamera, *Dancing Communities*, 39.

21. See Jill Dolan, *Utopia in Performance* (Ann Arbor: University of Michigan Press, 2005).

22. Maggie Nelson, *The Argonauts* (Minneapolis: Graywolf Press, 2015), 25.

15

"Oh No! Not This Lesbian Again"

THE PUNANY POETS QUEER THE
PIMP-HO AESTHETIC

Raquel L. Monroe

"How many of y'all saw the Real Sex segment?"

Lucky Seven, the Punany Poet's "Lesbian Laureate" confidently positions herself in the middle of the stage. Her baggy khakis hide the strap-on she always
wears during performances. A group of twenty-something, well-manicured,
trendy, black lesbians occupy the first four to five rows of the ninety-nine-seat
theatre. The women blind the poet with flashes from their cameras to demonstrate their admiration. The erotic dancer, Punany's Pearl, stands beside Lucky
Seven, twirling a cucumber in her hand, and precociously smiles at the audience.
A white G-string and matching bikini top barely cover the Pearl's b-cup breasts,
and leave little to the imagination. The entire Manhattan crowd responds to the
poet's question with appreciative applause, except for the disgruntled couple sitting behind me. Clearly disgusted by Lucky Seven's reappearance on the stage,
the woman shuffles in her seat, "Oh no, not this lesbian again; I don't want to
see her." She swiftly grabs her coat and purse. Her male partner rises and snarls,
"Let's go! We'll be sure to look into stuff before we come see it again." The couple
noisily exits the performance taking their homophobic nonsense with them.

Oblivious to The Disgruntled, Lucky Seven spits her rhyme, with Punany's
Pearl as her nimble sidekick. "Well this one's for y'all."

LUCKY SEVEN: Ice cube said put a sock on the pickle and I did. *(Lucky Seven
    slides a condom onto Punany's Pearl's cucumber.)*
    Ice cube said put a sock on the pickle and I did.
PUNANY'S PEARL *places the cucumber at her vagina.*

LUCKY SEVEN: Ice cube said put a sock on the pickle and I did.[1]
PUNANY'S PEARL *swivels her hips in time to Lucky's rhythmic chant.*

In "Cucumber Cu Cum Her," Lucky Seven and Punany's Pearl re-imagine rapper-turned-movie star Ice Cube's 1991 hit "Look Who's Burnin'." The duet's erotic condom demonstration literally and discursively propels lesbian sexuality and fantasy into commercial hip-hop's hyper-masculinist sphere. Their performance elucidates the absence of lesbian sexuality from safe sex/HIV prevention discourses.[2]

Jessica Holter created the Punany Project in 1995 after 32-year-old rapper Eric "Eazy-E" Wright died from AIDS-related complications.[3] Wright, the founder of the notorious West Coast "gangsta" rap group "NWA" (Niggaz With Attitude), launched the careers of Ice Cube and mega hip-hop producer Dr. Dre. At the time of Wright's death, Holter, an entertainment journalist for the *Oakland Tribune* and a spoken word artist, was shocked and dismayed by the hip-hop community's lackadaisical response to Wright's death. "It was like no one cared. I was backstage so I knew what was going on. People were still hitting it raw [having sex without condoms]," Holter explains in one of the many conversations we've had over the years.[4] She appropriated hip-hop aesthetics to introduce HIV/AIDS and sexual violence interventions and preventions to reach young disenfranchised black women and men that she deemed the most at risk for HIV/AIDS infection. To reach these groups Holter shaped the Punany Poet's performances to mirror the raw, raunchy, "hood" ontology of mid-1990s West Coast hip-hop that came to define hip-hop's commercial sound. Holter's exploration of the painful and pleasurable experiences of the "punany," a black colloquialism for "vagina," however, challenges the narrow representations of black female sexuality performed in hip-hop music videos. In male-dominated commercial hip-hop, the "punany" is a prop that provides pleasure for men. In the Punany Poets' performances, the punany is centered as a way to foreground the multifaceted pleasures and fantasies of queer and straight black women.

The provocative cucumber duet between Lucky Seven and Punany's Pearl allows women to occupy both the subject and object position, and to explore the depths of sexual pleasure. Lucky Seven appropriates the cucumber and offers up a female-bodied feminine masculinity that would never appear in commercial hip-hop. As the erotic dancer, Punany's Pearl reifies the controlling images of black women produced in the media and commercial hip-hop.[5] The dancer looks like the staged version of the "Video Ho" or "Video Vixen," but her dancing body refutes alignment with the essentialist construction of their identities. Within Punany performances, specifically when Holter pairs

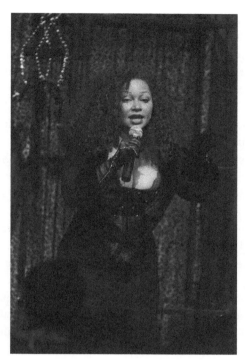

FIGURE 15.1 Jessica Holter, creator and artistic director of the Punany Poets. Photo courtesy of Jessica Holter.

Punany's Pearl with Lucky Seven, dancing bodies articulate queer spaces for black women to play with pleasurable explorations of femininity. The Pearl's body labors to imbue the erotic dancer—heretofore imagined as the disempowered, objectified, erotic dancer—with agency. Holter strategically uses the dancing body to appeal to the straight men and queer women in her audience. Considering her heterogeneous African American audience, Holter's somewhat diverse representation of lesbian sexuality is notable. Rather than adhere to the hyper-femme girl-on-girl or woman-with-woman sex acts commonly featured in commercial hip-hop videos—supposedly lesbian performances whose structures make explicit their performance for heterosexual men— she casts women whose performances of masculinity threaten to usurp the heteronormative dominance of straight men, and makes it possible for black women to indulge sexual fantasy and play typically reserved for men.

In *The Second Sin*, an evening-length performance of spoken word, erotic dance, and music, queer pimps and hos are two of the many archetypes lifted from the margins of disenfranchised black communities and inserted into the show. The final scene of the first act contextualizes the space from which

Lucky Seven and Punany's Pearl's intervention emerges. Holter performs under her alias, Ghetto Girl Blue, a promiscuous, bi-sexual "stripper type" continually mistreated by men. In her white faux fur jacket and too tight mini dress, Ghetto Girl Blue personifies the strung out sex workers that circulated on 1970s television shows like *Starsky & Hutch*. In this scene, Ghetto Girl Blue appears as the HIV positive sex worker "Ghetto Cinderella."[6] Lucky Seven is her complementary pimp in the closing scene in the first act. The figures in this scene also include singer/actress Kween, whose jeans and Forever 21-esque shirt help situate her as the quotidian self-love/self-righteous cis-gender female condemning the explicit sexuality on stage. Writer/poet DJ Blackmon, speaks to black women about sex and men in a familiar "sistah-next-door" tone. Her modest red dress and remarkable heels accentuate the homegrown knowledge she theorizes with the audience, similar to the ways black women chat around the kitchen table or at the hair salon. Holter always casts at least one erotic female dancer, so the Punanies always have a dancing Pearl. Her name in this performance is Michelle Brewer. Poet/erotic dancer S.L.A.M (Sexy Like a Muthafucka') and musician/writer Keno Mapp personify het-erosexual male perspectives on sex and sexuality. S.L.A.M, typically shirtless but fully clothed for this scene, is eye candy for the straight women in the audience. Juxtaposed against S.L.A.M's chiseled body, Keno's thin frame and longish curly hair frame him as the innocuous "artist" type. As archetypes of subaltern black identities, the performers converge onto an imagined ghetto street corner as prostitutes, pimps, lesbian stud whores, and Welfare Queens to present an evening of erotic poetry, dance, and song, not only about the pleasures of sexual intercourse but also the substance abuse, violence, and sexually transmitted diseases that might accompany intimate encounters.

Pleasure, joy, terror, and violence are the Punany Poets' intimate bedfel-lows. Through these dialogic engagements, the Punany Poets elucidate how the erotic lingers in the orgiastic space between life and death. Their erotic, humorous, and sometimes disturbing portrayal of inner city struggles high-light how in desperate conditions oppression and resistance unfold on and through the body. The Punany Poets' contentious depictions of disenfran-chised black women struggling to obtain subjecthood in a society that has simultaneously rendered them hyper visible and invisible support Saidiya Hartman's argument delineating the construction of black identity. Hartman contends that under the reign of slavery's terror, with no physical space for resistance, the enslaved used their bodies as the resistant site while simul-taneously enduring physical abuse.[7] The subjugation endured by enslaved Africans through forced public performances, beatings, rape, and the notion of "false will" greatly contributes to the formation of black identity. The bawdy performances of the Punany Poets reflect this delicate negotiation between joy and pain.

Debating Punany

Much of the Punany Poets' past and present success results from the repetitive airing of their appearance on HBO's *Real Sex 24* in 2000. Their sex-positive approach to HIV/AIDS intervention and prevention inspired my initial interest in the Punany Project.[8] The Punany Poet's five-city tour of *The Second Sin* and my analysis of their work intersect with the monolithic discourses about black men on the "down low" and the representations of black women in hip-hop videos circulating in the popular black press in 2004. The imagined threat of men secretly sleeping with other men and promiscuous women dancing for men ignited long-held black respectability politics. A hangover from the Progressive Era, the politics of respectability, wielded by black women's groups often affiliated with the Baptist church, mandated that all black bodies adhere to strict codes of conduct that mirrored the chaste, Victorian performance of sexuality and manners performed by their white counterparts.[9] Black respectability politics maintain a strangle hold on sexuality and identity formation in black communities.

In 2004, black respectability politics had a very public collision with black queer life and gender representation in hip-hop. J. L. King released his controversial book *On the Down Low: A Journey into the Lives of "Straight" Men Who Sleep with Men*, scandalizing much of black America. It demonized black men who sleep with other black men as the primary cause of soaring HIV infections in black women.[10] In turn, the down low rhetoric cast black women as passive victims unable to engage with sex in a safe manner. The rejection of black women as sexual and intimate agents in the discourse around the down low coincided with black feminist groups protesting the depiction of black women in commercial hip-hop. Also in 2004, members of Spellman College's Feminist Majority Leadership Alliance (FMLA) launched a historic feminist protest against rapper Nelly's appearance on their campus, a visit he made to advertise a bone marrow registration campaign. The female students drew particular attention to a scene in his video "Tip Drill" (2003) in which a member of his entourage slides a credit card between an erotic dancer's butt cheeks.[11] The Spellman protest incited the popular African American women's magazine *Essence* to launch a year-long "Take Back the Music Campaign," interrogating the representation of black women in music videos.[12]

Within some African American intellectual spaces, like those unfolding at Spelman and in newly published black popular press in the early 2000s, activists and intellectuals perceived the Punany Poets as sexual outlaws and betrayers of the race because of their salacious depictions of black women. The Poets' portrayal of black women as HIV positive sex workers, Welfare Queens, strippers, and lesbian pimps were antithetical to black feminists fighting for black women to be seen as fully realized beings, a conception that only had room to champion women in committed, heterosexual relationships that produced children. The Punany Poets' appearance on HBO in 2000 catapulted them into the throes of popular culture, resulting in bookings in small venues theaters across the country. On this tour, however, the Black Student Union at Colorado State University protested the Poets' appearance on their campus, and Howard University refused to book them, even though Howard hosted white playwright Eve Ensler's *Vagina Monologues*, which deals with similar sexually explicit content.[13] Young, black intellectuals could not stand for representations that ran the risk of reducing black women to their backsides. Unfortunately, this policing of women's bodies by these powerful protest groups only added the stereotype of black women as "victim," alongside "sexual object," to the list of possible characters for black women. This characterization denied black women pleasure in any sexual realm and also positioned black women as always pawns in a heteronormative drama. Furthermore, the gatekeepers of black intellectual discourse assigned deviancy to expressions of black female sexuality that failed to neatly articulate heteronormative dyads. The Punany Poets thrived in spite of this narrow perspective on pleasure and fantasy. As a collective of queer women and straight women and men, The Punany Poets challenge the idea that black women's pleasure is impossible and, if possible, only to be found within a heterosexual frame. "Cucumber Cu Cum Her," the duet between the dancing Pearl and the Lesbian Laureate, renders visible alternative, potentially subversive readings of black female sexualities. When Lucky Seven playfully rubs the cucumber against the Pearl's backside, while the dancer peeps over her shoulder to watch, they permit a queer reading of the Punany Project. My focus on the dancing in the duet discursively moves the background dancers/video hos/video vixens that Punany's Pearl personifies from the assumed passive periphery of hip-hop videos to the center of dance and gender studies. This shift constructs Punany's Pearl and the dancing bodies she signifies as agential subjects with power. In turn, Lucky Seven's performance as pimp declares masculinity and dominance as viable expressions of female sexuality. Together they emulate and re-imagine the reviled pimp and castigated vixen/ho personified in the hip-hop videos admonished by black feminists. Before I discuss "Cucumber

Cu-Cum-Her" as a whole, I analyze each character separately to elucidate how they function in the Punany Poet's *The Second Sin*.

Queering the Ho

The video begins. In slow motion, an ocean liner cruises into view. Bass booms. The camera glides over a single image of a woman, suspended in mid-air, rocking side to side. Her white bikini softly contrasts against her waist-length black hair, and caramel-colored skin. The slow motion angle captures the curves of her body—her breast, thighs, and hips—but her face fades as the camera cuts to the next scene. On the cruise ship, a shirtless black man rhythmically bounces to the beat. Champagne gushes from the bottles he holds in his outstretched arms. A gaggle of bikini clad women, variations of the first woman we saw, bounce behind him and another black man who raps fully clothed in beach attire. The camera cuts to slowly follow a woman's leopard-print bikini bottom that sways from side-to-side as she walks. Her butt leads us to more women in bikinis, nonchalantly dancing, lounging, and drinking. The camera dissects the women into only slender abs, voluptuous breasts, butts, and thighs. The camera next cuts to a woman luxuriating in a hot tub surrounded by other women, while the man with the champagne empties his bottle onto her face.

This is the opening scene of music mogul Jay Z's 2000 mega-hit "Big Pimpin'." The lyrics heard while the scene unfolds are as follows:

> You know I—thug 'em, fuck 'em, love 'em, leave 'em
> Cause I don't fuckin' need 'em
> Take em out the hood, keep em lookin good
> But I don't fuckin' feed em
> First time they fuss I'm breezin'
> Talkin bout, "What's the reasons?"
> I'm a pimp in every sense of the word, bitch
> Better trust, then believe 'em.[14]

The background dancers/models casually dance to lyrics that blatantly disregard their personhood. These images exemplify the representations of black women in hip-hop that enraged black women with a feminist consciousness in the same period as the Punany Poets began to tour their work. The camera angles and narratives staged in the opening moments of the video show how women in hip-hop videos are treated as dancing mannequins farmed for their body parts. The sentiments expressed in "Big Pimpin'"—its lyrics, filming, and stagings—define the commercial hip-hop scene at the turn of the twenty-first century: a fantastical sexual playground where young black men measure their success by the amounts of high-end bottles of champagne they could afford to dump on nearly nude women.

Vernacular references to the dancers as vixens and hos signify their maligned perception and consumption within the political economy of hip-hop. Yet, I contend that the black feminist analysis of the dancing bodies as passive commodities and mere props of misogyny elides the dancers' physical labor, usurps their agency, and suppresses further conversations and explorations of what else this body might do and does, and the pleasures of those watching and performing.

Punany's Pearl's dancing body significantly shifts the epistemologies of the often working-class, usually disparaged, erotic dancer from the defiled strip club into the political economy of popular culture. The libidinal labor the dancer/stripper exerts to gratify insatiable onlookers is no longer hidden in imagined dark, seedy conclaves where husbands and boyfriends sneak to fulfill their fantasies for available female flesh. She strategically deploys her dancing body to satiate the audience's desire for the familiar representation of black dancing bodies in music videos. Punany's Pearl and the video vixens provide the canvases upon which the Poets, the rappers, and their audiences project their fantasies. Just as the male rappers rely on the video dancers to personify their success, the dancing Pearl's body is paramount to the Punany Project. She provides their performances with the raunchy aesthetics of hip-hop upon which the Project relies. The pleasure she performs as she offers her flesh for consumption threatens to undo the patriarchal delineations of appropriate pleasure for women everywhere. She is a laborer who knowingly capitalizes on her sexual plurality. As the designated "ho" in the Poets' performances, she dances to fulfill the fantasies of *anyone*—not just straight men—who take pleasure in her dancing body, and she takes pleasure in her dancing as well.

Holter's first installment of the Punany Poets consisted of her and two female strippers performing at exclusive private parties for Oakland, California's hip-hop royalty. The "stripper type" had become a cultural mainstay in hip-hop videos, just as Punany's Pearl continues to be integral to the Punany Project. Still struck by the reaction to Eazy E's death, Holter knew that male hip-hop artists currently flirting with stripper culture in their videos would best receive her messages of safer sex when aroused by hypersexual, hyper-feminized dancers gyrating in their laps and kissing each other.[15] Holter chose to feature the black stripper character, even though the erotic dancer's abject body somewhat hinders the efforts black feminists expend to reimagine black women as more than the hypersexual objects they are characterized as in the white and hip-hop imaginary.[16] At the level of cultural institution, too, the emphasis on the stripper figure continues persistent problems. The limited roles available to black female artists in popular culture further problematize the centrality of the stripper. Young black dancers desiring to work in television and videos think they must be prepared to don a bikini, and straighten or extend their hair to secure employment. The years of dance and acting training many endure fades behind the bravado of an insecure rapper. Yet, the stripper's popularity also acknowledges her corporeality and lays bare the very real fantasies and desires of many women and men under-theorized in dance, and critical race and gender studies.

Within the Punany Project all of the poets rely on Punany's Pearl's nearly nude body to titillate their texts. Holter purposefully uses Punany's Pearl to seduce her audience in the first half of the show, so she can ease them into the "sexedutainment" post-intermission. By the time Punany's Pearl performs "Cucumber Cu Cum Her" with Lucky Seven, she has won over the audience with multiple appearances with the other poets. *The Second Sin* opens with Holter masturbating herself with a vibrator as Punany's Pearl undulates behind a scrim in a makeshift bathtub. The audience has to decide if the poet masturbates to the Pearl's current image or a memory of her. In both scenarios, her dancing exists as Holter's fantasy. Her dancing body signals that she is the one to watch, admire, learn from, and consume.

Later, Pearl performs as a fetish object for S.L.A.M, the erotic male dancer/poet who manipulates her as if she is an extension of his own body. S.L.A.M literally flips the dancer upside down and swings her between his legs in their duet to Prince's "Darling Nikki." In the song, Prince describes an encounter with a woman he met "in a hotel lobby masturbating to a magazine."[17] Again, Punany's Pearl personifies the fantasy, sitting with a magazine awaiting S.L.A.M's entrance onto the stage.

In the first half of *The Second Sin*, after dancing with/for Holter and S.L.A.M, the dancing Pearl controls the fantasy with her only solo performance. She teasingly spreads her legs, moves her black G-string aside, and eases a string of pearls out of her vagina, thus revealing the origins of her name. The women in the front row, who blinded Lucky Seven with flashes from their cameras at the beginning of this essay, relentlessly snap pictures, while other audience members gasp with delight, and spontaneously applaud the dancer's astonishing feat. Up to this point in the performance, they have experienced her as a malleable object in Holter's and S.L.A.M.'s fantasies. When the dancer "births" the pearls, she illuminates her subjectivity, and further toys with a patriarchal, heteronormative frame.

Holter determines with whom the dancer will perform, but her labor and skill are not lost on female audience members. After more than one performance, women approach me to ask if "she [Punany's Pearl] teaches classes?" The women recognize her salacious performance as artifice, something that can be taught and deployed when desired. If the dancer can seamlessly manipulate her body to perform as the object of both same sex and heterosexual desire, and hide things in her vagina and extract them at will, what else can she do? Punany's Pearl's dancing body elucidates the potential to actualize fantasies, and pleasure yourself, your mate, and anonymous voyeurs. She does not merely flip or refuse a script, as respectability politics demand black women do, but instead she takes on the script of black female sexuality in hip-hop, extending and expanding it to her own means. Her ability to reveal the labor she exerts to navigate seemingly boundless fantastical terrains reveals her as an intelligible dancing subject. Thinking of strippers/erotic dancers/video vixens as women, who knowingly and purposefully curate fantasies, differentiates them from the mindless, naïve, bikinied models I described to open this section. Punany's Pearl's erotic dancing body choreographs black feminist queer epistemologies and ontologies rarely performed within black popular culture.

As the hyper-feminized artifice exchanged between the Poets to enact their words, Punany's Pearl's excessive flesh reverberates beyond the strictures of what heteronormative politics deem appropriate performances of sexuality.[18] Holter, intimately aware of the politics of respectability in black communities, choreographs the final scene in the first act of The Second Sin to "check" the queerness performed in the first forty minutes. The "checking" illuminates attempts to discipline queer bodies, but within the Punany Project, the disciplining ultimately fails because Holter, her poets, and dancer, queer the hip-hop aesthetics that emerge from the margins of disenfranchised African American and Latinx communities. Punany's Pearl's performance with Lucky Seven's queer pimp further exploits this failure.

Queering the Pimp

In The Second Sin a fully clothed Punany's Pearl, along with the rest of the cast, close the first act on an imagined ghetto street corner where they play with "hood" stereotypes. In her poem "Shoes," poet D. J. Blackmon advises women to pick a good man like they would a good pair of shoes. Male poet Keeno performs his poem, "I Don't Want to Wear a Condom," as Punany's Pearl and songstress Kween drape themselves around S.L.A.M. The trio disgustedly snubs Lucky Seven who performs as the pimp to Holter's HIV positive sex worker Ghetto Cinderella. As S.L.A.M.'s accessories, Punany's Pearl and Kween reify the pervasive images of black women as interchangeable garnishes buttressing hyper hetero-black masculinity. S.L.A.M.'s assumed capacity to attract and please two women confirms and celebrates his pimp status as constructed within the representations of hyper black masculinity in hip-hop videos. The trio's open disdain for Lucky Seven as a butch pimp and Holter as a femme ho exemplifies the reception of black queers within factions of black communities. The two pimps side-by-side—S.L.A.M the metaphorical pimp and Lucky Seven the literal—elucidate the performative nature of gender, and how "Big Pimpin'" is a construct available to both men and women. Lucky Seven's masculinity extends the boundaries of blackness, imaged after heterosexual black male masculinity. Her presence in the scene demands revisions to truncated constructions of blackness and queerness.

Lucky Seven further complicates the performance of sexualities on this street corner with her solo performance "Stud Whore." Dressed in a "fresh to death" white suit complete with white fedora hat, Lucky Seven signifies the nostalgic representation of African American pimps popularized in 1970s Blaxploitation films and reinvigorated by rappers Jay Z, Snoop Dog, and 50 Cent, to name a few. In this particular performance, the poet demonstrates the fluidity of masculinity, and the paradoxical pleasure-pain matrix between sex and fantasy. She directs her rhyme toward male poet Keeno and female singer Kween who scoff and exit the stage with intertwined arms. She stares them off of the stage then flows,

> I remembered when it happened.
> My heart snapped into the lips cracking of a former lover . . .
> This piece left me, so I became a stud whore.
> Offering peace to any woman who opened her door to my piece.
> I reached inside her tomb,
> which had become the tomb
> of man's ejaculated bullshit. . . .
> I became the straight woman's sex slave. . . .
> A woman fucking women for money.
> (*She scans the audience until she finds a man to land her final*
>   *lyrical blow*).
> Don't you just love the irony
> that men are still trying to get with me?[19]

The audience responds with knowing "Umphs" and "Um hmms" to this melancholic performance. Solo, without Punany's Pearl's swiveling hips to project her fantasies onto or Holter's Ghetto Cinderella to pimp, Lucky Seven inhabits both the subject and object position. She is exploiter and exploited. As a "stud" she performs a hyper-masculinity with assumed dominance over women. But as a "whore," women use her for their own sexual gratification and disregard her personhood. As a "stud whore," she not only demonstrates the fluidity of sexual identities but also the vulnerability hyper-masculinity seeks to mask.

E. Patrick Johnson's postulations on black masculinity and its relationship to the formation of an authentic black identity delineate a clear line from notions of black male queerness and ineffectuality to the performance of pimpin' and hyper-masculinity that Lucky Seven appropriates. In "Manifest Faggotry," Johnson argues that Black Panther Eldridge Cleaver and Black Arts poet Amiri Baraka, both considerable architects of the 1960s Black Arts and Black Power movements, not only disavowed homosexuality but also aligned it with whiteness. In turn, their discursive moves suggested that to be queer is to be white. To be black and effective in the fight against oppression is to be straight and male.[20] Johnson explains:

> The representation of effeminate homosexuality as disempowering is at the heart of the politics of hegemonic blackness. For to be ineffectual is the most damaging thing one can be in the fight against oppression. Insofar as ineffectiveness is problematically sutured to femininity and homosexuality within a black cultural politic that privileges race over other categories of oppression, it follows that the subjects accorded these attributes would be marginalized and excluded from the boundaries of blackness.[21]

The architects of the Black Power and Arts movements considered women and effeminate men antithetical to the homogeneous black identity they constructed to fight against racism and classism. The kitchen and the bedroom were deemed vital spaces for women. Queer men deployed invisibility as a necessary strategy to protect themselves against ridicule and sanctioned violence. Visibility within the boundaries of blackness required intelligent and articulate choreographies of masculine virility and strength. Middle-class black men or black men with legible educations or access to resources were well suited to perform this limited construction of black masculinity. Black men, or more inclusively, black subjects with masculine gender expression who experienced severe economic and social disenfranchisement navigated toward hyper representations of heterosexual black masculinity—the pimp. Although pimps exist on the margins of an already marginalized community, their ability to create economic viability assures the subjects who embody the pimp visibility and credibility.

The obsession with "pimpin'" in commercial hip-hop best personifies how some black men employ hyper-masculinity to access white patriarchal ideals of what it means to be a "man." Historian Robin D. G. Kelley suggests that heterosexual black men celebrate the pimp for his hustle, style, and verbal charisma not his physical dominance over women. The articulation of the "pimp aesthetic" demonstrates how black men navigate economic oppression and racism that pathologize black masculinity.[22] The accumulation of "bling" and women evidences their success. Lucky Seven's performance with Punany's Pearl elucidates how pimpin's access to masculinity and its potential pleasures are not predetermined by sex.

"Cucumber Cu Cum Her," the queer duet, turns Ice Cube's rap "Look Who's Burnin'" on its misogynist head. In the song, Ice Cube chides a woman he runs into at the neighborhood "free clinic" for having an STD. The rapper relishes the woman's misfortune because she never gave him or "anyone who lived on the block" the time of day. According to Ice Cube, she deserves to be "burnin'" from something she probably caught from a "college boy."[23] "You should put a sock on the pickle and your pussy wouldn't be blowin' smoke signals," he tells the woman.[24] Like other rap songs in the 1990s, "Look Who's Burnin'" vilifies women as the carriers of HIV infection.[25] It also illustrates how the disenfranchised man from the hood launches his venomous attack and constructs his identity against those with access to upward mobility to mask his frustration related to his economic and social marginality. Lucky Seven and Punany's Pearl's performance of "Cucumber Cu-Cum-Her" repurposes the song, and their role-play as pimp and ho render visible multiple ways to explore fantasy and pleasure unavailable for women within the hip-hop aesthetic. Their performance appropriates heteronormative constructions of female sexuality. Together they choreograph a queer pimp-ho aesthetic:

PUNANY'S PEARL *faces the audience with the cucumber in her mouth*
   kneels and spreads her knees wide.
LUCKY SEVEN:
   Had to slow my role cuz cucumbers are kinda' fat.
   Big pickle made her relax
   'til she arched her back waaaaaaay back.
PUNANY'S PEARL *undulates her spine and arches back, until her head and*
   breasts disappear towards Lucky Seven who stands behind her, leaving the
   audience to gaze upon her ribcage, vagina, and thighs.
LUCKY SEVEN:
   She gave me more scratches than in my rap.
   You can call me, "Super Fly," "The Mack," or "Shaft"
   of cucumber
   cause orgasms to cum in multiples.

Super Fly (1972), *The Mack* (1973), and *Shaft* (1971), were popular Blaxploitation films with protagonists with the same names—Super Fly a cocaine dealer, The Mack a pimp, and Shaft a private detective. Like Lucky Seven, their relationship to a female companion or their ability to usurp the dominant structure renders their masculinity visible.

Lucky Seven's choreography of dominance as a pleasurable space for women to occupy supports Andreana Clay's contention that when queer women of color perform otherwise misogynist hip-hop lyrics they "construct new meanings of the text and become active consumers who change the context of sexuality and masculinity."[26] Ice Cube demanded, "Put a sock on the pickle." Lucky Seven playfully remixes the command to metaphorically "sock the pickle" with a cucumber and condom to celebrate black lesbian sexuality, revealing gender's performativity, and eroticize safe sex.

In her ethnographic study of the performances of masculinities on the dance floor in women of color, queer nightclubs in the San Francisco Bay area, Clay insists that black queer women, denied access to notions of womanhood within black communities, relate to the disenfranchised, outsider status of the "nigga" and "playa"—pimp, heralded and performed in commercial hip-hop culture. On the dance floor, black lesbians embody these reviled representations of black masculinity to infuse them with new meaning and reveal the performativity of these identities.[27] When a black lesbian performs a thugged out nigga identity bobbing her head, and mouthing the lyrics to a particular hardcore rap, she does so, not to perform her dominance, but to declare her "loyalty to this group, this identity and this community."[28] Like Lucky Seven, women who embody the playa pimp however, will dance the lyrics with their partners, particularly if they describe a sex act. Clay insists the playa-pimp persona offers black lesbians the opportunity to explore "their masculinity in relationships to the women that they love and have sex with" in a safe, exciting, normalized environment.[29] For Lucky Seven and Punany's Pearl, the Punany stage is said environment.

Conclusion: Discursive Shifts

On the Punany stage, lesbian stud whores and pimps, erotic dancers, HIV positive prostitutes, and Welfare Queens bump up against the heteronormative mores of pleasure and sexuality that condemn women for seeking, having, and enjoying sex outside of the confines of committed heterosexual relationships. Yet, their blackness and black working-class aesthetics position them outside of a queer politics defined by whiteness.

Cathy Cohen derides the queer movement for its construction of a straight/ queer dichotomy that fails to consider the vectors of oppression under-represented populations experience. In "Punks, Bulldaggers, and Welfare Queens," she rallies for queer politics that consider race, class, gender, and "the nonnormative and marginal positions of punks, bulldaggers, and welfare queens ... as the basis for progressive transformative coalition work."[30] My analysis of Jessica Holter's Punany Poets advances Cohen's vision for progressive queer politics. The strategic casting of the black bodies living on the fringes of society not only performs a sex positive approach to HIV/AIDS intervention and prevention but also queers notions of "black love" heretofore imagined and constructed solely within a heteronormative context to buttress black respectability politics. The Punany Poets' desires to represent, perform, and fulfill the erotic fantasies of black women while simultaneously addressing the violences perpetuated against us foregrounds the black female body, and our sexual, psychic, spiritual, and emotional health. The rare combination of lesbian and heterosexual couples and singles in their audiences provides opportunities for black women—black people, often separated by economic, religious, or other restrictions of our heterosexist, patriarchal economy—to see and support one another. The Punany Project answers Cohen's call for "transformative coalition work" with a resounding "We got this!"

I hope my reading of the Punany Project inspires dance scholars to shift the discourse within dance studies from critiques that relegate the erotic dancers as always already objectified to examine the ways this body labors to give and receive pleasure. The literary and media reduction of the dancing body to an unintelligent, sexualized object creates anxieties among dance scholars that leaves pleasure under-theorized in dance studies. Similar constructions of black women within the white imaginary hinder discourse around black female sexuality in African American studies. All of these assumptions prove problematic for black erotic dancers. They leave her body dancing in the winds of dismissed objectification, which supplants her labor and agency.

Theorizing how pleasure across or in concert with identities challenges the heterosexist stranglehold on pleasure and fantasy circulating in the pop culture imaginary. An analysis of pleasure will elucidate how erotic dancers skillfully morph and shift their identities to embody, negate, and produce the signifiers of pleasure that interpolate their dancing bodies. Dance scholars need to embrace the erotic dancers whose labor emboldens the sex work industry and much of popular culture. After all, many of our students work as go-go and erotic dancers to pay for their expensive dance degrees. Yet, as they learn about how local and global dance practices reflect political economies, their professional physical practice is reviled, or worse, ignored in dance research. If dance scholars remain silent, we dismiss a substantial portion of the field, and we allow postulations on pleasure to remain disembodied in the academy.

I realize the critique of erotic dancers is more nuanced than I give here, and that my discursive conflation of video vixens, erotic dancers, and Punany's Pearl into one identity fails to consider how they might be differently received and perceived in their perspective performances spaces. I maintain however, that the space these bodies occupy is more than "passive," "objectified," "ho." They signify queer epistemologies that render visible alternative avenues for explorations of pleasure. In the conclusion of "Cucumber Cu-Cum-Her" Lucky Seven and Punany's Pearl traverse an erotic terrain to encourage safe sex between female-bodied sex partners. The poet works toward her crescendo while the dancer displays more of her virtuosic skill.

LUCKY SEVEN:
> Latex slappin' double platinum
> I fucked her so good 'til she hit a high note.

PUNANY'S PEARL *drops to her knees, and faces the poet's pelvis with a mouthful of cucumber.*

LUCKY SEVEN:
> Then put my cucumber down her throat
> 'til she damn near choked.

PUNANY'S PEARL *slides the cucumber down her throat, tosses her head back, pumps her pelvis, and swallows more cucumber.*

LUCKY SEVEN:
> 'Til she damn near choked.

PUNANY'S PEARL *continues to pump and swallow.*

LUCKY SEVEN:
> 'Til she damn near choked
> off the cum juice as it oozes
> and she yells and screams my name,
> "Lucky Seven God Damn! God Damn!"
> *(The poet throws her head back, and extends her arms to the side in victorious jubilation and performative ejaculation).*

To remind the audience that their performance is a condom demonstration, Punany's Pearl quickly rises off of her knees, stands prim and proper next to Lucky Seven, flashes a broad and innocent smile, and delicately displays the cucumber as a winning prize. Lucky Seven replaces her rhythmic pattern with the matter-of-fact gleeful tone of a game show announcer.

LUCKY SEVEN.
Lucky Seven's warning:
Place a latex condom on top of a cucumber
before inserting into the vagina.
In other words, "sock the pickle."

The performers smile, and Punany's Pearl lightheartedly skips offstage bouncing her head from side to side. Lucky Seven skips and giggles off behind her. Their exits remove the pimp-ho layer of artifice from their sexual performance, leaving the audience with the image of two geeky teenagers delighting in an equally geeky joke.

Notes

1. Lucky Seven, "Cucumber." *The Second Sin.* Pantheon Theatre, NYC. March 24, 2004.
2. Katie Hogan describes how the representation of women and HIV/AIDS in literature and the media divides women into categories of "good" and "bad" or casts them as nurturing helpmates to men and children infected with HIV/AIDS to make the disease palpable to middle America. "Good" women contract the disease through blood transfusions or sex within a committed relationship with a male partner. "Bad" women are prostitutes or intravenous drug users infected by sex with multiple men or dirty needles. The discourse assumes lesbians do not have sex with men, and therefore are not at risk, and do not need intervention and prevention education. See Hogan, *Women Take Care: Gender, Race and the Culture of AIDS* (Ithaca, NY: Cornell University Press, 2001).
3. For an in-depth discussion on NWA, please refer to http://www.nwaworld.com/bio.shtml.
4. Holter, personal communication, July 5, 2006.
5. Patricia Hill-Collins asserts that Video Vixens, Mammies, Black Ladies, and Educated Bitches are the current identities for black women circulating in the media. See Patricia Hill-Collins, *Black Sexual Politics* (New York: Routledge, 2004), 138–39.
6. Holter's performance of the "Ghetto Cinderella" characterizes the limitations of the Punany Poets HIV/AIDS prevention efforts. The performance reifies antiquated ideas that sex workers are at greater risk for infection than women in monogamous relationships. Its limitations are beyond the scope of analysis in this chapter.
7. Saidiya Hartman, *Scenes of Subjection: Terror, Slavery, and Self-Making in Nineteenth-Century America* (New York: Oxford University Press, 1997).

8. Raquel L. Monroe, "Representin' the Forbidden: The Punany Poets, Black Female Sexuality, and HIV and Performance" (PhD diss., UCLA, 2006).

9. See Paisley Jane Harris, "Gatekeeping and Remaking: The Politics of Respectability in Women's History and Black Feminism," *Journal of Women's History* 15, no. 1 (2003): 212–20. For a comprehensive discussion on the impact respectability politics have had on HIV/AIDS prevention and intervention in black communities, and the construction of black female sexuality, see Cathy Cohen, *The Boundaries of Blackness: AIDS and the Breakdown of Black Politics* (Chicago: University of Chicago Press, 1999?); and Evelynn M. Hammonds, "Black (W)holes and the Geometry of Black Female Sexuality," in *Feminism Meets Queer Theory*, ed. Elizabeth Weed and Naomi Schor (Bloomington: Indiana University Press, 1997), 136–56.

10. For a nuanced discussion on King and the down low, see Jeffrey Q. McCune Jr., *Sexual Discretion: Black Masculinity and the Politics of Passing* (Chicago: University of Chicago Press, 2014).

11. See Rose Arce, "Hip-hop Portrayal of Women Protested: Movement Grows into National 'Take Back the Music Campaign,'" CNN.com, March 4, 2005, http://www.cnn.com/2005/SHOWBIZ/Music/03/03/hip.hop/.

12. For a detailed analysis of the campaign, see Shanara R. Reid-Brinkley, "The *Essence* of Res(ex)pectability: Black Women's Negotiation of Black Femininity in Rap Music and Music Videos," *Meridian's: Feminisms, Race, Transnationalism* 8, no. 1 (2008): 236–60.

13. Holter, personal communication, July 5, 2006.

14. Jay Z, "Big Pimpin'," from the album, *Vol. 3 . . . Live and Times of S. Carter*, 2000.

15. Holter, personal communication, November 3, 2003.

16. See bell hooks, *Ain't I a Woman: Black Women and Feminism* (Boston: South End Press, 1989).

17. Prince, "Darling Nikki" from the album *Purple Rain*, 1984.

18. Nicole Fleetwood's theorizations on what she calls "excess flesh," offers a generative framework by which to view how African American female artists, in this case erotic dancers, knowingly employ their jiggling flesh to ensure their visibility. Nicole R. Fleetwood, *Troubling Vision: Performance, Visuality, and Blackness* (Chicago: University of Chicago Press, 2011).

19. Lucky Seven, "Stud Whore," *The Second Sin*. Pantheon Theatre, NYC. March 24, 2004.

20. E. Patrick Johnson, *Appropriating Blackness: Performance and Politics of Authenticity* (Durham, NC: Duke University Press, 2003), 50–51.

21. Ibid., 51. Phillip Brian Harper complicates the narrative of queer black men within the Black Arts Movement. See Phillip Brian Harper "Eloquence and Epitaph: Black Nationalism and the Homophobic Impulse in Response to the Death of Max Robinson," *Social Text* 28 (1991): 68–86.

22. Mark Anthony Neal, *New Black Man* (New York: Routledge, 2006), 133.

23. Ice Cube, "Look Who's Burnin'" from the album *Death Certificate*, 1991.

24. Ibid.

25. In her article "AIDS Gets a Bad Rap," hip-hop cultural critic dream hampton launches an insightful critique against the Red Hot Organization-sponsored CD *America is Dying Slowly* (1996). hampton argues that the compilation of hip-hop artists dedicated to combating AIDS through music "placed the weight of the epidemic on the shoulders of its women, implying that it is the wanton appetites of groupies that spread HIV infection." See hampton, "AIDS Gets a Bad Rap," In *POZ* 17 (1996): 3, http://www.poz.com/articles/254_1816.shtml.

26. Andreanna Clay, "'I Used to be Scared of the Dick,'" in *Home Girls Make Some Noise: Hip Hop Feminism Anthology*, eds. Gwendolyn D. Pough, et al. (Mira Loma, CA: Parker Publishing, 2007).
     158.

27. Ibid., 155.

28. Ibid., 156.

29. Ibid., 158, 159.

30. Ibid., 22.

16

Choreographing the Chronic

Patrick McKelvey

Consider two scenes from *The BugChasers* (2007), a work of dance theatre conceived by Miami-based choreographer Octavio Campos, and devised in collaboration with members of his ensemble, Camposition.[1]

Two white leathermen face one another and interlock their legs. They lean down and back, retracing small circles on the floor with their heels as they spin one another around again and again. Quick at first, their pace slows, inversely proportional to the ecstasy that registers on their faces during this fuck that seems both exceptional and banal, at once routinized monogamy and an anonymous encounter. For all of his aggression and dominance—he spits in his bottom's face upon orgasm—the top struggles to support his partner: their entwined legs do not sufficiently anchor them. The bottom's harness remains untouched. He supports his partner instead through a huge sheet of plastic that begins at his brow and cascades over his shoulders like a bridal veil. The plastic extends into a sling that wraps around the top's lower-back, tethering him to his leather bride. The scene does not represent genital contact, but given the literal climax in the form of fluid exchange (saliva) and the sheer volume of the repurposed plastic sheet, the plastic cannot *not* suggest an enormous condom, holding the men who dance and fuck both inside and outside of its embrace. But does it support them or restrict them from moving (and fucking) otherwise? Is this gay marital bliss, the back room at a bathhouse, or both? We cannot decide.

A pageant unfolds twice to the melodies of Barry White's "Love's Theme" and Roberta Flack and Donny Hathaway's "Where is the Love?" Pageant 1: Six dancers donning various states of female drag, many complete with outlandishly colored wigs, stand parallel to one another in a sparse chorus line. Turned out at a slight angle, but still facing the audience, they repeatedly shift their weight into their upstage hips, a move both seductive and playful. They cross left over right as they move across the stage, slowly lifting their arms in gestures that alternate between domestic labor and aristocratic poise. They thread needles and shuttle them back and forth, they mime adjusting the glasses that they are not wearing, they allow their exposed forearms to linger, as if keeping perfect time while forgetting that they were supposed to be waving like royalty. Pageant 2: As snowflakes descend upon them, the ensemble repeats their previous pageantry, this time wearing little more than their dance belts and stockings. Some are top-less and others entirely naked, only residual makeup smudges remain from their drag exploits. The hip thrusts and hand gestures repeat as before. But rather than traveling in a straight line, they move in a circuitous loop. A seventh dancer lays akimbo as the artificial snow gathers around him. In exhaustion? In ecstasy?

Following two years of developmental workshops, *The BugChasers* pre-miered in 2007 at the Carnival Center for the Performing Arts at Miami Dade College. Campos's work explores the lives and desires of its titular figures, bugchasers: (primarily) queer men who deliberately pursue HIV. A series of loosely connected vignettes juxtapose live dancers with onscreen representations of porn, gay social media, and nature documentaries.[2] A lec-ture on the merits of safe sex fades into a lengthy monologue in which Max, one of the bugchasing protagonists, waxes both earnestly and parodically about gay male self-representation in cyberspace. Middle-class white parents repurpose the veil-scaffold-condom as an inverse quarantine tent in which to expose their children to the chicken pox virus and thus preempt its looming inevitability.

This essay mobilizes dance studies, queer disability studies, and perfor-mance studies in order to examine how bugchasers stage alternative tem-poralities of seroconversion. Seroconversion is the biomedical narrative by which a subject moves from one HIV status to another. Conventionally, such narratives are constructed by two consecutive HIV tests that produce different results. With rare exceptions, medical, popular, humanistic, and social sci-entific discourses represent seroconversion as having one possible permuta-tion: the HIV– subject becomes HIV+. Seroconversion should be understood as distinct from the event of infection. Whereas infection names the biological event in which someone acquires the virus, seroconversion names the socio-medical narrative process through which a subject comes to understand her-self as having a change in serostatus.

This essay argues that the inventive practices through which bugchas-ers represent seroconversion enact an alternative temporality of seroconver-sion. This temporality, the chronic, intervenes in dominant discourses about bugchasing, queer disability performance, and HIV/AIDS more broadly. I adopt a broad and flexible definition of choreography that addresses how the chronic is organized by and enacted within historical, theoretical, and critical discourses as much as by the dancers in Campos's ensemble. In order to demonstrate how chronic seroconversion is enacted across these various domains, I have organized the body of this essay into three sections. I begin by revisiting a now infamous moment in the history of HIV/AIDS dance by way of queer disability studies and performance studies before examining how journalists, queer theorists, and bugchasers themselves—and finally, Campos and his dancers—stage the temporality of seroconversion.

Queer Disability and Representability

In 1994, *The New Yorker* published "Discussing the Undiscussable," dance critic Arlene Croce's review of Bill T. Jones's *Still/Here*. Croce's piece would more accurately be labeled a "non-review" insofar as it elaborated a polemic about a work of dance theatre she had elected not to attend.[3] Croce alleged that *Still/Here* constituted "victim art," which she refused to watch because she would have been "forced to feel sorry" for the dancers onstage, many of who were living with illnesses including HIV/AIDS, then understood as terminal.[4] Her diatribe ignited a number of enduring debates regarding writing about art, identity politics, and the choreography of social difference.[5] Croce precipitates her dismissal of all "victim art" by listing a range of disabled performers who she "avoid[s]": "overweight dancers . . . old dancers, dancers with sickled feet, or dancers with physical deformities who appear nightly in roles requiring beauty of line."[6] Here, and elsewhere in her review, Croce adheres to what disability theorists call a "medical model" in which disability is understood as an individual problem located in a flawed body that demands "cure or rehabilitation."[7]

Croce mobilizes this medicalizing perspective in order to divest disabled people of their mimetic capacities, marking them as unable to represent anything other than their own impairment. "In theater," she writes, "one chooses what one will be. The cast members of *Still/Here*—the sick people whom Jones has signed up—have no other choice than to be sick."[8] Croce's aesthetic and political grievances against Jones concern his inclusion of performers who purportedly lack the autonomy to choose to be healthy (the possibility that disabled embodiment might be desirable is not on Croce's radar), and by extension, to choose to perform. To wit, she writes: "In theater, one chooses what one will be." In so doing, Croce participates within a long line of thinking in which disabled people are understood to challenge "American ideology" in terms of "the abstract principles of self-government, self-determination, autonomy, and progress" insofar as they are "imagined as unable to be productive, direct their own lives, participate in the community, or establish meaningful personal relations."[9]

To critique the ableist assumptions undergirding Croce's argument is not to suggest that we merely broaden our conception of autonomy to incorporate the agency of disabled people. Disability theorists (to say nothing of the entirety of poststructuralist thought) have long written off the possibility—or desirability—of the autonomous individual. Additionally, spectatorial encounters with performing subjects are always prone to what Nicholas Ridout terms "semiotic shudder[s]," the inability to decide whether the performing subject is producing a sign or failing to produce one.[10] Nevertheless, as Croce's review demonstrates, disability persists as an axis legislating who does and does not enjoy access to such autonomy. From her perspective, spectating disabled performers does not result in such indeterminacy: disabled performers constituted by the medical "fact" of their disablement, are mimetically incapacitated and cannot signify anything other than themselves.

Croce understands the capacity to represent difference to be differentially distributed along the lines of race, gender, sexuality, and ability. This line of thinking participates within discourses and practices long subject to analysis within the study of dance, performance, and disability. For example, dance scholar Susan Manning has argued that modern dance's feminist potential was contingent upon white female dancers performing racial difference, such as when dancers in Helen Tamiris's *How Long Brethren* (1937) donned "metaphorical blackface."[11] Cross-racial representation facilitated displays of mimetic prowess, enabling white womanhood to become the social location from which African American life could be represented. Within early American modern dance, then, mimetic capacity was understood to be predicated upon the purported neutrality of white dancers performing racial difference, and had the effect of obfuscating the performance labor of dancers of color. Performance theorist Rebecca Schneider contends that antitheatrical and antimimetic anxieties are always already gendered in their preference for the (supposedly masculine) original over the (purportedly feminine) copy.[12] Reading Manning and Schneider in tandem illuminates how the construction of certain subjects as privileged bearers of mimetic capacities requires constructing others not as subjects, but as objects of representation. Such a maneuver effectively renders those represented—but who do not themselves represent—as deprived of mimetic capacity. To return to Manning's example: black life could be represented on the concert dance stage, but it was white dancers, not black dancers, who represented those lives. For Croce, illness and disability might be viable themes for a dance work, so long as illness and disability was understood as proper to the characters represented and not by the "victims" doing the representing.

Disability does not merely offer another category of social difference across which mimetic capacity is unevenly distributed. Rather, the difference of disability proves foundational to understanding the distribution of such capacities across an expansive range of identities. Ellen Samuels argues that "fantasies of identification," efforts to "definitively identify bodies, to place them in categories delineated by race, gender, or ability status, and then to validate that placement through a verifiable biological mark of identity" emerged "at the turn of the [twentieth] century and has become even more powerfully instituted into the present."[13]

Notably, Samuels emphasizes that such fantasies "are haunted by disability even when disabled bodies are not their immediate focus, for disability functions as the trope and embodiment of true physical difference."[14] Theories of the social construction of gender, race, and sexuality continue to proliferate, but for many, disability—perhaps because of the endurance of the medical model—continues to be understood as the unmediated, the ontological, the real. Understandings of disability as "the embodiment of absolute difference" render disabled performers at the furthest remove from mimetic capacity, purportedly unable to play against the identity categories that they themselves inhabit. Croce reproduces this understanding when she contends that the dancers in *Still/Here* "have no other choice than to be sick," and thus, cannot signify anything other than their "victim" status. For Croce, as for others, disability can be represented but the disabled performer cannot represent.

HIV/AIDS enjoys enduring purchase in discussions about disability, mimetic capacity, and—to borrow Croce's language—choice. Consider, for example, the lead-up to the Americans with Disabilities Act (ADA) which, when it passed in 1990, became the most comprehensive piece of disability rights legislation in the history of the United States. The bill that became the ADA was debated at the height of the AIDS crisis, during which time the popular, medical, and moral imagination conflated HIV/AIDS with homosexual men. Judicial rulings earlier in the 1980s clarified that "contagious diseases," and by extension, HIV/AIDS, were protected under Section 504, the civil rights precursor to the ADA.[15] It is perhaps no surprise, then, that the specter of AIDS figured prominently in congressional debates about the ADA. As legal scholar Ruth Colker argues, the House minority report "characterized the ADA as a 'homosexual rights' bill even though homosexuals were specifically exempted from statutory coverage."[16] Colker goes on to cite the report's theatrical language: "We believe that the ADA is a homosexual rights bill in disguise."[17] The disproportionate impact of HIV/AIDS on queer communities makes these slippages between sexuality, disability, and HIV/AIDS somewhat predictable. But this suggestion that disability rights legislation might be queers in crip's clothing suggests how questions of performance and representation are central for considering the relationship between HIV/AIDS and disability more broadly.

Queer disability studies also offers a perspective from which to address HIV/AIDS in general and bugchasing in particular. In his foundational contribution, *Crip Theory*, Robert McRuer extends familiar claims that "homosexuality and disability clearly share a pathologized past" by arguing that "able-bodiedness, even more than heterosexuality, still largely masquerades as a nonidentity, as the natural order of things."[18] McRuer draws upon lesbian feminist poet and theorist Adrienne Rich to demonstrate how compulsory heterosexuality and "compulsory able-bodiedness" are mutually constitutive enterprises that deny the possibility that disabled embodiment and identity would ever be desirable, that someone would ever "choose" to inhabit or claim them. McRuer offers several examples of how these assumptions get articulated, but perhaps more effective—and affective—is his ventriloquization of the following question: " 'In the end, wouldn't you rather not be HIV positive?' "[19] He continues, "The culture asking such questions assumes in advance that we all agree: able-bodied identities, able-bodied perspectives are preferable and what we all, collectively, are aiming for."[20] To take seriously the subcultural practice of bugchasing is to denaturalize the presumptive superiority and desirability of seronegativity, and by extension, able-bodiedness. It is also to question Croce's assumptions that one would never "choose" (again, to use her language) disability, and that once one chooses disability, that there are no other choices to be made. As the following pages demonstrate, the bugchaser challenges the temporal logic that declares that in becoming HIV+, one necessarily does so "in the end."

The Age of the Chronic

I write this essay in an acutely different historical milieu than the one in which Croce was writing and in which Jones first staged *Still/Here*. In the twenty-odd years that have passed, the AIDS crisis has transformed into the AIDS chronic. My characterization of the relationship between AIDS and contemporary (biological and social) life as chronic is not a suggestion of the transcendence of AIDS or its waning relevance. The transformation of the crisis into the chronic is not a narrative of progress. The chronic describes the radical reconfiguration of the temporal structures in which the lives of people with HIV/AIDS—and queers and disabled people more broadly—are produced, experienced, and foreclosed. This temporal transformation becomes clearer, perhaps, when we consider the chronic not only relative to the crisis but also to the terminal.

Since the late 1990s, privileged populations with access to adequate medical care and insurance coverage have been able to live with HIV as a chronic illness managed through persistent pharmaceutical intervention, rather than an illness that necessarily advances to AIDS and terminates with death. Certainly, the ability to experience HIV/AIDS as chronic rather than terminal is unevenly distributed along lines of race, class, and geography. But the move from the crisis/terminal to the chronic is a transformation that both references and exceeds the material realities of people living with HIV/AIDS. However unrealized for under-resourced communities and populations targeted by profound forms of structural violence, the very possibility that HIV/AIDS might be experienced as chronic operates with persuasive force regarding how lives might be lived. My investment in "the chronic" as a category emerges not only from the term's medical usages but also from recent interest within queer theoretical work on temporality. Elizabeth Freeman provocatively examines the chronic's temporal and diagnostic connotations:

> To say that something is chronic used to be to say that it is timeish, about time, that it takes time as its primary subject or material. . . . Yet in medical parlance, chronicity means something more than that: it defines a condition as ongoing, subject to relapse and remission. . . . It is important to keep in mind that this model . . . was a shift away from stigmatizing models of moral failure, and even from their relentless plot of decline.[21]

The AIDS chronic might have had its founding moment with the release of advanced antiretroviral (ARV) therapies in the late 1990s, but this chronic era includes a number of other developments alongside these pharmacological advancements. The advent of widespread social media for men who have sex with men—from websites like ManHunt and Adam4Adam to more recent cell phone applications like Grindr and Scruff—have proven crucial. These outlets have ushered in the chronic not because of their roles in facilitating live sexual encounters (or not), but because of how they have multiplied the ways in which users might identify their serostatus, an act of identification once imagined to only have two possibilities: HIV– and HIV+. For example, Adam4Adam asks users to list their HIV Status—"Don't Know, Negative, Positive, and Undetectable"—and also allows them to leave the field blank.[22]

These options are one of many means through which serostatus has been decoupled from resolute binarism. The emergence of the new category of "the undetectable" has proven especially important in loosening the grip of the HIV+/HIV− binary. To become undetectable, someone who has previously tested HIV+ must achieve, through pharmaceutical intervention, a viral load that cannot be detected through blood work. "Undetectable" does not signify the absence of HIV, but an inability to register the quantity of viral antibodies present within a given threshold. This threshold is variable and subject to change based upon both testing location and advancements in bloodwork testing practices.

The emergence of "undetectable" as both a medical diagnostic and as a social category of serostatus identification is important for thinking about the temporality of seroconversion. Because the categories of undetectable and HIV+ are mutually compatible, one might simultaneously claim both serostatuses. That the undetectable person inhabits (at least) two serostatuses decouples the act of serostatus disclosure from the enunciation of a single, identifiable truth. In the early twenty-first century, serostatus disclosure has become the nadir of the Foucauldian confession, the act through which the truth of the subject is both revealed and consolidated, the significance of which becomes increasingly clear with regards to establishment of criminal statutes for nondisclosure.[23] The proliferation of possible—and sometimes overlapping—serostatuses that one might disclose, then, is a politically charged development.[24] The emergence of the category of undetectable makes possible the understanding that one can move between different serostatuses after the initial diagnostic moment. For reasons of pharmaceutical efficacy, changing testing technologies, or the political or social context of disclosure, one might move between claiming HIV+ and undetectable serostatuses, or one might claim them simultaneously.

Bugchasing, the sexual practice represented in Campos's choreography, is one form of queer kinship and intimacy that has emerged in tandem with the technological, pharmaceutical, and political developments that constitute the chronic.[25] Definitions of bugchasing are perhaps as varied as the people who have attempted to define it, each of whom differently emphasize matters of history, intent, and context. But most of these definitions share an understanding of bugchasing as a subcultural practice through which (primarily) gay men deliberately pursue HIV. The practices through which one might chase HIV vary, but usually include condomless sex with an expansive repertoire of sexual partners, sometimes limited to those who identify as HIV+. Internal ejaculation, anonymity, quantity, and viral potency are often valued over the quality, duration, or "safety" of the sexual encounter.

Still, questions about what constitutes bugchasing proliferate. On Internet communities such as *Breeding Zone* and *BugShare,* users debate what constitutes the practice, identifying it with or in contradistinction to the practice of barebacking (condomless sex) more generally. How important is intentionality? Is the person who regularly pursues condomless sex but who is ambivalent about the possibility of seroconversion a bugchaser in the same way as the person who foregrounds seroconversion as the ultimate goal of their sexual practices? How do access to health insurance and plans to pharmaceutically intervene upon infection affect one's status as a bugchaser? Can someone who takes PrEP (pre-exposure prophylaxis) that minimizes the risk of infection, still chase? With what frequency must one get tested for HIV in order for their status as a chaser to be legitimized?

Many of these questions index the relationship between changes in practices of queer intimacy and changes in biomedicine since the late 1990s. These questions share investments in the relationship between modes of producing knowledge about one's own serostatus (the HIV test) and practices of communicating that knowledge, whether that be a verbal utterance, a deliberate silence, the sharing of medical paperwork, mutual rapid testing, or modes of bodily fashioning, such as tattooing. These attempts to distinguish between the real bugchaser and the imposter bolster serostatus as truth, and they do so relative to normative and biomedically supported narratives of that truth's singularity and meaningfulness: the event of seroconversion moves one from one register of truth, "being" HIV−, to another register of truth, "being" HIV+. Yet bugchasing undermines these narratives of singularity, linearity, and truth.

This essay attends to how Octavio Campos's dance theatre piece *The BugChasers* (2007) choreographs bugchasing through an engagement with Internet social networking and hook-up sites for bugchasers. Bugchasers have figured prominently within disparate fields of aesthetic and cultural production since the early 2000s. These works include Louise Hogarth's documentary film *The Gift* (2003), Showtime's *Queer as Folk* (2000), and Dakota Chase's young adult novel *Changing Jamie* (2008), but I attend to Campos's piece and queer Internet media because they similarly challenge dominant understandings of the temporality of seroconversion. In the series of exposés printed about bugchasers in the popular press, critics have mobilized these Internet communities as their primary evidence for the problem that bugchasers purportedly present to contemporary queer politics. Many critics do not account for the fact that these Internet communities are practices of representation, effectively treating these websites as transparent documentation of precedent sexual encounters and scripts for future execution. Other critics, however, focus upon these websites as exclusively representational with little to no relationship to lived sexual practice.

Linear narratives of seroconversion became persistent across alarmist representations of the bugchaser. Consider one of the first major exposés on bugchasing published by *Rolling Stone* in 2003. In "Bug Chasers: The Men Who Long to Be HIV+," Gregory Freeman established ethical and narrative tropes that would soon become conventional in journalistic (and quasi-journalistic) accounts.[26] The essay oscillates between intrigue and disgust as it establishes bugchasing as a practice that warrants attention because of the threat that it poses to public health. Freeman juxtaposes interviews with public health workers, AIDS Service Organizations (ASOs) administrators, and two self-identified bugchasers alongside excerpts from online personal ads in which bugchasers explicate their desires for "hot poz load[s]" and "poison seed."[27] He analogizes the irresponsible behavior of bugchasers to the institutions and activists who he believes failed to adequately respond to the emergence of bugchasing with empirical research and public awareness campaigns targeted at eradication. Freeman repeatedly emphasizes the inevitability of seroconversion as the primary reason men find bugchasing to be an attractive pursuit. Freeman distributes the figure of the bugchaser across two interview subjects, each of whom experiences one of the two temporal relationships to the chase that Freeman thinks are possible: one man who successfully seroconverted and is now filled with remorse, and a second still gleefully engaged in the chase.

Responses to the exposés took a number of forms, as mainstream gay pundits and queer theorists alike weighed in on the matter. Andrew Sullivan and Dan Savage immediately took Freeman to task for his irresponsibly poor research, but saved the brunt of their attack for bugchasers themselves.[28] Savage castigated gay men for everything from "having anal sex on the first date" to—it gets better—reviving the sexual culture of risk that "laid out the welcome mat for HIV in the 1970s."[29] Tim Dean, David Halperin, and Gregory Tomso did not lag far behind in introducing bugchasing to queer studies, sometimes investing the practice with a utopian political promise in contradistinction to the alarmist responses of mainstream critics.[30] Tomso, for example, celebrates bugchasers' collective resistance to neoliberal imperatives of self-care.

Despite their range of political and ideological perspectives, these writers all reify the temporality of the chase—and seroconversion in general—as uncompromisingly linear. Tim Dean writes, "seroconversion is something that happens only once. It holds a unique status, somewhat akin to losing one's virginity," effectively reproducing narrow conceptions of sex long contested within feminist studies.[31] Halperin insists that seroconversion is the event *par excellence*: "there is nothing episodic about the event of HIV transmission: it happens only once."[32] That queer theorists committed to challenging representations of bugchasers as pathological produce unidirectional narratives suggests how deeply entrenched normative understandings of the temporality of seroconversion are. These linear narratives bolster seroconversion's discursive and affective power to govern queer life as "the event." This risks rendering people with HIV passive bystanders to whom the disease happens, rather than subjects who can inhabit life with HIV in any number of different directions. Certainly, this passivity might hold some promise to the extent that it departs from narratives that blame people with HIV for the "behavior" that results in seroconversion. But this also risks evacuating bugchasing, and the AIDS chronic, of history. The figure of the bugchaser, who purports to choose seroconversion, enacts his seroconversion again and again. In so doing, he challenges seroconversion's singular eventfulness and its historical indexicality. That is, he chronically repeats his entrance into the chronic, investing HIV/AIDS with a history even as he empties the historicity of his own seroconversion. The bugchaser, the subject who insists on becoming HIV+, points to the possibility that things might be otherwise.

Chasing the Chronic

When bugchasers first appear explicitly in Campos's work, they provocatively contest linear constructions of the chase. Two ensemble members, Matt and Ron, stand center stage and inform the audience that they are both bugchasers. Ron never speaks, but Matt continues, "Before, we couldn't give two shits about our future."[33] They narrate their concerns with the future as emerging alongside (rather than dissipating because of) their self-identification as bugchasers. In so doing, they upend popular assumptions regarding what drives one to chase. They conceive the future as a sexual utopia in which they can "fuck anytime we want, anywhere we want, anyone we want" without being haunted by the possibility of seroconversion. They frame bugchasing as a means of embracing the future rather than a way to curtail its very possibility. While *The BugChasers* hesitates to legitimize this resiliently optimistic conception of an HIV+ future, this scene constructs the chase as the reconfiguration, rather than the foreclosure, of a future.

Campos's incorporation of reproductive themes and language also encourages thinking about bugchasing as something other than a rejection of life, endurance, and futurity. At one point, Matt announces that "the hot thing about toxic cock is every man who leaves his seed in you LIVES in you forever. I carry the 'ghosts' of so MANY hot men in me." This projection of viral inheritance into the future—which users in online bugchasing communities often analogize to male pregnancy—renders the temporality of the chase irreducible to the refusal of a future. Bugchasers' appropriation of heteronormative temporal structures of reproduction and futurity establishes the possibility of multiple, intersecting temporalities that govern the logic of the chase. Without some irony, they repurpose the virus—conventionally associated with illness, if not death—as a source for affirming and sustaining life.

This rhetoric of pregnancy and inheritance might seem to bolster the linear temporality of seroconversion rather than challenging it. Yet the chronicity of the chase appears in high relief by foregrounding the route to such a future. Matt comes out as a bugchaser by declaring, "I am a chaser. I am a successful chaser. I am now HIV+."[34] In this procession of speech, Matt revises his initial identification, "I am a chaser," with a declaration of his success, "I am a successful chaser," and then concludes by disclosing his new serostatus, "I am now HIV+," as evidence of that success. Initially, the structure of this speech might seem to adhere to a linear narrative of seroconversion that is ubiquitous within representations of chasing. But note the grammatical construction of this speech. The slippages between the present tense and past acts and identifications insist that we reconsider the temporality of the chase. Matt does not narrate his transformation from being a chaser to being HIV+, but instead details a list of coterminous identifications. Matt's grammatical slippage between past and present suggests that each of these statements offer a different account of naming and describing himself, rather than a series of replacements in his progression from one subject position to another. He both "is" a chaser and "is" HIV+. What, then, of the temporality of seroconversion?

This seeming temporal misstep—this movement in which chasing and seropositive identities exist simultaneously—refuses the linear narrative often attached to bugchasing. It confirms instead the chronic temporality that characterizes the chase. To sustain the chase as a chase, bugchasers must perform themselves as if HIV− in order to produce the serodiscordance (at least one HIV+ partner and one HIV− partner) the chase requires. Irrespective of the outcome of that encounter, chasing requires that the bugchaser perform as if HIV−, as if his previous attempts at seroconversion necessarily failed. In concert with the known or unknown biomedical truth of his serostatus, the bugchaser chronically stages his serostatus as if HIV−. In so doing, the bugchaser renders undecidable his success or failure at "becoming" HIV+. This commitment to, rather than anxiety about, the undecidable proffers a unique contribution to debates about disability, sexuality, and mimetic (in)capacity more broadly.

The opening scene of *The BugChasers*, titled "The French Kiss," stages mimetic failure as constitutive of—rather than anomalous within—chasing as an erotic and social practice. The scene opens with a woman named Natasha lip-synching and playfully dancing opposite a red shoe. She plucks a young man named Joshua from the audience in order to teach him her choreography. When Joshua proves unable to replicate the routine, Natasha stops the music and proceeds to assault him violently, using the red shoe as a weapon.[35] Like Natasha herself, the scene performs a pedagogical function. It teaches audiences to look for mimetic failure and the stakes that attend it. This staging of Joshua's mimetic failure proves noteworthy for two reasons. First, this scene introduces an individual's capacity for imitation as requisite for entrance into queer community. Second, this scene locates Natasha and Joshua within two different theatrical registers, evincing each performer's respective capacity for mimetic representation. Natasha, an expert in the queer theatricality of lip-synching, emerges as the arbiter of success and failure, while Joshua, the untrained spectator, fails at imitative practice. Of course, Joshua is not really an unprepared spectator plucked haplessly from the audience, but an actor playing the role of a spectator turned failed actor/dancer. This staging of mimetic failure as a product of representation renders undecidable the relationship between success and failure. This predicament is perhaps not entirely different from that of Matt, who chronically stages his pursuit of seroconversion as failed in order to sustain the chase as a chase.

The throughline of *The BugChasers* is less, in Campos's words, "the stupid things people do in order to fit in," than it is a persistent staging of mimetic failure. For example, one scene alludes to how the medical realities of illness and disability animate spectatorial anxieties about a performer's mimetic capacity. In this scene, Michael comically announces a competition for audience members to participate in: "Join the Camposition Poz, Poz, POZ contest. Three cast members are HIV+. If you can guess which ones, just fill out the ballot in the lobby, drop it in the fish bowl and you just might win dinner for two to Chili's."[36] Not only does such a game play with spectator's varied beliefs in the degree to which the HIV+ body is legible as such, it also asks them to grapple with their own complex feelings about disability and mimetic capacity. Who in the ensemble is playing "against" his own serostatus? This would constitute a theatrical maneuvering not terribly dissimilar from that performed by the character of Matt, who both *is* a chaser and *is* HIV+, who replays through the theatrical scenario of the chase the act of achieving the serostatus he has already acquired. And for whom in the ensemble does the theatrical frame of the event—appearing in a work of dance-theatre called *The BugChasers*—ironically thwart the act of disclosing their own serostatus as actually constituting an act of disclosure? What do we make of the emphasis on the ocular "proof" of serostatus not only in terms of the surface of the body and its movement, but relative to other bodies moving on stage and relative to the spoken act of disclosure? But the piece is not remotely interested in answering the questions it introduces. Instead, it parodies the visual intelligibility of serostatus, the game of chance that one enters by playing this game, and the potential rewards of such a gamble: the suburban embarrassment of dinner for two at a chain restaurant.

Elizabeth Freeman highlights how the language of chronicity can sometimes to be used to evacuate historicity. Something that is chronic cannot be helped, it merely is. Chronic: it has been. Chronic: it remains. Chronic: it will continue to be. Yet to articulate the transformation of the AIDS crisis into the AIDS chronic is not only to chart a historical shift, but to invest the temporality of seroconversion with a history. Written in the last days of 1994, Croce's attack on Bill T. Jones's *Still/Here* preceded by two years the development of advanced ARV therapies that animated the transformation of the AIDS crisis into the AIDS chronic. Croce's construction of victim art was inflected with anxieties not only about the ethics of watching ill bodies "suffer" on stage but also the ethics of spectating bodies in the process of dying. For Croce, Jones's performers were irredeemably oriented toward death, and anxieties about temporality—HIV/AIDS status as terminal—informed her non-review. By turning to the bodily repertoire of bugchasing as it circulates online and in Campos's *The BugChasers*, I hope to have restored to the chronic a sense of historicity.

But what can the bugchaser's theatrical play, his location between success and failure, his chronic staging of the chronic, be understood to do? The chaser relentlessly pursues that which is biomedically authored as HIV+, both in terms of the identities of his sexual partners and the subject position he hopes eventually to inhabit himself. It would seem disingenuous, then, to suggest that chasers pose challenges to regimes of medicalization. Bugchasers are conversant with the biomedical authorship of serostatus. They are not flippantly dismissive of regimes of medical authority, but rather they betray investments in and attachments to it. I argue instead that the bugchaser's undecidable relationship to mimesis, his chronic staging of his serostatus which may or may not be biomedically conferred, resonates with the efforts of Elizabeth Freeman and others to rethink the privileging of the political capacity of rupture and transgression within feminist historiography and queer theory.[37] Yes, the bugchaser challenges linear narratives of seroconversion by restaging himself as HIV– after a "successful" conversion so that the chase can continue. But he also composes a chase from a series of conversions (however successful, however failed) that are emphatically linear. The undecidability of the shape of the chaser's chronic journey matches his undecidable relationship to mimetic capacity, whether disclosures are theatricalizing his serostatus or authenticating them. Returning to Robert McRuer's *Crip Theory* description of the incessant, if unspoken affirmation of compulsory able-bodiedness may prove illuminating: "In the end, wouldn't you rather not be HIV-positive?"[38] The affect and political potential of the bugchaser within the queer and crip times of the chronic lies less in encouraging a reevaluation of seroconversion as necessarily undesirable, than in his contestation of the foregone conclusion that in becoming HIV+, one necessarily does so "in the end."

Notes

1. Camposition/Octavio Campos, "The Bugchasers_OUT!," YouTube 8:35, January 12, 2008, https://youtu.be/7VzXxhEjofA?list=UUGXghbJ8hS-jGH9AEdeHoMA. All movement description and analysis in this essay is based upon this recording.
2. Michael Yawney and Matthew Glass, *The BugChasers* Synopsis/Script, October 22, 2007, unpublished manuscript. Hereinafter cited as Synopsis/Script.
3. Arlene Croce, "Discussing the Undiscussable," in *The Crisis of Criticism*, ed. Maurice Berger (New York: New Press, 1998).
4. Ibid., 17.
5. Ibid., 29. *The New Yorker*'s publication of "Discussing the Undiscussable" in 1994 sparked responses from artists and academics alike. See Joyce Carol Oates, "Confronting Head-On the Face of the Afflicted," in *The Crisis of Criticism*, ed. Maurice Berger (New York: New Press, 1998). Carol Martin, "High Critic/Low Arts," in *Moving Words: Re-Writing Dance*, ed. Gay Morris (New York: Routledge, 1996). Petra Kuppers, *Disability and Contemporary Performance* (New York: Routledge, 2003). David Roman, "Not-about-AIDS," *GLQ: A Journal of Lesbian and Gay Studies* 6, no. 1 (2000): 1–28.
6. Ibid., 17.
7. Tom Shakespeare, "The Social Model of Disability," in *The Disability Studies Reader*, ed. Lennard J. Davis (New York: Routledge, 2013), 214–21.
8. Ibid., 16.
9. Rosemarie Garland Thomson, *Extraordinary Bodies: Figuring Physical Disability in American Literature and Culture* (New York: Columbia University Press, 1997), 46.
10. Nicholas Ridout, *Stage Fright, Animals, and Other Theatrical Problems* (Cambridge: Cambridge University Press, 2006), 66.
11. Susan Manning, "Black Voices, White Bodies: The Performance of Race and Gender in *How Long Brethren*," *American Quarterly* 50, no. 1 (1998): 24–46.

12. Rebecca Schneider, *Performing Remains: Art and War in Times of Theatrical Reenactment* (New York: Routledge, 2011).

13. Ellen Samuels, *Fantasies of Identification: Disability, Gender, Race* (New York: New York University Press, 2014), 2, 9.

14. Ibid., 3.

15. Lennard Davis, "Flat Earth, Deaf World," in *Enabling Acts: How the Americans with Disabilities Act Gave the Largest US Minority Its Rights* (Beacon: Boston, 2015), 76–99, at 80.

16. Ruth Colker, *The Disability Pendulum: The First Decade of the Americans with Disabilities Act* (New York: New York University Press, 2005), 50.

17. Ibid., 51.

18. Robert McRuer, *Crip Theory: Cultural Signs of Queerness and Disability* (New York: New York University Press, 2006), 1–32, at 1.

19. Ibid., 1–32.

20. Ibid., 8.

21. Elizabeth Freeman, "Hopeless Cases: Queer Chronicities and Gertrude Stein's 'Melenctha,'" *Journal of Homosexuality* 63, no. 3 (2016): 329–48.

22. Adam4Adam website, Registration Step 5. http://www.adam4adam.com.

23. Michel Foucault, *The History of Sexuality, Volume 1: An Introduction* (New York: Vintage, 1978).

24. See David Oscar Harvey, "Red, Red, Red: An Essay/Film in Eleven Parts," *Women's Studies Quarterly* 40, nos. 1–2 (2012): 320–30.

25. Within the context of communities of queer men, HIV/AIDS has long been the springboard for the innovation of new and innovative means of sexual practice. For example, Douglas Crimp's "How to Have Promiscuity in an Epidemic" chronicles queer efforts to promote new forms of intimacy in the face of a (then, almost necessarily) deadly virus. Crimp and others attribute the invention of safe(r) sex to gay men and define that term in a capacious manner irreducible to the use of condoms or abstinence: including watersports and sex acts which deprivileged genital contact. These modes of queer intimacy responded not only to the persistence of the virus and its disproportionate impact on gay male communities but also to a broader national morality in which all practices of sexual intimacy between two (or more) men—with or without condoms or other prophylactics—were seen to be inviting infection. While the figure (or terminology) of the bugchaser would not enter popular parlance until the late 1990s, the idea that queer men were willfully infecting themselves does not significantly depart from popular discourses on AIDS and sexual morality in the 1980s. See Douglas Crimp, "How to Have Promiscuity in an Epidemic," in *Melancholia and Moralism: Essays on AIDS and Queer Politics* (Cambridge, MA: MIT Press, 2004).

26. Gregory Freeman, "Bug Chasers: The Men Who Long to Be HIV+," *Rolling Stone*, January 23, 2003.

27. Ibid.
28. Andrew Sullivan, "Sex- and Death-Crazed Gays Play Viral Russian Roulette!," *Salon*, January 24, 2003; Dan Savage, "Bug Chasers," *Savage Love*, January 30, 2003.
29. Savage, "Bug Chasers."
30. Timothy Dean, *Unlimited Intimacy: Reflections on the Subculture of Barebacking* (Chicago: University of Chicago Press, 2009); David Halperin, *What Do Gay Men Want?: An Essay on Risk, Sex, and Subjectivity* (Ann Arbor: University of Michigan Press, 2008); Gregory Tomso, "Bug Chasing, Barebacking, and the Risks of Care," *Literature and Medicine* 23, no. 1 (2004): 88–111; Gregory Tomso, "Viral Sex and the Politics of Life," *South Atlantic Quarterly* 107, no. 2 (2008): 265–85.
31. Dean, *Unlimited Intimacy*, 52.
32. Halperin, *What Do Gay Men Want?*, 28.
33. Synopsis/Script, 5.
34. Ibid.
35. Ibid., 1.
36. Ibid., 7.
37. Freeman, "Hopeless Cases."
38. McRuer, *Crip Theory*, 8.

17

Expressing Life Through Loss

ON QUEENS THAT FALL WITH A FREAK TECHNIQUE

Anna Martine Whitehead

▶ "Memory Loser"
▶ in conversation with Anna Martine Whitehead

Friday afternoon, opening day.

A few members from the 2013 iteration of Keith Hennesy's *Turbulence (a dance about the economy)* recline on each other in a small studio on the third floor of the Abrons Art Center in New York's Lower East Side. A couple of white queers, a couple of Black queers, of varying ages and body types, all looking cute and cool and eager. We are here at the American Realness festival to dance a piece about collective ecstasy and unsustainable structures, but first we are here to talk to filmmaker Marin Sander-Holzman. The conversation goes like this (paraphrased):

MARIN: Audiences who haven't seen you sometimes assume that you are just these freaks from San Francisco. What they don't realize is each dancer in this show actually has a very specifically honed craft; you bring specialized skills to the project.

ME: But also, we *are* these freaks from San Francisco.

A moment of shared understanding overcomes us: our "specifically honed craft"—our virtuosity—might be irreducibly "freak"-ish, if we can think of that term beyond the pejorative and consider it as a life practice.

(I do not carelessly attach the term *freak* to the facts and fictions of queer, Black, and othered life. Indeed, the etymology of that word bears striking similarities to the ways both queer performance and Black life are conceptualized contemporarily. First appearing in the sixteenth century and deriving from the Old English *frician* "to dance," the term *freak* was used by the white Europeans with the power to name things to describe someone of "capricious notion," "sudden turn of mind," "bold," or "gluttonous" disposition.[1] These early definitions are decidedly ambivalent and connote a turn away from all that is associated with normativity and predictable reason: sensuality, creativity, oppositionality. I employ the term here as a signifier of queer Blackness in the context of anti-Black capitalist heteronormative patriarchy. The term is relational, and in this way also supposes a loss of the safety and access that privilege affords. Through relatively bold and capricious living, queers have experienced the extreme losses that have plagued Black folks and people of color for centuries: access to family, employment, healthcare, political protection, and so on. I use the term *freak* to suggest both a devastating lack of hegemonic protection and a legacy of sensuous and spirited cultural inventiveness.)

We are at the Abrons. Later on that same evening as the interview, Emily (who is white) and I (who am Black and mixed-race) practice scaling a two-story window on the side of the theater with a single Spanset hung from a railing. Our lighting designer approaches us laughing, happy to recognize us.

"Oh, it's you! From down the street I thought you were a couple of performance artists or something!"

This moment of interpolation makes us recognizable as individuals, as un-subjects. We are apparently not performance artists, not the people who might fall from the roof: we are merely us. In that instant there is a collapse of the impulse to climb a wall, the potential failure of falling, and the performance of self in which Emily and I are compulsively engaged. It is a taste of freedom. Indeed, we could have fallen in the very next moment, leading to a chain reaction of minor and major catastrophes for both the company and the theater. Yet our potential to fall did not seal our identities as the fallen (at least, not this time), either because the lighting designer was positive we wouldn't fall, or—more likely—she was certain we'd done this a thousand times before. The certainty of our thousand times before—and our easy conjuring of that certainty—was our taste of freedom.

I don't mean to say that freedom is the impossibility of collapse. Freedom is the moment of recognition that collapse is not only inevitable, but critical as well as continuous. Freedom is the moment you might have fallen but have everyone convinced otherwise. We do not stop collapsing. Freedom is at once the fall, the performance of not falling, and the awareness of all that comes after (without knowing what—except more falling— comes after).

Freedom is unsustainable. We would that very night return to the inside of the theater where one of the women in our company would be physically assaulted during the evening; a few of us would dance our variegated Black and queer and gender non-conforming bodies for a mostly white audience; we would all climb trapezes and perform fake and real healings and shake and shout and generally read as freaks from San Francisco. This was the work. Where we felt freedom on the balcony, we returned to the stage to present our-selves as "food for fantasy," to recall Bill T. Jones.[2] Freedom from the burden of subjection offers itself as merely a fleeting taste, but this we already knew. Our familiarity with loss prepared us for the loss of freedom, too.

Still, it was nice to momentarily be recognized as ourselves, rather than being pathologized through misrecognition. That recognition comes on the back of a [recurring] queer turn in performance and art in general—toward the fallible, un-categorical, un-marketable, and, by extension, the proximal to death. These markers of a life lived outside of capital are, perhaps discon-certingly, accumulating value. To exist outside the laws of capital—to be bold and creative and at-risk—are simultaneously life-affirming and indicative of potential social as well as corporeal death. These moves are increasingly registering as a burgeoning field called "queer performance" and implicating performance in general. This development of the field facilitates our ability to safely express loss as an arts practice, even while it attempts to codify a ges-tural language that pivots on the wildness of danger and grief.

The conceptualization of freedom as un-marketability does not originate with the development of queer cultural practice: this freedom is rooted in ontologies of Blackness whose roots are entangled in queer and trans* ways of knowing. The compulsion to embellish an expectation of failure and collapse that is always already presumed in the case of both Black and/or queer bodies is a queer Black freakish practice.

In thinking about practice, I struggle with the distinctions between re-sistance, survival, and art.[3] I hope to circumvent any confusion by defining queer/Black legacies of cultural production as the aggregate and often ephem-eral activities that reject violent erasure, that are both borne of and resulting in a collective consciousness. José Muñoz points toward these gestic legacies of what he deems survival in his interrogation of Kevin Aviance's vogue moves. Muñoz rightly identifies Aviance's vogue patterns as multivalenced "store-houses of queer history and futurity ... ephemera that are utterly necessary."[4] I want to consider Aviance and vogue in general within the larger wheelhouse of queer performance, not only as a vessel for queer temporality but also as a racialized expression of a somatic relationship to gravity and an extreme proximity to loss.

It is a particularly queer racialization Muñoz names. Queer in its illegibility, nonwhite in its mysteriousness: something fantastical and forever in the process of becoming material. I am interested in that materiality and its potential. I want to frame, for instance, Aviance's Machiavellian dip as a Black act—unable to bring anything but racialized realness—in that it literally reproduces a virtuosic collapse (giving over to the spirit), resurrects, and collapses again. (This virtuosity exists alongside and in conjunction with the inherent Blackness of vogue and its Africanist origins.)

I like the lack of temporal or even geographic fixity in the term "racialized realness." It provides me with the freedom to repeatedly recollect the plunge of the young African woman en route to the New World—the one who hoists herself atop the stern rail of her slavers' ship and throws herself over. I am encouraged to remember her Black body as one in the throes of queer collapse, and to identify my remembrance of her as a further queering; another compulsory resurrection-to-death narrative with an undeniable materiality like Aviance's dip. Racialized realness: that moment of embodying survival, and resistance, and performance. To me, these Coriolis spirals—a force moving in the opposite direction of the force of its frame—which resurrect and collapse, on repeat, through history's retelling and through live re-performance, are necessarily Black and could be nothing other than queer.[5] Outside of the debate around revolutionary resistance and radical survival, I see the spiral—or the revolution—as an iterative somatic compulsion toward the freedom that we know. The practice of turning against the frame is the freak technique Marin and I were grasping at in our interview: the enduring habit of transforming oneself through significant loss into something desirable, vulnerable, and fierce.

On Collectivity and Collapse, or All My Friends Have Poor Posture

Sunday, Super Bowl night, around 1 a.m.

Seven cops are bursting through the front door of our two-bedroom home, startling me from my sleep in the main room. Max is staggering out of his bedroom, groggy.[6] Flashlights everywhere and I cannot see, and no one has announced they are the police. Here is a semi-automatic rifle and here is a man's voice barking questions, ordering me to forget about putting on clothes, just get out of bed and face the wall. Lil, female-bodied like me, is pulled out of their bed and ordered to stand in the bathroom as Max, a Black cisgender man, is handcuffed and led out. Something about "we'll release him; it's for your own safety," and we don't understand this because Max is our friend and partner and the yelling police are the strangers who have just broken into our home. Something about someone in the neighborhood with a weapon (is it a semi-automatic?), and then something else about a burglary—no cop seems clear—and meanwhile several cops have broken from the pack to raid our neighbor's bungalow just north of us. Within a half hour it is announced it was a false alarm, Max is released; he comes walking back up the driveway to us and the cops are already gone.

This is how it happened. Afterward, we shook. Max repeatedly bit his lip. Our neighbors' bodies strained and their faces and particularly their eyes had become slack from post-trauma exhaustion. Lil sobbed. I have never seen Yemi's body look the way it did for those next nine hours: without bones. Their rib cage and shoulder girdle melted away and their spine struggled to hold up all the muscles. Yemi's skin sagged off their spine like this; even their cheekbones pulled downward. I don't remember what I did with my body; I do not know how I looked; I avoided mirrors. We all shook for a long time.

In another instant, a year and a half prior, I had witnessed these same somatic reactions to trauma in the bodies of other friends after the tragic death of April, who climbed and fell from a downtown building after struggling through mental illness and being refused healthcare without insurance and in possession of a gender non-conforming body. April had been a housemate, a best friend, co-organizer, and/or lover to many of us—their untimely evacuation from our community of the living hit hard and wrought its effects unmistakably across our bodies. It would seem that indescribable loss finds its way most intensely to the parts of the body above the waist—sinking everything into the sacrum and lower lumbar, making the hips heavy and tilted. Zones of trauma develop: the fingers to the forearm extensors; the chest, shoulders, traps, jaw and cheekbones; the eyes, cheeks, and forehead a third.

To answer the impossible question, "How does one make their eyes empty?" study the face of someone who has experienced violent loss. The tailbone pulls at the eyes, seems to pull them out and deep down into the heels. The emptiness of the eyes belies a confused grief, an affect that can be circuitously applied to the shape of emptiness created by a hollowing of the space between the deltoids and the ilium. The post-trauma empty-body shape might suggest that muscular composure is at least partly circumscribed by the body's aptitude at turning trauma into cellular tissue—a refusal to relinquish trauma. When we are shocked by unintelligible violence, that muscle memory is dislodged from its quiet holding patterns inside our bodies. Or, if we are repeatedly shocked so that the violence becomes normalized, the hollowed and heavy body becomes the normative body.

The body molds itself around loss; it carries the burden of danger and grief. There are so many possible outcomes to physically holding that feeling, and only one of those is to continue standing. There are other options, more dynamic and more interesting to me in these moments of disaster: to fall down, to get back up, to fall under the weight of sorrow again, to get back up. To shake to keep from crying. To fly to keep from drowning. Freedom is the release of tension under weight paired with the appearance of bearing no weight at all. That is our bold and capricious freedom practice, our freak technique.

Everything to Know about Living I Learned from Falling Queens

Arthur Jafa once described to me his notion of a b-boy as someone who makes falling down look fly. "We can't help them beating us down to the ground, but we can make the descent look good."[7] It is not hard to draw the conceptual links between the b-boy's fly fall and the practice of falling fabulously epitomized in the vogue suicide dip. The breaker moves in ways a body is not supposed to move: seemingly emerging from the ground and flying up into the air, breaking itself into pieces and collapsing back downwards onto arms, neck, stomach. Similarly, the voguer prances fiercely, challenging the room with her materiality: its significations and slippages. The voguing body—like the breaking body—is an otherworldly body unleashed, moving against the rules of gender and physics before exploding into collapse with wild grace onto her one leg. Both the break and the dip are a sharp turn away from European-derived movement language in which the body labors to present order, to stiffen and rise. Both the break and the dip offer to audiences the desire, the challenge, the contagion of collapse.

In this context, it is also small wonder that breaking and voguing, and HIV/AIDS and crack (and its associated neoliberalized wave of incarceration) all originated or otherwise found their stronghold within the same ten-year period, in New York (in the case of breaking and voguing, mostly uptown), among people of color (mostly Black). It is not surprising that dance forms that embellish collapse should enter the popular gestural lexicon at the same time that multiple epidemics (AIDS, crack, and incarceration) were terrorizing the popular imaginary. And it is not hard to understand why these moves were advents of Black communities, since Black folk have been dancing joy through danger, loss, and grief for so long.

Black cultural production, iterated as urban street breaking in the 1970s, necessarily developed in tandem with queer of color gestic space-making at the ball. Although she does not reference dance specifically, Cathy Cohen makes a strong argument for the reconsideration of queerness as always already racialized due to its relationship to hegemony. Cohen argues that a queer subject is the individual facing the threat of ideological and normalizing violence. The queer subject is she whose materiality as a dying and/or brutalized body functions as a critical component in the production of the state.[8] In this way, we are all at-risk of becoming queer subjects, certainly none more so than she who is Black. Sharon Holland also contends "the space of death is marked by blackness and is therefore always already queer."[9] According to Holland and Cohen, the tools we use to identify blackness are further employed to create queer subjects. I would argue that we make and un-make ourselves using these very interpolative tools. So many of the ways we know how to be expressively queer come from the same places we learned how to move as Black folks and people of color, queer and otherwise; when we learned the performance of Blackness, we were learning queer performance, too. These ways of knowing are sharpened through the persistent practice of virtuosic descent, which itself reflects an unencumbered relationship to gravity that is the privilege of the oppressed.

I want to sit with this idea of loss as a generative constraint in queer Black and freakish expressive culture. Beyoncé Knowles (who owes everything to queer Black expressive pageantry) was interviewed after her infamous tumble at the Amway Arena in 2007.

LOLA OGUNNAIKE FOR CNN: "When you're falling, what are you thinking?"
BEYONCÉ KNOWLES: "I just kept thinking, *You better get up.* I was like, *Just go for it—do it harder.* Whenever I do something like that, I always perform really, really hard . . . I just go crazy."

Indeed, we know about this: going hard, collapsing, going crazy, enduring, keeping the wig on, keeping the lip-synch tight. We are all enlivened by disaster and our continuation over and past it, by enduring through what Sara Jane Bailes calls the "compromised circumstance," then incorporating that gesture of compromise into our own movement language.[10] The pull toward gravity, the concave shoulder girdle, the still or slack body, a raging or falling body, a breaking body, a body dancing ambivalence, a body untethered to reality. These become the buoyant body, the leaping body, the grooving body. These are re-presentations of the queer Black life, the life curved around loss. This is what we know how to do: make meaning out of our heavy movement to make ourselves more alive.

There is little else as real as watching a femme break her legs to dip, or watching Jesse as he went into a panic atop a rafter during a performance of *Turbulence*, or watching Yemi recover her posture and go on to help build a movement against anti-Black police violence. At first I thought Jesse's fear was a put-on; he'd climbed that high and higher so many times. But this time his body had lost its taught rigidity, and his arms were flailing in a disordered way that betrayed the terror suddenly overtaking him. I also thought it was a put-on when a notice showed up on social media that my friend April had gone missing—but that, sadly, turned out to be too real as well. The realness of these near-collapses or utter collapses is made undeniable by subsequent resurrections that disrupt the straight narrative of rise-and-fall. The femme returns upright, broad and powerful, stilettos and all (fall-to-rise). Jesse shouted at us from the rafter, "I'm not joking," and, with our help, he descended, and then he exited the room to calm down (rise-to-fall-to-fall). April turned out to have died, which we did not expect, and then we sang their favorite song in a cavernous house full of candles for about two weeks, and now we make art and get tattoos about them, even years later (I am still figuring out the narrative structure of this one).

The queer folk dance of death, the Africanist dance familiar to all disenfranchised people, though more familiar to some than others, rejects any Western compositional paradigm (beginning-middle-crescendo-dénouement). It is something more like fall-fall-rise-rest-rise-rest-fall or rise-fall-rise-fall-rest-rest-snap, and so on. A-B-A-B-C-B-C is no longer applicable in the freak technique. It is a practice around and through loss, a scary dance, and a sorrowful one, too—as sad as it is ecstatic, as ecstatic as it is subtly complex. And perhaps more than providing a context in which our right to life can be named, these dances exist for us to remind ourselves that we are alive in the first place. The freak technique is an embodied promise: to get down with the lowness of death as boldly as we groove to a life yet unknown.

Notes

1. Douglas Harper, *Online Etymology Dictionary*, 2001–2014, http://www.etymon-line.com/index.php?term=freak.
2. Henry Louis Gates Jr., "The Body Politic of Bill T. Jones," *New Yorker*, November 28, 1994, 117.
3. The links between the compulsions to make art and to live and to struggle are sewn into indigenous and African ontologies. The differentiation between these compulsions is debated elsewhere and is particularly well-articulated by Omise'eke Tinsley and Christina Sharpe, "Queering Slavery Working Group," March 27, 2014, https://www.youtube.com/watch?v=Jw-iD0Gqybs.

4. José Muñoz, *Cruising Utopia: The Then and There of Queer Futurity* (New York: NYU Press, 2009), 81.

5. I am also wary of the potential violence we do to our historical subjects when we claim the right to queer them. But I want to leverage Holland's positing of queer as a signifier of a relationship to death, see Sharon Patricia Holland, *Raising the Dead: Readings of Death and (Black) Subjectivity* (Chapel Hill, NC: Duke University Press, 2000), 179; and Fred Moten's argument about power and the fundamental violence of language. "This violence is intrinsic to art making," said Moten during a recent talk he gave at the Roy and Edna Disney/CalArts Theater. "The problem is not the fundamental violence of language, but the regulation of the deployment of said violence" (Fred Moten, lecture given at Roy and Edna Disney/CalArts Theater, March 20, 2014).

6. All names changed at the request of those discussed.

7. Arthur Jafa, conversation with the author, 2012.

8. Cathy Cohen, "Death and Rebirth of a Movement: Queering Critical Ethnic Studies," *Social Justice* 37, no. 4 (2011–2012): 126–32.

9. Holland, *Raising the Dead*, 180.

10. Sara Jane Bailes, *Performance Theater and the Poetics of Failure: Forced Entertainment, Goat Island, Elevator Repair Service* (New York: Routledge, 2011).

References

Ahlgren, Angela K. "Butch Bodies, Big Drums: Queering North American Taiko." *Women and Music: A Journal of Gender and Culture* 20 (2016): 1–26.

Albright, Ann Cooper. *Choreographing Difference: The Body and Identity in Contemporary Dance*. Middletown, CT: Wesleyan University Press, 1997.

Banerji, Projesh. *Dance in Thumri*. New Delhi: Abhinav Publications, 1986.

Banes, Sally. *Dancing Women: Female Bodies on Stage*. New York: Routledge, 1998.

Berlant, Lauren, and Michael Warner. "Sex in Public." *Critical Inquiry* 24, no. 2 (1998): 547–66.

Boyd, Nan Alamilla. *Wide Open Town: A History of Queer San Francisco to 1965*. Berkeley: University of California Press, 2003.

Briginshaw, Valerie. *Dance, Space and Subjectivity*. New York: Palgrave, 2001.

Brinkley, Shanara R. Reid. "The *Essence* of Res(ex)pectability: Black Women's Negotiation of Black Femininity in Rap Music and Music Videos." *Meridian's: Feminisms, Race, Transnationalism* 8, no. 1 (2008): 236–60.

Buckland, Fiona. *Impossible Dance: Club Culture and Queer World-Making*. Middletown, CT: Wesleyan University, 2002.

Burt, Ramsay. *The Male Dancer: Bodies, Spectacle, Sexualities*. 2d ed. New York: Routledge, 2006.

Burt, Ramsay. "The Performance of Unmarked Masculinity." In *When Men Dance*, edited by Jennifer Fischer and Anthony Shay, 150–67. New York: Oxford University Press, 2009.

Butler, Judith. *Bodies that Matter: On the Discursive Limits of "Sex."* New York: Routledge, 1993.

Butler, Judith. *Gender Trouble: Feminism and the Subversion of Identity*, 10th anniversary ed. New York: Routledge, 1999.

Butler, Judith. "Performative Acts and Gender Constitution: An Essay in Phenomenology and Feminist Theory." *Theatre Journal* 40, no. 4 (1998): 519–31.

Butler, Judith. *Speech Acts: A Politics of the Performative*. New York: Routledge, 1997.

Campbell, Alyson, and Stephen Farrier. "Introduction." In *Queer Dramaturgies: International Perspective on Where Performance Leads Queer*, edited by Alyson Campbell and Stephen Farrier, 1–26. London: Palgrave Macmillan, 2015.

Case, Sue-Ellen. "Towards a Butch-Femme Aesthetic." *Discourse* 11, no. 1 (1988): 55–73.

Chakravorty, Pallabi. *Bells of Change: Kathak Dance, Women and Modernity in India.* Kolkata: Seagull Books, 2008.

Chatterjee, Sandra, and Cynthia Ling Lee. "Solidarity—Rasa/Autobiography—Abhinaya South Asian Tactics for Performing Queerness." *Studies in South Asian Film and Media*, The Body: Indian Theatre Special Issue, 5, no. 1 (2013): 129–40.

Chauncey, George. *Gay New York: Gender, Urban Culture, and the Making of the Gay Male World.* New York: Harper Collins, 1994.

Cheng, Meiling. *In Other Los Angeleses: Multicentric Performance Art.* Berkeley: University of California Press, 2002.

Claid, Emilyn. *Yes? No! Maybe—: Seductive Ambiguity in Dance.* London: Routledge, 2006.

Clay, Andreanna. "'I Used to be Scared of the Dick': Queer Women of Color and Hip-Hop Masculinity." In *Home Girls Make Some Noise: Hip Hop Feminism Anthology*, edited by Gwendolyn D. Pough, Elaine Richardson, Aisha Durham, and Rachel Raimist, 148–65. Mira-Loma, CA: Parker Publishing, 2007.

Cohen, Cathy J. *The Boundaries of Blackness: AIDS and the Breakdown of Black Politics.* Chicago: University of Chicago Press, 1999.

Cohen, Cathy. "Death and Rebirth of a Movement: Queering Critical Ethnic Studies." *Social Justice* 37, no. 4: 126–32.

Cohen, Cathy. "Punks, Bulldaggers, and Welfare Queens: The Radical Potential of Queer Politics?" In *Black Queer Studies: A Critical Anthology*, edited by E. Patrick Johnson and Mae G. Henderson, 21–51. Durham, NC: Duke University Press, 2005.

Collins, Patricia Hill. *Black Sexual Politics: African Americans, Gender, and the New Racism.* New York; Routledge, 2004.

Crenshaw, Kimberle. *Demarginalizing the Intersection of Race and Sex: A Black Feminist Critique of Antidiscrimination Doctrine, Feminist Theory and Antiracist Politics.* London: Routledge, 2009.

Crimp, Douglas. "How to Have Promiscuity in an Epidemic." In *Melancholia and Moralism: Essays on AIDS and Queer Politics*, by Douglas Crimp. Cambridge, MA: MIT Press, 2004.

Croft, Clare. "Feminist Dance Criticism and Ballet." *Dance Chronicle* 37, no. 2 (2014): 195–217.

Currah, Pasiley, and Susan Stryker. "Introduction." *TSQ: Transgender Studies Quarterly* 1, nos. 1–2 (2014): 1–18.

Cvetkovich, Ann. "White Boots and Combat Boots: My Life as a Lesbian Go-Go Dancer." In *Dancing Desires: Sexualities On and Off the Stage*, edited by Jane Desmond, 315–348. Madison: University of Wisconsin, 2001.

D'Emilio, John. *Sexual Politics, Sexual Communities: The Making of a Homosexual Minority in the United States, 1940–1970.* 2d ed. Chicago: University of Chicago Press, 1998. First published 1983 by University of Chicago Press.

de Lauretis, Teresa. "Queer Theory: Lesbian and Gay Sexualities—An Introduction." *differences: A Journal of Feminist Cultural Studies* 3, no. 2 (1991): iii–xviii.

Dean, Timothy. *Unlimited Intimacy: Reflections on the Subculture of Barebacking.* Chicago: University of Chicago Press, 2009.

defrantz, thomas f. "Blacking Queer Dance." *Dance Research Journal* 34, no. 2 (2002): 102–5.

defrantz, thomas f. "Foreword: Black Bodies Dancing Black Culture-Black Atlantic Transformations." In *EmBODYing Liberation: The Black Body in American Dance*, edited by Dorothea Fischer-Hornung and Alison D. Goeller, 11–16. Hamburg: Lit, 2001.

Desmond, Jane. "Introduction." In *Dancing Desires: Sexualities On and Off the Stage*, 3–32. Madison: University of Wisconsin, 2001.

Dolan, Jill. *The Feminist Spectator as Critic.* Ann Arbor: University of Michigan Press, 1988.

Dolan, Jill. *Utopia in Performance: Finding Hope at the Theater.* Ann Arbor: University of Michigan Press, 2005.

Doty, Alexander. *Flaming Classics: Queering the Film Canon.* New York: Routledge Press, 2000.

Doty, Alexander. *Makings Things Perfectly Queer: Interpreting Mass Culture.* Minneapolis: University of Minnesota Press, 1993.

Duberman, Martin. *The Worlds of Lincoln Kirstein.* New York: Alfred A. Knopf, 2007.

Duggan, Lisa. *Sapphic Slashers: Sex, Violence, and American Modernity.* Durham, NC: Duke University Press, 2000.

Dyer, Richard. *White.* London: Routledge, 1997.

El-Tayeb, Fatima. *European Others: Queering Ethnicity in Postnational Europe.* Minneapolis: University of Minnesota Press, 2011.

Eng, David L., with Judith Halberstam and José Esteban Muñoz. "Introduction: What's Queer about Queer Studies Now?" *Social Text* 23, nos. 3–4 (2005): 1–16.

Engebretsen, Elisabeth L. *Queer Women in Urban China: An Ethnography.* New York: Routledge, 2014.

Fanon, Franz. *Black Skin, White Masks.* London: Pluto Press, 1986.

Fleetwood, Nicole R. *Troubling Vision: Performance, Visuality, and Blackness.* Chicago: University of Chicago Press, 2011.

Foster, Susan Leigh. "The Ballerina's Phallic Pointe." In *Corporealities: Dancing Knowledge, Culture, and Power*, edited by Susan Leigh Foster, 1–24. London: Routledge, 1996.

Foster, Susan. "Choreographies of Gender." *Signs* 24, no. 1 (1998): 1–33.

Foster, Susan. "Choreographies of Protest." *Theatre Journal* 55, no. 3 (2003): 395–412.

Foster, Susan. *Choreographing Empathy: Kinesthesia in Performance.* New York: Routledge, 2010.

Foster, Susan Leigh. "Closets Full of Dances." In *Dancing Desires: Sexualities On and Off the Stage*, edited by Jane C. Desmond, 147–207. Madison: University of Wisconsin, 2001.

Foucault, Michel. *The History of Sexuality*, Volume 1: *An Introduction*. New York: Vintage, 1978.

Freeman, Elizabeth. "Hopeless Cases: Queer Chronicities and Gertrude Stein's 'Melenctha.'" *Journal of Homosexuality* 63, no. 3 (2016): 329–48.

Garafola, Lynn. "The Travesty Dancer in Nineteenth-Century Ballet." *Dance Research Journal* 7, no. 2 (1985): 35–40.

Garcia, Cindy. "'Don't leave me, Celia!': Salsera Homosociality and Pan-Latina Corporealities." *Women & Performance: A Journal of Feminist Theory* 18, no. 3 (2008): 199–213.

Gates, Henry Louis, Jr. "The Body Politic of Bill T. Jones," *New Yorker*, November 28, 1994, 117.

Gere, David. *How to Make Dances in an Epidemic: Tracking Choreography in the Age of AIDS*. Madison: University of Wisconsin Press, 2004.

Goldman, Andrea S. *Opera and the City: The Politics of Culture in Beijing, 1770–1900*. Stanford, CA: Stanford University Press, 2012.

Gopinath, Gayatri. *Impossible Desires: Queer Diasporas and South Asian Public Cultures*. Durham, NC: Duke University Press, 2005.

Graff, Ellen. *Stepping Left: Dance and Politics in New York City, 1928–1942*. Durham, NC: Duke University Press, 1997.

Halberstam, Jack. *The Queer Art of Failure*. Durham, NC: Duke University Press, 2011.

Halberstam, Judith. *In a Queer Time and Place: Transgender Bodies, Subcultural Lives*. New York: New York University Press, 2005.

Halperin, David. *One Hundred Years of Homosexuality and Other Essays on Greek Love*. New York: Routledge, 1990.

Halperin, David. *Saint = Foucault*. New York: Oxford University Press, 1995.

Hamera, Judith. *Dancing Communities: Performance, Difference, and Connection in the Global City*. New York: Palgrave, 2007.

Hammonds, Evelynn M. "Black (W)holes and the Geometry of Black Female Sexuality." In *Feminism Meets Queer Theory*, edited by Elizabeth Weed and Naomi Schor, 136–56. Bloomington: Indiana University Press, 1997.

Harper, Phillip Brian. "Eloquence and Epitaph: Black Nationalism and the Homophobic Impulse in Response to the Death of Max Robinson." *Social Text* 28 (1991): 68–86.

Hartman, Saidiya. "Venus in Two Acts." *Small Axe* 26.12, no. 2 (2008): 1–14.

Henderson, Mae G., and E. Patrick Johnson. "Introduction." In *Black Queer Studies: A Critical Anthology*, edited by Mae G. Henderson and E. Patrick Johnston, 1– 20. Durham, NC: Duke University Press, 2005.

Herring, Scott. *Another Country: Queer Anti-urbanism*. New York: New York University Press, 2010.

Hogan, Katie. *Women Take Care: Gender, Race and the Culture of AIDS*. Ithaca, NY: Cornell University Press, 2001.

Holland, Sharon Patricia. *Raising the Dead: Readings of Death and (Black) Subjectivity*. Durham, NC: Duke University Press, 2000.

hooks, bell. *Ain't I a Woman: Black Women and Feminism*. Boston: South End Press, 1989.

Hubbs, Nadine. *The Queer Composition of America's Sound*. Berkeley: University of California Press, 2004.

Hughes, Holly, and David Roman. *O Solo Homo: The New Queer Performance*. New York: Grove Press, 1998.

Hunt, R. Justin. "Queer Debts and Bad Documents: Taylor Mac's Young Ladies Of." In *Queer Dramaturgies: International Perspectives on Where Performance Leads Queer*, edited by Alyson Campbell and Stephen Farrier, 210–227. London: Palgrave Macmillan, 2015.

Jiang, Jin. *Women Playing Men: Yue Opera and Social Change in Twentieth-Century Shanghai*. Seattle: University of Washington Press, 2009.

Johnson, David K. *The Lavender Scare: The Cold War Persecution of Gays and Lesbians in the Federal Government*. Chicago: University of Chicago Press, 2004.

Johnson, E. Patrick. *Appropriating Blackness: Performance and Politics of Authenticity*. Durham, NC: Duke University Press, 2003.

Johnson, E. Patrick. "'Quare' Studies, or (Almost) Everything I Know about Queer Studies I Learned from My Grandmother." In *Black Queer Studies: A Critical Anthology*, edited by E. Patrick Johnson and Mae Henderson, 124–57. Durham, NC: Duke University Press, 2005.

Jones, Bill T., and Peggy Roggenbuck Gillespie. *Last Night on Earth*. New York: Pantheon Books, 1995.

Juhasz, Suzanne. "Queer Swans: Those Fabulous Avians in the *Swan Lakes* of Les Ballets Trockadero and Matthew Bourne." *Dance Chronicle* 31, no. 1 (2008): 54–83.

Khubchandani, Kareem. "Lessons in Drag: An Interview with LaWhore Vagistan." *Theatre Topics* 25, no. 3 (2015): 285–94.

Kolb, Alexandra. "Nijinsky's Images of Homosexuality: Three Case Studies." *Journal of European Studies* 39, no. 2 (2009): 147–71.

Krishnan, Hari. "From Gynemimesis to Hypermasculinity: The Shifting Orientations of Male Performers of South Indian Court Dance." In *When Men Dance*, edited by Jennifer Fischer and Anthony Shay, 379–91. New York: Oxford University Press, 2009.

Kuppers, Petra. *Disability and Contemporary Performance*. New York: Routledge 2003.

Kuppers, Petra. "Vanishing in Your Face: Embodiment and Representation in Lesbian Dance Performance." *Journal of Lesbian Studies* 2, nos. 2–3 (1998): 47–63.

Kwan, SanSan. *Kinesthetic City: Dance & Movement in Chinese Urban Spaces*. New York: Oxford University Press, 2013.

Loots, Lliane. "'You Don't Look like a Dancer!'": Gender and Disability Politics in the Arena of Dance as Performance and as a Tool for Learning in South Africa." *Agenda* 29, no. 2 (2015): 122–32.

Love, Heather. "Introduction." *GLQ* 17, no. 1 (2011): 1–14.

Lugowski, David M. "Queering the (New) Deal: Lesbian and Gay Representation and the Depression-Era Cultural Politics of Hollywood's Production Code." *Cinema Journal* 38, no. 2 (1999): 3–35.

Manalansan, Martin F. *Global Divas: Filipino Gay Men in the Diaspora: Perverse Modernities*. Durham, NC: Duke University Press, 2003.

Manalansan, Martin F., IV, Chantal Nadeau, Richard T. Rodriguez, and Siobhan B. Sommerville. "Queering the Middle: Race, Region, and a Queer Midwest." *GLQ: A Journal of Lesbian and Gay Studies* 20, nos. 1–2 (2014): 1–12.

Manning, Susan. *Modern Dance, Negro Dance: Race in Motion*. Minneapolis: University of Minnesota Press, 2004.

McBride, Dwight A. *Why I Hate Abercrombie & Fitch: Essays on Race and Sexuality*. New York: New York University, 2005.

McCune, Jeffrey Q., Jr. *Sexual Discretion: Black Masculinity and the Politics of Passing*. Chicago: University of Chicago Press, 2014.

McRuer, Robert. *Crip Theory: Cultural Signs of Queerness and Disability*. New York: New York University Press, 2006.

Meduri, Avanthi. "Multiple Pleasures: Improvisation in Bharatanatyam." In *Taken by Surprise: A Dance Improvisation Reader*, edited by Ann Cooper Albright and David Gere, 141–50. Middletown, CT: Wesleyan University Press, 2003.

Meyer, Richard. *Outlaw Representations: Censorship & Homosexuality in Twentieth-Century American Art*. Oxford: Oxford University Press, 2002.

Moore, Mignon R. "Lipstick or Timberlands? Meanings of Gender Presentation in Black Lesbian Communities." *Signs: Journal of Women in Culture and Society* 32, no. 1 (2006): 113–29.

Muñoz, José Esteban. *Cruising Utopia: The Then and There of Queer Futurity*. New York: New York University Press, 2009.

Muñoz, José Esteban. *Disidentifications: Queers of Colors and the Performance of Politics*. Minneapolis: University of Minnesota Press, 1999.

Muñoz, José Esteban. "Gesture, Ephemera, and Queer Feeling: Approaching Kevin Aviance." In *Dancing Desires: Choreographing Sexualities On and Off the Stage*, edited by Jane C. Desmond, 423–44. Madison: University of Wisconsin Press, 2001.

Nash, Jennifer C. "Re-thinking Intersectionality." *Feminist Review* 89 (2008): 1–15.

Neal, Mark Anthony. *New Black Man*. New York: Routledge, 2006.

Noriega, Chon. "'Something's Missing Here!': Homosexuality and Film Reviews during the Production Code Era, 1934–1962." *Cinema Journal* 30, no. 1 (1990): 20–41.

Novack, Cynthia Jean. *Sharing the Dance: Contact Improvisation and American Culture.* Chicago: University of Chicago Press, 2009.

Pollack, Howard. "The Dean of Gay American Composers." *American Music* 18, no. 1 (2000): 39–49.

Puar, Jasbir K. "Global Circuits: Transnational Sexualities and Trinidad." *Signs: Journal of Women in Culture and Society* 26, no.1 (2001): 1039–65.

Puar, Jasbir. *Terrorist Assemblages: Homonationalism in Queer Times.* Durham, NC: Duke University Press, 2007.

Reagon, Bernice Johnson. "Coalition Politics: Turning the Century." In *Home Girls: A Black Feminist Anthology*, 2d ed., edited by Barbara Smith, 343–56. Camden, NJ: Rutgers University Press, 2000: 343-56.

Reddy, Vasu, and Judith Butler. "Troubling Genders, Subverting Identities: Interview with Judith Butler." *Agenda: Empowering Women for Gender Equity: Special Issue: Sexuality in Africa* 18, no. 62 (2004): 115–23.

Risner, Doug. "Rehearsing Heterosexuality: 'Unspoken' Truths in Dance Education." *Dance Research Journal* 34, no. 2 (2002): 63–78.

Rivera-Servera, Ramón. "Choreographies of Resistance: Latina/o Queer Dance and the Utopian Performative." *Modern Drama* 47, no. 2 (2004): 269–89.

Rivera-Servera, Ramón. *Performing Queer Latinidad: Dance, Sexuality, Politics.* Ann Arbor: University of Michigan Press, 2013.

Rofel, Lisa. "Grassroots Activism: Non-Normative Sexual Politics in Post-Socialist China." In *Unequal China: The Political Economy and Cultural Politics of Inequality*, edited by Wanning Sun and Yingjie Guo, 183–93. New York: Routledge, 2013.

Roman, David. "Not-About-AIDS." *GLQ: A Journal of Lesbian and Gay Studies* 6, no. 1 (2000): 1–28.

Roman, David. "Theatre Journal: Dance Liberation." *Theatre Journal* 55, no. 3 (2003): 377–94.

Roof, Judith. *Come, as You Are: Sexuality and Narrative.* New York: Columbia University Press, 1996.

Roorda, Eric Paul. "McCarthyite in Camelot: The 'Loss' of Cuba, Homophobia, and the Otto Otepka Scandal in the Kennedy State Department." *Diplomatic History* 31 (2007): 723–54.

Samuels, Ellen. *Fantasies of Identification: Disability, Gender, Race.* New York: NYU Press, 2014.

Savigliano, Marta. "Notes on Tango (as) Queer (Commodity)." *Anthropological Notebooks* 16, no. 3 (2010): 135–43.

Sedgwick, Eve Kosofsky. *Epistemology of the Closet.* Berkeley: University of California Press, 1990.

Sedgwick, Eve Kosofsky. "Queer and Now." In *The Routledge Queer Studies Reader*, edited by Donald E. Hall and Annamarie Jagose with Andrea Bebell and Susan Potter, 3–17. New York: Routledge, 2013.

Sedgwick, Eve Kosofsky. *Tendencies*. Durham, NC: Duke University Press, 1993.

Sommerville, Siobhan. "Queer." In *Keywords for American Studies*, edited by Bruce Burgett and Glenn Hendler, 182–90. New York: NYU Press, 2007.

Spillers, Hortense. "Mama's Baby, Papa's Maybe: An American Grammar Book." *Diacritics* 17, no. 2 (1987): 64–81.

Stoneley, Peter. *A Queer History of the Ballet*. New York: Routledge, 2007; repr. New York: Routledge, 2009.

Streb, Elizabeth. *How to Become an Extreme Action Hero*. New York: Feminist Press, 2010.

Streitmatter, Rodger. *Outlaw Marriages: The Hidden Histories of Fifteen Extraordinary Same Sex Couples*. Boston: Beacon Press, 2012.

Thomson, Rosemarie Garland. *Extraordinary Bodies: Figuring Physical Disability in American Literature and Culture*. New York: Columbia University Press, 1997.

Tolentino, Rolando B. "Macho Dancing, the Feminization of Labor, and Neoliberalism in the Philippines." *The Drama Review* 53, no. 2 (2009): 77–89.

Vogel, Shane. *The Scene of Harlem Cabaret: Race, Sexuality, Performance*. Chicago: University of Chicago Press, 2009.

Walters, Suzanna Danuta. *The Tolerance Trap: How God, Genes, and Good Intentions are Sabotaging Gay Equality*. New York: NYU, 2014.

Warner, Michael. *Fear of a Queer Planet: Queer Politics and Social Theory*. Minneapolis: University of Minnesota Press, 1993.

Weinberg, Jonathan. "Substitute and Consolation: The Ballet Photographs of George Platt Lynes." In *Dance for a City*, edited by Lynn Garafola with Eric Foner, 128–51. New York: Columbia University Press, 1999.

Wilson, James. *Bulldaggers, Pansies, and Chocolate Babies: Performance, Race, and Sexuality in the Harlem Renaissance*. Ann Arbor: University of Michigan Press, 2010.

Wolf, Stacy. "'Defying Gravity': Queer Conventions in the Musical *Wicked*." *Theatre Journal* 60, no. 1 (2008): 1–21.

Wolf, Stacy. "'Never Gonna Be a Man/Catch Me If You Can/I Won't Grow Up': A Lesbian Account of Mary Martin's Peter Pan." *Theatre Journal* 49, no. 4 (1997): 493–509.

Wong, Deborah. "Taiko and the Asian/American Body: Drums, *Rising Sun*, and the Question of Gender." *World of Music* 42, no. 3 (2000): 67–78.

Wong, Yutian. *Choreographing Asian America*. Middletown, CT: Wesleyan University Press, 2010.

Yoon, Paul J. "Asian Masculinities and Parodic Possibilities in Odaiko Solos and Filmic Representations." *Asian Music* (2009): 100–130.

Young, Iris Marion. *On Female Body Experience: "Throwing Like a Girl" and Other Essays*. New York: Oxford University Press, 2005.

Index